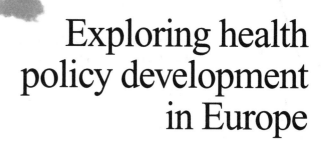
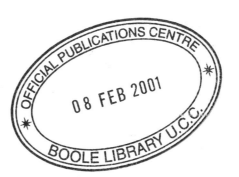
Exploring health policy development in Europe

WHO Library Cataloguing in Publication Data

Exploring health policy development in Europe / edited by Anna
Ritsatakis ... [et al.]

(WHO regional publications. European series ; No. 86)

1.Health policy – trends 2.Policy making 3.Health for all
4.Evaluation studies 5. Europe I.Ritsatakis, Anna II.Series

ISBN 92 890 1352 4   (NLM Classification: WA 540)
ISSN 0378-2255

Text editing: Frank Theakston
Cover design: Sven Lund

World Health Organization
Regional Office for Europe
Copenhagen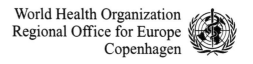

Exploring health policy development in Europe

Edited by: Anna Ritsatakis
Ruth Barnes
Evert Dekker
Patsy Harrington
Simo Kokko
Peter Makara

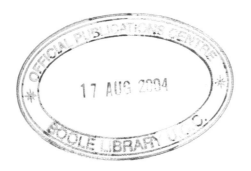

WHO Regional Publications, European Series,

ISBN 92 890 1352 4
ISSN 0378-2255

PRINTED IN FINLAND

Contents

Foreword

This book provides a detailed and comprehensive review of health for all policy development in the WHO European Region until 1996. It covers all of the Member States in the Region, bringing together information from a wide range of sources. The study on which the book is based draws together some of the main policy lessons from over 20 years of experience in Europe. Particular attention is paid to health for all as a value-driven policy framework and, more specifically, to the types of policies and programmes that have been adopted to bring those values to life in a variety of policy contexts. Exploring health policy development in Europe identifies some of the future challenges for policy-makers throughout the Region, such as increasing inequities in health, social exclusion, demographic changes, rising expectations and the rapidly expanding developments in information and technology.

Despite rather different economic, political and social environments, more than half of the European Member States have developed health policies in accordance with the health for all framework, and a broad basis of support for this approach has been created. This was evident at the forty-eighth session of the WHO Regional Committee for Europe, in Copenhagen in September 1998, when all 50 active Member States passed a resolution approving the revised regional health for all policy for the 21st century as a "guiding framework for health policy development in Member States", and commended this framework to both the Member States and to other international bodies as a framework for health policy development.

I am convinced that this book will provide a strong basis for the further development of target-setting for the promotion of equity in health in Europe. WHO's newly established European Centre for Health Policy in Brussels is already taking this work further. I should like to express my continued support for this type of health policy analysis, and look forward to seeing in future publications the development of many of the issues raised here.

J.E. Asvall
WHO Regional Director for Europe

Prologue

Following the 1994 WHO European Health Policy Conference, a number of policy-makers expressed their interest in a publication that would capture the practical experience of WHO Member States in formulating and implementing health for all policies. A series of discussions between some key players in the development of national health policies – Dr Ruth Barnes, Dr Evert Dekker, Dr Peter Makara and Dr Simmo Kokko – and the WHO Regional Office gave rise to the present study.

Exploring health policy development in Europe examines countries' experience since the early 1980s in using the WHO European health for all policy framework as a guide to developing comprehensive policies for health. The study addresses the process by which countries have sought to put into practice the health for all principles of equity, participation and intersectoral action. The intention in doing this was to gain new knowledge that would assist WHO in fulfilling its mandate to support Member States in developing health for all policies.

Given the complexity and scope of the task, it was realized early on that the first attempt should provide a broad record of the main developments, followed by a more in-depth analysis of individual aspects at a later stage. Indeed, the study has uncovered a wealth of material that will support the continued development of health for all as a flexible policy framework, and has provided a valuable learning experience for the further refinement of policy analysis skills. But it also leaves many questions.

Chapter 1 sets the context and purpose of the study and the methods used, indicating the sources of the information. These included feedback from a checklist sent to all Member States, case studies, written policy documents, key players in the policy development process in countries, documentation from Regional Office activities, and the personal experience accumulated by the authors.

Chapter 2 presents 13 case studies describing the health for all process in 10 European countries. The countries were selected to give a reasonable geographical coverage and to include those of different sizes, political and administrative organization, and health care systems. Care was also taken to ensure a mix of both comparative newcomers to health for all and countries with longer experience.

One of the main sources of information was the checklist sent to all Member States, requesting information on the formulation and implementation of general and issue-specific health policy documents. Brief country profiles were also prepared and are given in the annex. Part of the interest of following policy processes is in the endlessly changing policy environment. In certain countries, some of what is described here has already progressed further or is under review.

Each of the health for all principles was examined from the standpoint of the policy instruments used to promote them. The results of this analysis are outlined in Chapter 3. Given the tremendous breadth and complexity of the area covered, it was not possible to report in detail on each country's experience, but rather to give an overview and samples of the variety of experience in the Region.

Finally, in Chapter 4, we explore the changing policy environment in which countries will be called upon to develop policies for health in the future, referring to trends such as globalization, increasing decentralization of power, new technologies and changing patterns of social support. The chapter identifies some of the factors that facilitate or inhibit the achievement of a smooth policy development process, and outlines a system for putting health at the centre of development.

This book is intended as the first in a series that will report on studies aimed at expanding the knowledge and research base for health policy analysis. Work has already started in relation to policy development issues, such as the methodology for target-setting and health impact assessment, coordinated by the European Centre for Health Policy in Brussels. Considerable interest in similar issues has also recently been shown by the European Union, as it moves towards developing a policy for public health.

We hope that this publication will be of use to those in health administrations who have an interest in, or are in a position to influence, health policy development, to their colleagues in other sectors and departments whose work may impinge on health, and to decision-makers at national, regional and local levels who must take action for health and development. It is also hoped that much of the material presented will also reach a wider readership, and provoke some of the interest and discussion necessary for democratic decision-making.

Owing to the principal authors having other commitments, including the setting up of the European Centre for Health Policy in Brussels, the finalization and publication of the study took longer than expected. This, of course, made the task of all those contributing to the process very much more difficult. We would like to thank in particular the following people for their patience and support: all the named authors, who gave generously of their time and effort to prepare case studies; Birthe Havn, Programme Assistant for the Country Health Policies Programme, who was responsible for keeping track of the various texts over that long period; the staff of the Publications unit – David Breuer, Pamela Charlton, Gill Nissen and Frank Theakston – who had to deal with a very complex manuscript and endless references; Wendy Enersen, who performed a miracle in finalizing the typeset book; and Chris Riley and Liz Mesthenaiou, who were among the colleagues and friends who took the time and trouble to read and comment on parts of the text.

Having reached the end of this long task, we already know that we need to start again, looking at new developments. We trust we can rely on the continued support of colleagues across Europe to keep tracking, sharing and learning from country experiences.

Anna Ritsatakis
Head, European Centre for Health Policy

Contributors[a]

Ruth Barnes	Senior Health and Health Policy Analyst in the Economics and Operational Research Division at the Department of Health in England, with responsibility for analytical support to the development of a health strategy for England, including comparative analysis of health policy development in Europe.
Conxa Castell	Head, Chronic Diseases Prevention Section, Department of Health, Catalonia, Spain, with responsibility for health for all policy development in Catalonia for chronic diseases.
Evert Dekker	From 1985 to1994, coordinator of health policy at the Netherlands Ministry of Health, with responsibility for general health policy development and mental health policy.
Gül Ergör	Assistant Professor of Public Health, with responsibility for training provincial managers on health for all policy implementation in Turkey.
Vilius Grabauskas	Professor and Rector, Kaunas Medical Academy, and chair of a task force responsible for developing the National Health Programme in Lithuania; at the international level, chair of the Standing Committee of the WHO Regional Committee for Europe.

---

[a] The positions and responsibilities given for each of the contributors are those that obtained at the time of writing.

Per Haglind

City Medical Officer, Gothenburg, Sweden, with responsibility for preparing public health reports and providing expert support in public health to the city council and local district councils.

Lena Rydin Hansson

Executive Officer, County Health Policy, Östergötland, Sweden, with responsibility for developing regional health policy and strategies and resource allocation.

Patsy Harrington

Short-term Professional, WHO Regional Office for Europe, with responsibilities related to the activities of the Country Health Policies Programme and the Regions for Health Network.

Simo Kokko

Head of Research and Development at STAKES, Finland, a government research and development centre for social welfare and health with particular interest in primary care.

Diana McInnes

Branch Head in the Health Promotion Division at the Department of Health, England, with responsibility for coordinating and monitoring the development of a health strategy for England.

Peter Makara

Director of the WHO Collaborating Centre for Central and Eastern Europe at the Hungarian National Institute for Health Promotion, responsible for health strategy development in Hungary.

Willy Nilsson

Epidemiologist in Gothenburg, Sweden, with responsibility for health for all indicators, preparing public health reports and providing expert support in epidemiology to the city council and local district councils.

Zafer Öztek

Professor of Public Health and consultant to the Ministry of Health of Turkey on health for all policy development, and editor of the draft national health policy document for Turkey.

Bosse Pettersson

Senior Health Promotion Adviser at the National Institute of Public Health, Sweden, with responsibility, *inter alia*, for monitoring and evaluation of the health for all targets.

Anna Ritsatakis

Regional Adviser for Country Health Policies and Equity in Health at the WHO Regional Office for Europe, and at present head of WHO's European Centre for Health Policy in Brussels.

Lluís Salleras	General Director of Public Health of the Department of Health of the Autonomous Community of Catalonia, Spain, responsible for the formulation of Catalan health policy.
Ricard Tresserras	Head of the health and health education programmes in Catalonia, Spain, with responsibility for health for all policy development for chronic diseases.
Morton Warner	Director of the Welsh Health Planning Forum (later the Welsh Institute for Health and Social Care), with responsibility for developing health policy and strategies in the Principality of Wales.
Birgit Weihrauch	Head of the Division of Health Policy and Health Protection in the Ministry of Women, Youth, Family and Health of North Rhine-Westphalia, Germany.
Ray G. Xerri	Director of the Department of Health Policy and Planning of Malta, with responsibility for health policy development and management of reforms in the health care sector.

1

Using the health for all framework to explore the development of health policy in the European Region of WHO

Creating a common basis for understanding

Speaking the same language

The study focused on the process of developing policies for health in Europe between the early 1980s and 1996. It is important to remember that some of the main policy terms used in the study may be understood differently in different countries and languages. For example, the English language distinguishes between politics and policy, but many other European languages do not. The need to create a basis for common understanding of policy terms became apparent during the preparations for the 1994 ministerial-level European Health Policy Conference (1–6) organized by the WHO Regional Office for Europe in collaboration with the European Commission and the Council of Europe, in which representatives from 46 countries took part.

The glossary (7) prepared for the Conference defines a policy as agreement or consensus on issues to be addressed in order to achieve a desired result or change. In other words, a policy is an agreement on goals and objectives, the priorities between these objectives and the main policy directions for achieving them. A goal refers to the long-range aims of society and is usually expressed in rather general terms. In the international literature and in many national policy documents, *goal* is frequently used interchangeably with *objective*, although according to United Nations usage (8), an objective is more specific than a goal and is an aim that can be partly achieved during a planning period. A distinction is sometimes made between primary and secondary objectives, with primary objectives relating directly to welfare – for example, improving public health – and secondary objectives being one of the means of achieving the primary objective – in this case, for example, improving public health by providing safe drinking-water. A target is an intermediate result towards the achievement of goals and objectives; it is more specific, has a time horizon and is frequently, though not always, quantified. So a target relating to the above objective would be to ensure that a certain percentage of the population has access to safe drinking-water by the year 2002. Reflecting this, a logical planning framework, for example, should use SMART targets: Specific, Measurable, Accurate, Realistic and Time-limited *(9)*.

A strategy is broad lines of action to achieve goals and objectives *(10)*. This includes identifying suitable points of intervention and ways of ensuring that numerous sectors are involved, considering the range of political, social, economic, managerial and technical factors that affect the strategy and defining the possible constraints and ways of dealing with them.

Public policies manifest themselves in many ways and are not always in the form of a policy document or text *(11)*. A policy may evolve as the result of administrative decisions: small incremental steps are taken that move towards implicit objectives, or "muddling through" *(12)*. Policies may be formally expressed through, for example, a constitution, the preamble to other legal documents and regulations, the platforms of political parties or explicit policy papers.

Policy-making means choices, and everyone makes them

All countries formulate policies and plan for the future. This might appear to be self-evident. The discussion at European health policy conferences over the years, however, shows that top-level decision-makers in the health sector have shifted back and forth in their thinking. For example, participants from 25 countries at the European Conference on National Health Planning held in Bucharest in 1974 apparently felt comfortable in defining planning for health as making "optimal use of all the scarce national resources available for the improvement of health (or health status) over a given period, whether those resources lie within the so-called health sector or outside it" *(13)*. Ten years later, at a similar European-level conference organized in The Hague, several countries initially resisted using the words *policy-making* and *planning* in relation to the processes and management of their health systems. They felt that such terms were inappropriate in their pluralistic systems and were more relevant for centrally planned economies. It was considered quite a breakthrough when they accepted a recommendation that "the term 'health planning and management' should be understood to comprise all purposeful approaches to promoting health and improving the equity, effectiveness, efficiency and quality of health systems" *(14)*. Following the changes in Europe after 1989, some countries in the eastern part of the Region took a similar position. In the initial years of the transition, they seemed to consider that they no longer needed policies and plans since they were now introducing pluralistic systems.

One explicit expression of government policy with which most people are familiar is the annual budget, which determines how much public money is to be spent for which purposes and how the necessary revenue will be raised. All countries use targets of various types as a routine part of public sector activity, although they may not be explicitly labelled as such. For example, most countries record the number of infants who die before reaching one year of age. If the ratio of deaths to live births is simply used to describe a given situation, then it is no more than an indicator. If, however, a decision is made to take action to achieve a certain ratio within a certain period of time, this is a quantified target.

A political process

Whether implicit or explicit, intuitive or based on scientific evidence, quantified or not, policy-making and target-setting constitute a political process (see Box 1.1). According to Ham *(15)*, "What goes on inside the black box of decision-making is not a rational, logical process in which information and research determine policy outcomes. It is a highly political process in which power and entrenched interest are the main driving force". The evidence gathered in this study shows that chance can also play

---

Box 1.1. Policy-making

Policy-making means making choices to bring about change.
Regardless of the approach and methods used, it is a political process.

Goal	A long-term general aim or aspiration.
Objective	Frequently used interchangeably with the term goal; usually more specific and can be partly achieved during the planning period.
Policy	An agreement or consensus on the issues, goals and objectives to be addressed, the priorities among those objectives and the main directions for achieving them.
Strategy	Broad lines of action to achieve the goals and targets, including: • identifying suitable points of intervention • ways of ensuring involvement of relevant partners • a range of political, social, economic, managerial and technical factors • constraints and how to deal with them.
Target	An intermediate result towards the achievement of goals and objectives, that is: • more specific than an objective • has a time horizon • frequently, but not always, quantifiable.

---

an important role, as it affects the broader socioeconomic environment and the people who happen to be in positions to make a difference. No wonder so many languages do not distinguish between policy and politics.

Global objectives for health – birth of the health for all policy

How the health for all movement started

In 1977, the World Health Assembly defined a global goal or objective for health when it decided that governments and WHO should aim in the coming decades for the "attainment by all citizens of the world by the year 2000 of a level of health that will permit them to lead a socially and economically productive life" *(10)*. This launched a new approach to health policy-making that became known as health for all by the year 2000. As the name suggests, the focus was on health rather than health care. The term *all* referred to the promotion of equity in health, and defining a time horizon for this objective signalled the intention to secure accountability for health.

A global strategy for health for all was launched in 1979 through a resolution endorsing the report and declaration from the International Conference on Primary Health Care held in Alma-Ata in 1978 *(16)*. The resolution invited WHO Member States "to act individually in formulating national policies, strategies and plans of action for attaining this goal, and collectively in formulating regional and global strategies" *(17)*. Twelve global targets were set, and a system for monitoring progress towards achieving them was agreed. It was clarified from the start that this was "not a separate 'WHO strategy', but rather an expression of individual and collective national responsibility, fully supported by WHO" *(17)*. Setting global targets for health, such as eradicating certain communicable diseases, was nothing new, but it was the first time that such a broad approach had been taken.

Why was the health for all movement initiated at that time?
The health for all movement partly reflected a broader concern in the United Nations family for a stronger focus on equity and intersectoral action. The benefits of economic growth were not reaching all segments of society, and the processes of growth and change were having positive, negative, unexpected and unknown consequences. In recognition of this, the United Nations General Assembly launched an international development decade in 1971–1980, stating that "the ultimate objective of development must be to bring about sustained improvement in the well-being of the individual and bestow benefits on all. If undue privileges, extremes of wealth and social injustice persist, then development fails in its essential purpose" *(18)*. The United Nations and other international organizations were searching for more integrated approaches to development planning and more appropriate indicators of social development *(19)*.

As might be expected, these shifts in policy focus reflected what was happening in the Member States. The rapid economic growth and technological advances of the 1960s had allowed increasing spending on health care and an optimism that many of the main challenges to public health could be brought under control. Nevertheless, by the 1970s concern was growing throughout the world that, despite these advances, people's health was not as good as it could be, and health care spending seemed to be a bottomless pit *(20)*. A particularly influential event at this time was the release of the Lalonde report *(21)* in Canada in 1974, which offered a new approach to policy analysis based on a health field concept. Next door, the Surgeon General produced the first report on health promotion and disease prevention in the United States, which established broad goals for improving health *(22)*, and this was followed by *Promoting health/preventing disease. Objectives for the nation (23)*. Researchers were questioning what could reasonably be expected from medical care *(24)*, especially expensive hospital care, and Finland had been spearheading a strong shift towards primary health care from the early 1970s *(25)*.

The policy climate was also influenced by those who had been students in the 1960s and who had by then entered the workforce, including the public services, bringing with them a reinforced sense of solidarity. Three dictatorships in southern Europe had fallen, reflecting hopes of new beginnings. The time was ripe for a new vision for health.

Developing a strategy and targets for health for all in the European Region of WHO

Europe hesitates but then carves a distinctive path

At first, there was some hesitation in Europe following the adoption of the global policy for health for all, partly because of the belief that this policy was not appropriate for industrialized countries, and partly because approaches to planning differed, especially between eastern and western Europe. Broadly speaking, in the countries in the western part of the region, health planning still meant planning for health care services on the basis of demand for and allocation of resources, whereas health planning in the countries in the eastern part of the Region was part of an overall process of development planning that relied heavily on norms and standards fixed at the central level and focused on inputs and outputs *(26)*.

Thus, the World Health Assembly adopted the health for all resolution in May 1977, but at the twenty-seventh session of the Regional Committee for Europe the following September it was still very much business as usual. According to the Regional Director at that time, Dr Leo A. Kaprio *(27)*, although the Regional Committee members believed in the principles of health for all, they thought that it was not relevant to Europe. In 1978, however, a global meeting on primary health care at Alma-Ata *(16)* changed the attitude in Europe. A large number of people came directly from Alma-Ata to the Regional Committee meeting in London, bringing with them fresh impressions that totally changed the feeling in the Regional Committee. Implementing immediately one of the recommendations from the Alma-Ata meeting, the Regional Committee set up the Regional Health Development Advisory Council, thus making the European Region the first WHO region to do so.

So the political and complex consultation process for formulating a health strategy and targets on a European level was set in motion with the then 32 Member States. The chairperson of the Regional Health Development Advisory Council at that time and until 1984 was the late Professor Brian Abel-Smith, who was also the main author of the strategy finally developed. The strategy adopted in 1982 recognized possible conflicting interests of social and economic sectors but stated unequivocally that "health development both contributes to and results from wider socioeconomic development" *(28)*, and that special efforts would be needed to improve the health of the underprivileged. The strategy consisted of "three main elements: the promotion of lifestyles conducive to health, the reduction of preventable conditions, and the reorientation of the health care system to cover the whole population". The strategy tentatively provided for a system of monitoring and evaluation and called for detailed targets to be defined for its implementation, and work for this had already begun. "Never before had the countries of the Region agreed to adopt a single health policy as a common basis for subsequent development, both in individual Member States and in the Region as a whole." *(29)*

Like-minded thinking

The health for all approach was reinforced by related activities at both the international and local levels and especially through discussions of health promotion that led to the Ottawa Charter for Health Promotion in 1986 *(30)*, and the development of new concepts such as healthy public policy. Over the years, this approach also influenced the work of other international organizations. By 1991, for example, the Council of Europe had formally adopted the health for all approach, and the *World development report 1993: investing in health (31)*, on which WHO collaborated closely with the World Bank, clearly showed the influence of health for all. Parallel to these activities, the Brundtland report *(32)* had drawn attention to the need to take account of the interrelationships between people, resources, environment and development. Although the report referred to health only in passing, it was based on values similar to the health for all approach, outlining the tremendous social inequity prevailing and the need for participation in decision-making.

A distinctly European flavour

The health for all process in Europe was unique, as no other WHO region initially developed specific regional targets for health for all. Another important characteristic of the European process was that political legitimacy of the targets was sought right from the start, both at the regional level through the Regional Committee for Europe and within many of the countries that later adapted the targets to their own needs. For example, Finland and the Netherlands were the first in Europe to develop national policies for health for all, and these were discussed in their parliaments in 1985 and 1986, respectively. In contrast, the national objectives in the United States, for the first round at least, were scientific targets developed by experts and not given political legitimacy *(23)*.

Developing the concepts

The present global and regional renewal of health for all *(33,34)* makes detailed examination of the history of these developments in Europe more valuable. Dr Kaprio describes excellently the process of formulating the targets, which began with a discussion of what was meant by targets for health and the scientific basis for defining such targets. There was substantial consultation with the Member States on the formulation of targets, both within the Regional Committee and by correspondence requesting feedback on the process.

By 1982, the Member States had agreed that the targets for Europe should be:

- directed towards a significant health problem;
- reliable (expressing a reduction of the identified problem);
- realistic;
- simply and clearly expressed;
- quantified as far as possible (making progress measurable);
- relevant to the regional strategy for health for all;
- politically acceptable; and
- meaningful and attractive to the public, politicians, administrators and professionals.

The basis on which the targets were to be defined was to be related to:

• the magnitude of the problem;
• past trends in its development;
• the expected magnitude and nature of the problem at the set target date if nothing were done;
• the effectiveness of proposed actions in dealing with the problem; and
• the situation on the target date if the actions were carried out as proposed.

Hundreds of experts from all parts of Europe worked with the WHO Regional Office for Europe to present 82 targets for the Regional Committee to consider. These were eventually reduced to a set of 38 targets, which were adopted unanimously in 1984. A brief comparison of these targets and of the commonly accepted definitions given above shows that some of the targets were in fact objectives. The lack of consistency in the terms used should perhaps not be surprising since this was a new way of working for many in the health sector.

Commitment and accountability
The 38 targets were not legally binding, but Member States agreed to use them to help set similar national priorities and targets. Equally importantly, they agreed to participate in a process of monitoring their individual and collective progress towards achieving the 38 European targets, using over 200 quantitative and non-quantitative indicators, 65 of which were defined as "essential". The Member States have already carried out the monitoring exercise five times (1984/1985, 1987/1988, 1990/1991, 1993/1994 and 1996/1997), which clearly indicates their seriousness of purpose, since the results of the process are published in regular reports *(35,36)*. In 1996 *(37)* it was agreed that basic health statistics should be reported annually and that national coordinators should be appointed in countries to ensure direct transfer of these data to the Regional Office, that information normally collected through relatively frequent surveys should be fed into the process every 3 years, and that every 6 years there should be a full-scale evaluation of health for all. The country data for the health for all indicators are now available on disk and on the Internet.

Some countries were already developing national health policies based on the principles of health for all even before the regional targets were finalized and adopted. By 1989, just before the fall of the Berlin Wall and the rapid changes in the countries in the eastern part of the Region, 17 of the 32 Member States had formulated or were preparing national health for all policy documents *(38)*.

The health for all movement slowed down in the late 1980s and early 1990s, as the political and economic changes in central and eastern Europe and a strong focus on health care reform in many countries took centre stage. In accordance with the agreed regional process, however, the Consultative Group on Programme Development and the WHO Regional Committee for Europe agreed in 1989 that an update of the targets was timely but that the basic structure should stay the same. The Regional Committee approved a revised set of targets for health for all in 1991 *(39)*. The six major themes of the first set of targets for health for all were retained: promoting equity in health, actively participating communities, a focus on health promotion and disease prevention, reorienting the health system towards primary health care and collaborating for health across sectors and cooperation across national frontiers. An explicit concern with ethics was added. This was the situation when the present study began.

The approach and values of the regional policy for health for all

Oriented towards outcome
The health for all policy was and is about improving and protecting health. It is therefore oriented towards outcome. The health for all paradigm recognizes that health outcome can only be influenced by affecting the prerequisites for health, such as income, education, nutrition, employment and housing and how people behave, and by providing appropriate health care.

An intersectoral approach
The health sector must be concerned with the policies of other sectors and with how these in turn affect lifestyles, the environment (in the broadest sense of the social, economic and physical environments) and health care demands. The weight given to changing the socioeconomic situation in which people live and work, changing behaviour or providing services differs at any given time or place. The aim is to invest in whatever brings the greatest health gain.

Outward-looking
The policy for health for all has shifted the focus from input to health care to concern with outcome in terms of health status. This means that the health sector has to be outward-reaching rather than inward-looking. Since the beginning of the health for all movement, it has been stated that health should be seen as an integral part of socioeconomic development. As shown in Chapter 4, intersectoral action for health increasingly entails not only accounting for how actions in other sectors may affect health status, reduce hazards to health and improve the services that deal with ill health and rehabilitation, but also considering how the health sector can contribute to achieving developmental objectives in sectors other than health.

Seeking new alliances and acquiring new skills
Formulating polices for health can be traced back to ancient times. Management by objective has also been discussed since the 1950s in other social and economic planning circles, but the emergence of the objective-led approach to health for all in Europe presented many people in the health field with a totally new way of thinking and working for which they were not prepared. More than a decade later, some countries still have difficulty coming to terms with this approach in practice.

This is partly understandable. Attempting to influence the determinants of health requires not only new thinking but new skills and tools to work with new partners in a range of new settings. In this regard, many countries still lack the essential capacity and skills to manage the formulation and implementation of policies and strategies based on health for all.

A continuous and complex process

Policy-makers wishing to develop a health for all policy are faced with a wide array of possible strategic directions and policy options for action in many sectors. It is a complex process. Indeed, achieving intersectoral action for health has perhaps proved more complex than had originally been anticipated.

As with any other type of policy development, developing policies for health for all is a continuous process of assessing the situation, formulating policy, implementing, monitoring, evaluating and revising, as shown in the classic policy development model in Fig. 1.1. In real life, the process is never as neat and linear as this. Different parts of the process are usually going on at the same time.

Fig. 1.1. Developing policy

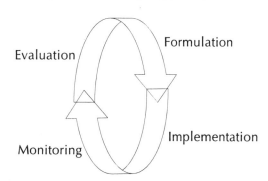

Providing the ethical framework

The health for all policy is based on clear values and policy principles. These define some of the boundaries within which decisions must be taken but do not necessarily make the challenges less complex.

Promoting equity in health is the underlying principle of the health for all policy. Public participation in decision-making is both an essential means of developing such a policy and one of its intended outcomes. Together, these principles provide the political or ethical framework for the health for all approach. A framework of values is essential to any policy-making process *(40)*. In effect, this circumscribes the range of policy options that are considered politically acceptable. A framework of values limits the policy choices open and thus ensures that the range of possible planning options is not too wide to handle.

Promoting equity in health

All aspects of a health for all policy should be based on promoting equity in health. Not all differences in health status are inherently inequitable. The term inequity has an ethical dimension. It refers to differences that are unnecessary and avoidable and that are considered unfair and unjust. The health differences that are considered unnecessary and unfair vary from country to country and from time to time.

A WHO discussion paper *(41)* identified the main determinants of health differences and the extent to which these are attributable to biological variation and free choice, for example, or to a situation or life circumstances that are mainly outside the control of the individuals concerned. Two other WHO documents discussed how socieconomic inequality can be measured *(42)* and what policies and strategies *(43)* might be implemented to promote equity in health.

Whitehead *(41)* gives the following working definition of equity in health:

> Equity in health implies that ideally everyone should have a fair opportunity to attain their full health potential and, more pragmatically, that no one should be disadvantaged from achieving this potential, if it can be avoided.

Distinguishing between equity in health and equity in access to health care is useful for policy purposes. Whitehead *(41)* defines equity in access to health care as:

- equal access to available care for equal need
- equal utilization for equal need
- equal quality of care for all.

This implies that everyone is equally entitled to the available services, that services are fairly distributed throughout a country based on health care needs and ease of access in each geographical area and that the barriers to access are removed. Such barriers might be financial, social, organizational and cultural. Equal quality of care implies not only that everyone can expect the same high standard of professional care but that the care is socially and culturally acceptable.

Participation in decision-making
The 1985 book outlining the health for all targets *(29)* states that "health for all will be achieved by the people themselves. A well informed, well motivated and actively participating community is a key element for the attainment of the common goal". This assumes that people have a right to participate in decisions that affect their health, not only their individual health but that of the society in which they live, and that they should be enabled to do this. This is an issue of human rights, democratization and a well functioning civic society. The process of developing health for all policy should ensure that the people affected by the policy and those responsible for implementing it participate broadly in making decisions and in evaluating the impact of decisions.

In the glossary *(7)* prepared for the 1994 European Health Policy Conference, participation is defined as the active involvement of people working together in some form of social organization in the planning, operation and control of health resources and services at the local and national levels.

In the process of developing health policy, participation requires involving policy-makers and other partners in all sectors of society that influence the determinants of health. It requires involving health professionals, both as the providers of care and as employees in an important economic sector, and the public as individuals, members of groups and communities and as users of health and other services. It means broad involvement at all stages of the cycle of policy development shown in Fig. 1.1, and not only in the implementation stage, as many seem to believe.

Even when there is political will to promote wide participation in decision-making, which is not always the case, such participation can be difficult to achieve. The most obvious challenges include:

- ensuring that the various partners involved speak the same language;
- understanding and respecting the culture, values and objectives of possible partners in the policy process and of the target groups for the policy;
- creating mechanisms and processes to facilitate participation;
- ensuring that appropriate and accessible information is available, especially for certain vulnerable groups; and
- building capacity, skills and opportunity for participation.

The business world offers examples of understanding different organizational cultures (44), and people carrying out market research have long understood that selling products requires different techniques to reach different segments of the population. In many countries, however, the health sector has perhaps been slow in picking up such lessons and techniques from other sectors. Experts have been wary of accepting that the perception of health problems by those who live with the problems is just as valid as their own, although there have been some encouraging attempts at participatory research (45). Health professionals are not always comfortable with sharing knowledge, which they can sometimes view as dissipating their power. Nevertheless, there have been some laudable and imaginative attempts to empower the non-experts. These include the Citizens' Jury in Wales (46) and other parts of the United Kingdom, the use of health facilitators in Östergötland County, Sweden (47), and towns in the Healthy Cities movement (48), which have tried to elicit the opinion of people who have difficulty in communicating and participating because of such factors as age, language or mental capacity.

Policies for health for all are determined by their values. At every stage of the policy process (formulation, implementation, monitoring and evaluation) and between all sectors collaborating (such as education, housing and employment), the impact of policy on equity in health and participation in decision-making must be taken into account.

A radical and ambitious change in approach
Whether or not they were fully aware of the wider implications at the time, in 1984 the WHO European Member States adopted a policy based on clear ethical principles of promoting equity in health and participation in decision-making, which could only be implemented through a radical shift in focus (Box 1.2). It is an ambitious undertaking by any standard.

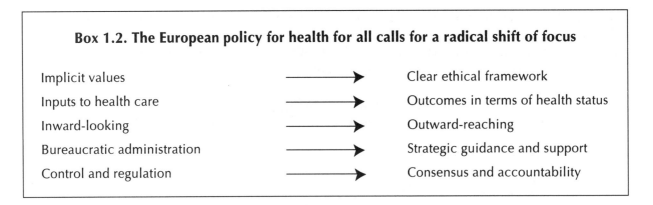

Box 1.2. The European policy for health for all calls for a radical shift of focus

Implicit values ⟶ Clear ethical framework

Inputs to health care ⟶ Outcomes in terms of health status

Inward-looking ⟶ Outward-reaching

Bureaucratic administration ⟶ Strategic guidance and support

Control and regulation ⟶ Consensus and accountability

Moving to the twenty-first century

Renewed health for all policies at the global level *(33)* and in the European Region *(34)* were developed in 1998. The basic approach remains unchanged, but the policies advocate strengthening commitment to aiming for the highest attainable level of health as a fundamental right. Considering health as a human right also entails greater sensitivity to issues of gender. The principle of sustainability, long promoted in the environmental sector, is now also emphasized in the renewed health for all policy. The importance of making health central to human development is strongly reiterated. Finally, in view of the need for greater efforts, an attempt has been made in both the global and regional health for all policies to define more clearly the role of WHO and its Member States.

Why analyse the development of health policy in Europe?

Policy is analysed for two main reasons: to describe policy or to provide information useful in making policy *(15,49)*. In carrying out this study, we were interested in both reasons. We hoped to gain more knowledge of policy development in Europe in order to use this information in supporting our Member States in making policy.

We would also endorse the view expressed by Dunn that "the aims of policy analysis extend beyond the production of 'facts'; policy analysts seek also to produce information about values and preferable courses of action. Policy analysis therefore includes policy evaluation as well as policy advocacy" *(50)*.

Why try to cover the whole of Europe?

The WHO European Region comprises 51 vastly differing Member States, varying from about a quarter of a million inhabitants in Iceland to almost 148 million in the Russian Federation. These Member States include some of the richest and the poorest countries in the world. For every 1000 live births, fewer than 4 infants die in Finland compared with 46 in Tajikistan. Thus it could justifiably be asked why so many and such different countries should be included in one study (see Fig. 1.2).

Fig. 1.2. The European Region of WHO

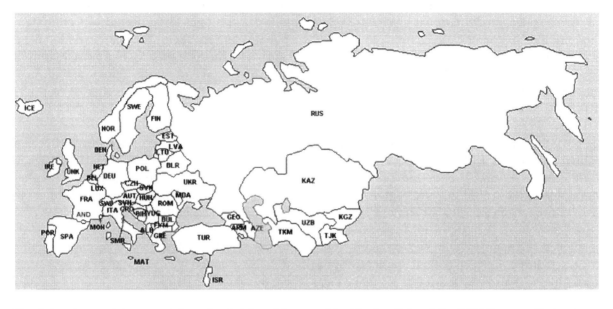

The designations and the presentation of material on this map of the Member States of the WHO European Region (as at 31 July 1997) do not imply the expression of any opinion whatsoever on the part of the World Health Organization concerning the legal status of any country, territory, city or area or of its authorities, or concerning the delimitation of its frontiers or boundaries. Dotted lines represent approximate border lines for which there may not yet be full agreement.

First, something can always be learned by escaping from the confines of parochialism to examine international experience, comparing one's own situation and challenges with those of others. Second, the key to the health for all policy is promoting equity in health not only within countries but between countries. An ethical standpoint therefore requires concern with what is happening in all Member States.

Third, the study of the experience of developing policy was recommended as a follow-up to the 1994 European Health Policy Conference; the Member States have thus mandated such a policy analysis.

Why analyse health policy from a health for all perspective?

Health policy development could equally well be examined from numerous perspectives, such as the roles of the partners in the policy process, the mechanisms for policy development and the events influencing the process. Taking a health for all perspective and using the framework described below greatly widened the scope of the study, thus causing more problems than a narrower perspective would have. The increase in the number of European Member States following the events of 1989 had already widened the field, so why did we take a broad health for all perspective, which vastly widened the scope?

We chose to take a health for all perspective for strong reasons. The 51 European Member States adopted the revised 38 health for all targets for Europe in 1991. Following the European Health Policy Conference and the Copenhagen Declaration of 1994 *(1)*, a resolution was brought to the Regional Committee in 1995, urging "all countries to continue to assess their policies and strategies for health and to take the necessary action to ensure that they are fully in line with the health for all approach" and encouraging "the use of national health for all policy frameworks in countries of central and eastern Europe and the newly independent states to guide international organizations, investors and donors towards addressing priority areas and concerns in their collaborative programmes" *(51)*.

The governments of the European Member States have therefore strongly reaffirmed their belief in the health for all approach, through the Regional Committee for Europe, twice since 1991. In May 1998, the World Health Assembly endorsed the renewed global policy for health for all, and the Regional Committee approved the revised regional policy in September 1998. Exploring policy development across Europe from a health for all perspective therefore appears to be both relevant and timely.

The choice of frame of reference is therefore linked to the WHO mandate to support and encourage Member States to develop national policies for health for all. Although we have tried to be as objective as possible, it is also important that we make clear where our interests lie *(52)*.

Why focus on the processes of developing policy?

The WHO Regional Office for Europe and the European Member States have a long history of examining the determinants of and the factors that influence health and the main causes of death and disease, and of considering ways of influencing those factors. This experience was embodied in the regional strategy for health for all. Much less, however, has been done to examine the processes by which such health policies are developed, the policy environments in which this takes place and the factors that seem to facilitate or hinder such processes.

The WHO evaluation of progress towards health for all in the European Region assesses progress in the Region target by target. Countries' replies concerning their progress in implementing the policy target (target 33) provide valuable information on the development of health for all policy. This information has been taken into account in this study. The overall monitoring process is not designed, however, to analyse experiences in countries in depth. This study is intended therefore to complement and expand on the monitoring exercise, and its preliminary results have already been fed back into the monitoring process *(36)*.

There are many new partners in analysis of health policy. A number of excellent comparative studies have been published recently. The one from the Organisation for Economic Co-operation and Development *(53)* focused more on health care, as did the work carried out by the Regional Office for Europe in preparation for the WHO Conference on European Health Care Reform in Ljubljana in 1996 *(54)*. A 1995 European Union study *(55)*, focusing mainly on health care reform, takes a somewhat wider public health approach but covers only the

12 countries that were members before 1995. There is therefore an obvious gap in the relevant literature regarding the processes of health policy development, and thus ample reason for carrying out this study *(56)*.

This study is not intended as an academic exercise. Health for all is itself an approach or process, and continuously developing it requires a deeper understanding of how it works or does not work.

The reasons for carrying out the study

The aims and purpose of this study reflect WHO's mandate to actively encourage and support countries to harmonize their actions with the health for all approach and the recommendations of the 1994 European Health Policy Conference. The aims of the study were therefore defined as being:

- to contribute to the ongoing elaboration of the health for all approach to developing health policy;
- to systematize the information available on the processes of health policy development and to provide the basis for continuous monitoring, which is essential for further analytical work; and
- to identify nationally (and, to some extent, subnationally) specific features as well as common features between countries and possibly patterns or trends.

The purpose of doing this was:

- to provide Member States with a better understanding of the health for all approach as it has been developed in countries in the European Region;
- to offer some benchmarks by which countries can compare their own progress;
- to identify possible problems of which policy-makers need to be aware, based on experience in countries;
- to provide the Regional Office with more in-depth information on the implementation of health for all development in the Member States in order: to improve its own capacity to support countries; to use this information for updating the strategy for health for all; and to enhance its capacity for working with other organizations; and
- to provide a learning experience for the further refinement of policy analysis skills.

The intended target groups for the study are mainly people working in health administrations who are interested in or can influence the development of health policy at the national, regional and local levels, as well as other people working in the health sector. Much of the material presented is also expected to be useful for other purposes, especially for trainers and students in educational institutions.

How the study was carried out

A team effort
A study of this breadth, both geographically and in scope, required participation by people with a wide knowledge of Europe and from different disciplines. This was achieved by establishing a steering group

composed of two WHO staff members and four other experts from Finland, Hungary, the Netherlands and the United Kingdom, who are also the editors of this publication. The members of the steering group are very diverse in basic training and have followed careers in public health and policy analysis. They include a geographer, a physician, two sociologists, a social planner and a business graduate.

The steering group met to establish the process for the study. It met a further three times to assess the case studies, to brainstorm on the interpretation of the initial results and to assess the progress of the study. It also made comments and recommendations for revising the initial drafts of the study.

The approach adopted

According to Heidenheimer et al., "comparative policy analysis occupies a middle ground between 'pure research' of a theoretical nature and 'applied science' directed towards the nuts and bolts of detailed problem solving" *(57)*. We have tried to reach a middle ground by taking a pan-European view, while offering information of use to individual countries and by balancing the obvious constraints of touching only the surface of a vast body of knowledge and hoping to identify areas for immediate follow-up.

The approach included trying to throw light on and interpret what has happened. There has been no attempt at this stage to examine the outcome for health status of these policy developments, or to carry out any causal analysis.

Evidence from many sources

Using evidence from many sources allowed much of the information to be confirmed by cross-checking, although this was not always possible. The main sources used were:

- evidence from written documents, including national policy documents, statistical reports and other published studies;
- information provided by key actors in the process of developing policy in countries, either by talking to them, which Milio *(52)* has strongly recommended as a means of understanding the process, or from their participation in and papers presented at scientific meetings and related activities;
- information from WHO Regional Office for Europe activities such as staff travel reports and the work of related programmes and networks; and
- the experience accumulated by the editors both from working in policy development at the national and local levels in their own countries and as consultants supporting policy development in other countries.

What is included in the study

The steering group decided that, if possible, all countries in the European Region should be covered on one of two levels described below. The steering group also felt that the analysis should include policy developments in European countries from the early 1980s, when the health for all policy was adopted.

To contain the study within the limits of the time and resources available, the main focus was on examining written health policy documents and the processes by which they were developed. This should not be interpreted as meaning that health policy can only be expressed through such documents. This restriction was intended only for the practical purposes of this study.

Compiling the information

In order to begin to systematize the data available on the process of developing health policy, a questionnaire was sent to all Member States requesting information on general and issue-specific health policy documents and on other activities designed to affect health. This was entered in a database set up for this purpose, using a commercial database program that is designed to be easily updated.

The information compiled was to be presented in two ways. Invited authors prepared in-depth case studies on a country or region. The criteria for the selection of the countries and regions to be included as case studies were:

- reasonable geographical coverage from the north, south, east and west;
- a mix of experience, including comparative newcomers to the health for all scene and countries with a longer exposure to the process; and
- examples of countries of different sizes, political and administrative organization and health care systems.

Brief profiles were prepared for the countries not covered by a case study.

The case studies provide a more in-depth analysis of health policy development than could be inferred from the broad overview of all Member States obtained through the questionnaires and country profiles. Although the authors were asked to follow a common framework based on the principles of health for all, the case studies were intended to be flexible and to provide a more subjective assessment by the authors. They were asked to qualitatively assess the processes and the forces facilitating and inhibiting the development of policies for health based on a health for all approach in a country or region. Their draft contributions were subjected to peer review and revised accordingly. With one exception, the case studies were not submitted for government approval

The country profiles were prepared in one of two ways. For countries for which the Regional Office had substantial information in its databases or from the publications of other international organizations, a draft was prepared and submitted to the ministry of health for revision and approval. Little information was available on some countries; in such cases the governments were asked to write the profiles. In the countries of central and eastern Europe and the newly independent states, the WHO liaison officers played a strong role in either providing the information or encouraging others to do so. In both cases, the health ministries approved the final text.

Design of the questionnaire and case studies and development of a framework for analysis

Since we were examining health policy from a health for all perspective, the principles and characteristics of health for all – including promoting equity, public participation, intersectoral policies on lifestyles, the environment and health care, reorientation to primary health care and an orientation towards health outcome – provided the overall analytical framework for the structure of the questionnaire, the case studies and the country profiles.

For each of the health for all principles or characteristics, respondents were asked which of the following policy instruments they were using and to give examples of these:

- research and information
- health education and awareness-building
- consultation and negotiation
- structural, administrative and management measures
- financial measures
- legislation and regulation
- human resource development, including education and training
- monitoring and evaluation of the process
- other.

Together with the questionnaire, a list of definitions of the health for all principles and of terms that might create confusion was sent out with the covering letter. These included, for example, the difference between health education and awareness-building and between consultation and negotiation (see Box 1.3).

These definitions were reiterated in the text of the questionnaire, which also included examples of possible policy instruments that might be used for implementing each of the health for all principles or characteristics.

The set of possible policy instruments used was a further refinement of a similar set of policy instruments used previously in a WHO review of Finland's health for all policy *(25)* that had provided a framework for analysis. The *Handbook for process evaluation in noncommunicable disease prevention (58)* prepared for the WHO Countrywide Integrated Noncommunicable Diseases Intervention (CINDI) programme uses a slightly different list for analytical purposes: policy development and coordination; legislation and regulation; marketing and organizational development; public education and mass media, community mobilization; preventive practice guidelines, professional education and involvement; monitoring, evaluation and research; and international collaboration. Each of these is then broken down further.

To assess how far the actions proposed in policy documents are carried out in practice, respondents were also asked whether the action was planned, was being implemented or had been completed.

Box 1.3. Definitions of health education, awareness-building, consultation and negotiation

Health education	Activities designed to facilitate changes in health-related behaviour and attitudes to health.
Awareness-building	Using information about health and available channels such as the mass media, and settings such as the city, school and workplace, to disseminate such information in order to create or change perceptions regarding the need for policy actions.
Consultation	Dialogue between policy-makers and other persons or groups that allows for an exchange of information and feedback.
Negotiation	Means for settling disputes whereby each party declares its desires and attempts to obtain as much as possible by making concessions to the other side, displaying its purposes or looking for trade-offs.

Respondents to the questionnaire were mainly officials in ministries or departments of health in a position to have the official view of policy developments. The authors of the case studies had more mixed backgrounds, including academics and researchers.

Strengths and limitations of the methods used

Setting up a database
Much of the information was collected by means of a questionnaire, structured according to a framework based on the health for all principles and the suggested set of policy instruments. This facilitated the structuring of a database along the lines of this matrix. Although this is by no means considered complete, it has allowed initiation of a unique type of database that offers great potential for further systematizing information about the process of developing policy.

The case studies
The case studies were prepared by people who had first-hand knowledge, having been involved in the processes they were describing. This allowed for valuable insight into what had actually happened and why. Being involved and committed to a process does not always allow policy-makers to stand back and be critical of that process, however, which means that there can be a trade-off between getting the insider's view and gaining a sufficiently critical view of weaknesses. In the case studies that have managed to give a balanced view of a national experience, there is at least as much to be learned from the mistakes and failures as from the successes.

The questionnaire provided a framework for systematizing policy information but was rather compli-cated to complete. Defining the various terms and categories of information facilitated the process of responding. Nevertheless, not all items could be defined in sufficient detail to preclude inconsistency in how countries categorized information in their replies.

Perhaps more importantly, the questionnaire referred to a very broad range of issues and to a long period of time. Completing it required quite a serious commitment from respondents. To the extent that the respondents were committed, a great deal of historical information has now been preserved. The respondents must, however, have been tempted to give a limited number of examples.

Referring to the health for all principles as part of the framework for analysing the process of policy development facilitates a focus on whether countries are really trying to bring about change or whether they are simply paying lip service to sensitive issues such as equity and public participation in decision-making. Using a set of possible policy instruments (or of possible strategies, as has been done in the CINDI handbook *(58)* also offers the opportunity of investigating perspectives on policy development that have been given little focus so far. Such an approach, however, presents important difficulties in categorizing the various policy proposals and actions.

Attempting to take a broad overview of a process as complex as the development of policies for health for all in 51 Member States is extremely ambitious, and it was not feasible to go into a great deal of depth in some areas of obvious interest. The advantage of this method of working is that it allows a broad-brush view of the whole picture and creates the potential for continued study and follow-up of individual elements and areas of concern.

The written sources of information used are reliable in that they reflect stated public policies. In view of the position and experience of the respondents, the information on the policy processes and the thinking behind these and on how they are being implemented are as reliable as similar qualitative data. The approach used therefore ensures that the information received is reliable and of high quality.

The main weakness of the approach lies in the information not received. Given the breadth of the issues covered, there is considerable potential for underreporting, and the relationship between information received and information not received is important.

The assessment, further development and revision of the methods used in carrying out the study are discussed in Chapter 4.

References

1. HARRINGTON, P. & RITSATAKIS, A., ED. *European Health Policy Conference: opportunities for the future. Vol. 1. Overviews and outcomes*. Copenhagen, WHO Regional Office for Europe, 1995 (document EUR/ICP/HFAP 94 01/CN01(I)).

2. HARRINGTON, P. & RITSATAKIS, A., ED. *European Health Policy Conference: opportunities for the future. Vol. 2. The policy framework to meet the challenges: intersectoral action for health.* Copenhagen, WHO Regional Office for Europe, 1995 (document EUR/ICP/HFAP 94 01/CN01(II)).

3. HARRINGTON, P. & RITSATAKIS, A., ED. *European Health Policy Conference: opportunities for the future. Vol. 3. Implementing policies for health at country, regional and city levels.* Copenhagen, WHO Regional Office for Europe, 1995 (document EUR/ICP/HFAP 94 01/CN01(III)).

4. HARRINGTON, P. & RITSATAKIS, A., ED. *European Health Policy Conference: opportunities for the future. Vol. 4. Health care reforms for health gain.* Copenhagen, WHO Regional Office for Europe, 1995 (document EUR/ICP/HFAP 94 01/CN01(IV)).

5. HARRINGTON, P. & RITSATAKIS, A., ED. *European Health Policy Conference: opportunities for the future. Vol. 5. Health challenges in central and eastern Europe and the newly independent states.* Copenhagen, WHO Regional Office for Europe, 1995 (document EUR/ICP/HFAP 94 01/CN01(V)).

6. *European Health Policy Conference: opportunities for the future. Report on a WHO Conference.* Copenhagen, WHO Regional Office for Europe, 1995 (document EUR/ICP/HFAP 94 01/CN01).

7. *Terminology for the European Health Policy Conference. A glossary with equivalents in French, German and Russian.* Copenhagen, WHO Regional Office for Europe, 1994 (document).

8. *U.N. correspondence course in social planning. Lecture No. 3.* New York, United Nations, Social Development Division, 1972.

9. *Logical framework approach. A flexible tool for participatory development.* Copenhagen, Danida, 1996.

10. *Formulating strategies for health for all by the year 2000: guiding principles and essential issues.* Geneva, World Health Organization, 1979 ("Health for All" Series, No. 2).

11. RITSATAKIS, A. *Framework for the analysis of country (HFA) policies.* Copenhagen, WHO Regional Office for Europe, 1987 (document ICP/MPN 032).

12. LINDBLOM, C.L. Still muddling, not yet through. *Public administration review*, **39**: 222–233 (1979).

13. *European Conference on National Health Planning, Bucharest, 12–16 March 1974.* Copenhagen, WHO Regional Office for Europe, 1974 (document EURO 4107).

14. *Planning and management for health. Report on a European Conference.* Copenhagen, WHO Regional Office for Europe, 1986 (EURO Reports and Studies, No. 102).

15. HAM, C. Analysis of health policy – principles and practice. *Scandinavian journal of social medicine*, **46**(Suppl.): 62–66 (1991).

16. *Alma-Ata 1978: primary health care.* Geneva, World Health Organization, 1978 ("Health for All" Series, No. 1).

17. *Global strategy for health for all by the year 2000.* Geneva, World Health Organization, 1981 ("Health for All" Series, No. 3).

18. Resolution 2681 (XXV) of the General Assembly of the United Nations. *In: Yearbook of the United Nations.* New York, United Nations, 1970, p. 586.

19. WOOD-RITSATAKIS, A. *Unified social planning in the Greek context.* Athens, Centre for Planning and Economic Research, 1986 (Studies 23).

20. ABEL-SMITH, B. & MAYNARD, A. *The organization, financing and cost of health care in the European Community*. Brussels, Commission of the European Communities, 1978 (Social Policy Series, SEC (78)3862).

21. LALONDE, N. *A new perspective on the health of Canadians*. Ottawa, Health and Welfare Canada, 1974.

22. *Healthy people. Report of the Surgeon General*. Washington, DC, US Department of Health and Human Services, 1979.

23. *Promoting health/preventing disease. Objectives for the nation*. Washington, DC, Department of Health and Human Services, 1980.

24. MCKEOWN, T. *The role of medicine: dream, mirage or nemesis?* London, Nuffield Provincial Hospitals Trust, 1976.

25. *Health for all policy in Finland*. Copenhagen, WHO Regional Office for Europe, 1991 (document EUR/FIN/HSC 410).

26. MCLACHLAN, G., ED. *The planning of health services: studies in eight European countries*. Copenhagen, WHO Regional Office for Europe, 1980.

27. KAPRIO, L.A. *Forty years of WHO in Europe. The development of a common health policy*. Copenhagen, WHO Regional Office for Europe, 1991 (WHO Regional Publications, European Series, No. 40).

28. *Regional strategy for attaining health for all by the year 2000*. Copenhagen, WHO Regional Office for Europe, 1982 (document EUR/RC30/8 Rev.2).

29. *Targets for health for all*. Copenhagen, WHO Regional Office for Europe, 1985 (European Health for All Series, No. 1).

30. Ottawa Charter for Health Promotion. *Health promotion international*, **1**(4): iii–v (1986) and *Canadian journal of public health*, **77**(6): 425–430 (1986).

31. WORLD BANK. *World development report 1993: investing in health*. Oxford, Oxford University Press, 1993.

32. WORLD COMMISSION ON ENVIRONMENT AND DEVELOPMENT. *Our common future*. Oxford, Oxford University Press, 1987.

33. *Health for all in the twenty-first century*. Geneva, World Health Organization, 1998 (document A51/ 5).

34. *HEALTH21: the health for all policy framework for the WHO European Region*. Copenhagen, WHO Regional Office for Europe, 1999 (European Health for All Series, No. 6).

35. *Health in Europe. The 1993/1994 health for all monitoring report*. Copenhagen, WHO Regional Office for Europe, 1994 (WHO Regional Publications, European Series, No. 56).

36. *Health in Europe 1997. Report on the third evaluation of progress towards health for all in the European region of WHO (1996–1997)*. Copenhagen, WHO Regional Office for Europe, 1998 (WHO Regional Publications, European Series, No. 83).

37. *Framework for the third evaluation of progress towards health for all in the European region of WHO (1996–1997)*. Copenhagen, WHO Regional Office for Europe, 1996 (document EUR/RC46/ inf.Doc./2).

38. *Consultation of countries with national health for all policy documents. Report on a WHO Meeting.* Copenhagen, WHO Regional Office for Europe, 1990 (EUR/ICP/MPN 040).

39. *Health for all targets. The health policy for Europe.* Copenhagen, WHO Regional Office for Europe, 1993 (European Health for All Series, No. 4).

40. LINDBLOM, C.E. *The policy-making process.* Englewood Cliffs, NJ, Prentice-Hall, 1968.

41. WHITEHEAD, M. *Concepts and principles of equity and health.* Copenhagen, WHO Regional Office for Europe, 1990 (document EUR/ICP/RPD 414 7734r).

42. KUNST, A.E. & MACKENBACH, J.P. *Measuring socio-economic inequalities in health.* Copenhagen, WHO Regional Office for Europe, 1994 (document EUR/ICP/RPD 416 12234).

43. DAHLGREN, G. & WHITEHEAD, M. *Policies and strategies to promote equity in health.* Copenhagen, WHO Regional Office for Europe, 1992 (document EUR/ICP/RPD 414(2) 9866n).

44. WINSEMIUS, P. Intersectoral negotiation. *In*: Taket, A.R., ed. *Making partners: intersectoral action for health.* The Hague, Ministry of Welfare, Health and Cultural Affairs, 1990, pp. 29–37.

45. SVENSSON, P.-G. & STARRIN, B., ED. *Health policy development for disadvantaged groups.* Oslo, Scandinavian University Press, 1992.

46. KIRCK, M. *Genomics: setting an agenda for regional health care.* Copenhagen, WHO Regional Office for Europe, 1998 (Regions for Health Network, Leading Edge Series, No. 4, document EUR/ICP/POLC 05 02 02 (4)).

47. HANSSON, L.R. Developing and implementing a regional HFA policy – the Östergötland experience. *In*: Harrington, P. & Ritsatakis, A., ed. *European Health Policy Conference: opportunities for the future. Vol. 2. The policy framework to meet the challenges: intersectoral action for health.* Copenhagen, WHO Regional Office for Europe, 1995 (document EUR/ICP/HFAP 94 01/CN01(II)), pp. 141–168.

48. TSOUROS, A.D., ED. *World Health Organization Healthy Cities project: a project becomes a movement. Review of progress 1987 to 1990.* Copenhagen, FADL Publishers and Milan, SOGESS, 1991.

49. WALT, G. Policy analysis: an approach. *In*: Janovsky, K., ed. *Health policy and systems development. An agenda for research.* Geneva, World Health Organization, 1996.

50. DUNN, W.N. *Public policy analysis: an introduction,* 2nd ed. Englewood Cliffs, NJ, Prentice-Hall, 1993.

51. *Resolution EUR/RC45/R4 of the WHO Regional Committee for Europe.* Copenhagen, WHO Regional Office for Europe, 1995 (document EUR/RC45/REC/1).

52. O'NEILL, M. & PEDERSON, A.P. Building a methods bridge between public policy analysis and healthy public policy. *Canadian journal of public health,* **83**(Suppl.1): S25–S30 (1992).

53. *The reform of health care systems: a review of seventeen OECD countries.* Paris, Organisation for Economic Co-operation and Development, 1994 (Health Policy Studies, No. 5).

54. SALTMAN, R.B. & FIGUERAS, J. *European health care reform: analysis of current strategies.* Copenhagen, WHO Regional Office for Europe, 1997 (WHO Regional Publications, European Series, No. 72).

55. ABEL-SMITH, B. ET AL. *Choices in health policy – an agenda for the European Union.* Aldershot, Ashgate, 1995.

56. KING, G. ET AL. *Designing social inquiry – scientific inference in qualitative research*. Princeton, Princeton University Press, 1994.

57. HEIDENHEIMER, A.J. ET AL. *Comparative public policy – the politics of social choice in America, Europe and Japan*, 3rd ed. New York, St Martin's Press, 1990.

58. *Handbook for process evaluation in noncommunicable disease prevention*. Copenhagen, WHO Regional Office for Europe, 1999 (document EUR/ICP/IVST 01 02 10).

2

Case studies

This chapter presents a set of case studies showing how the health for all approach was implemented in countries at national, regional and city levels. These are drawn from across Europe, and include those where the policy environment has been quite stable and others that have experienced considerable social, political and economic change. Although each took its own way towards health for all, there are many common elements in these accounts.

Finland is a pioneer in health for all policy development. The first Finnish health for all strategy was discussed by Parliament in 1985. This was reviewed by an international group and revised in the early 1990s, and a second revision is now in progress.

Germany is a federal country where the main responsibility for health lies at the level of the regions. North Rhine-Westphalia, the largest of the German Länder, presents the way in which targets for health were developed and indicates the value of sharing international experience through a WHO network of regions.

Hungary is a country in transition, which started well ahead of the field in taking a health promotion approach in the late 1980s. Somehow this momentum was lost in the changes that followed, so that at present there is no national health for all policy framework.

Lithuania found that regaining independence provided political impetus, and a degree of cross-party cooperation provided dedicated public health experts with the necessary support to persevere in a new approach to health policy development. In this way, effective use was made of local assets despite continuous changes in the political leadership.

Malta is an island in the Mediterranean that showed how a European-level health policy could be adapted to local conditions, and how smallness and the consequent broad responsibilities of government departments may be turned to advantage in promoting intersectoral action for health.

The Netherlands, a country with a pluralistic health sector and a long tradition of trying to reach consensus among many partners, attempted the complex health for all approach with mixed results. One of the enduring outcomes has been a strong focus on exploring the extent and causes of inequalities in health and investigating possible interventions to reduce the gaps.

Spain comprises 17 autonomous regions, which have followed rather different paths towards health for all policy development. Catalonia provides one example where an enthusiastic attempt was made to put health policy formulation and target-setting for health on a sounder evidence base. An economic downturn did not make the going easy.

Sweden now has a special Commission considering the formulation of national targets for health. Sweden demonstrates how complementary approaches can be taken at national level, at regional level (exemplified here by the county of Östergötland) and at city level (exemplified by Gothenburg), based on a well rooted democratic tradition.

Turkey, a country with a rather centralized administrative system, embarked on an attempt to mobilize a broad debate on health priorities. Some of the methods used were innovative, but were hampered by the problem faced by many countries: that of keeping up the health for all momentum in the face of pressure to focus on health care issues.

The United Kingdom undertook – parallel to health care reforms that sometimes seemed to dominate the scene – the development of policies based on health for all in the countries that make up the United Kingdom, firstly under a conservative and then under a socialist government. Case studies presented here from England and from Wales show how a long-term process gathered momentum, even when inequities in health had to be called "variations" in official documents.

These case studies were prepared by people who took an active part in the processes that they describe, giving them the special advantage of first-hand knowledge. Some of their statements are refreshingly frank as they set out the facilitating and inhibiting factors in taking a health for all approach. Whether or not their compatriots share their qualitative assessment, it is hoped that these unique insights into the policy development process will provoke further discussion and analysis, to the benefit of countries now embarking on a similar process.

The process of developing health for all policy in Finland, 1981–1995

Simo Kokko

Introduction

Finland constitutes a special case in country health policies, being among the first European countries to develop a national policy for health for all, and also because Finland's health policy was reviewed in a unique process by an international review group commissioned by the WHO Regional Office for Europe in 1990–1991.

This case study takes a broad look at trends in Finland's health policy and assesses the process of working towards health for all from the perspective of the economic difficulties in Finland in recent years.

Other processes are relevant to health policy in Finland besides the documented national policy for health for all. For example, since 1993 there has been a very radical shift from centralized state planning and intervention to extreme decentralization. This shift is remarkable and rare in international comparison; for example, 455 municipalities with an average of 10 000 inhabitants now have the main operative public responsibility for health.

A deep economic recession in 1991–1994 seriously shook the foundations of Finland's Nordic welfare state; unemployment was very high even after the economy turned around (the peak was 19% in 1993; in 1996 the rate was 16%). The whole political scene is being reoriented. The legitimacy of the core principles of the Finnish health and social services and social security benefits is being tested. In addition, the mass media are questioning the legitimacy of state involvement in public health and health protection and the related legislative and restrictive measures.

The Finnish health care system is being challenged by the promises of the market economy, competition and orientation towards patient demands. These approaches are very different from the orientation towards need – as perceived or deduced from epidemiological studies – that comprised the information basis of Finland's strategy for health for all.

The following text focuses on the 1987 document *Health for all by 2000 – the Finnish national strategy (1)*. Other documents discussed include a report by a WHO health policy review group, *Health for all policy in Finland (2),* and a revised version of Finland's strategy for health for all from 1993 *(3)*.

Two ongoing policy processes are closely associated with the work towards health for all: a pilot project, the health for all municipalities project *(4)* and the policy line given highest priority by the Ministry of Social Affairs and Health, a reform of the service structure *(5)*, which is a national policy project aimed at promoting the reorientation of health care services towards primary and other ambulatory services. The relationships between these documents and the processes behind them are explained in the next section.

Finland's health policy process from 1981 to 1995

Background

The public sector became responsible for health in all the Nordic countries, in contrast to the more pluralistic countries of central Europe. This can best be explained by the origin of the public sector in the Nordic countries. Before the twentieth century, the Lutheran Church and the civil administration were integrated, and only later did the non-ecclesiastical public sector institutions emerge. Care of those in special need was therefore gradually transferred to the public sector. The national cultures were relatively homogeneous, and the state and other public sector authorities have had unchallenged respect in these countries until recently. The public authorities therefore became policy-makers and also integrated the financing and provision of health services.

Until the 1960s, health policy in Finland was directed towards the processes of overall construction of a nation that first became independent in 1917. The health challenges were typical of that era: tuberculosis, nutrition problems, and services that were underdeveloped in a very large country with a predominantly rural and agrarian population. Population-level studies on nutrition in Finland were international pioneers. The nutrition of children was studied; the country needed strong citizens to build the country and defend it, if necessary. After the Second World War, a peculiarly Finnish public health approach was built based on the institution of *neuvola* (literally translated "the advisory place"). Pregnant women and mothers of young babies and schoolchildren were monitored and advised. A network of (at the time) modern hospitals was built in the 1950s.

In the 1960s, Finland began to realize that the patterns of health problems were changing. Health care services were intensively developed and expanded in the 1960s. Epidemiological and other population-level studies began to contribute to the thinking behind health policy. The ideas of prevention with the help of modern methods, such as screening, strengthening of primary care and targeting resources by need, rose to the top of the health policy agenda.

This gave rise to the approach of the 1970s, which some historians might characterize as the state-led, command-and-control era in health policy and the development of health services. A competing interpretation would say that this was a time of high regard for the experts. The expert institutions and individuals in Helsinki knew best what needed to be done. In Finland, command and control was a special relationship between the centralized state authorities and the municipal providers of health services. All service providers had to submit their rolling five-year plans to the state to be approved. The state had various ways of communicating what could be approved and what could not. Only after approval would the state pay its agreed half of the actual costs of health services. The municipalities rarely offered services financed independently of the state subsidy system.

Primary health care services expanded rapidly in the 1970s. A new law in 1972 based the public provision of primary health care on health centres. This legislation gave new preventive services official or even legal status, including occupational health services, student health, organized family planning and organized measures related to common risk factors for chronic diseases in the population. The 1970s were also a time of epidemiological studies in Finland: for example, the North Karelia project (6) and wide population-level studies by the National Pensions Institute (7,8). Finland passed a law restricting and controlling tobacco smoking in 1977. Nutrition policies were developing rapidly because of the national interest in heart disease.

Initiation of the Finnish process for health for all

Finland became active in WHO, mainly through active individuals: Finnish experts became involved in developing the WHO strategy for health for all in the late 1970s. Finland's health policy of the 1970s and WHO's policy on health for all had much in common, especially the emphasis on reorienting health services towards primary care and the determined interest in preventive services and later in health promotion.

Finland's health policy experts had been involved in drafting the European strategy for health for all. In 1982, WHO and Finland signed an agreement in which Finland became a pioneer country for WHO in developing a national strategy for health for all. One of the reasons Finland was chosen was its experience in developing primary health care in the 1970s. Nevertheless, Finland's health policy development had been relatively monosectoral until then, despite the obvious opportunities for engaging and integrating other sectors at the state, provincial and municipal levels.

The decision of the leading health policy-makers in Finland to launch the process for health for all was both an ambitious attempt to do things differently and also an acknowledgement of the fact that continuing to expand health services would not necessarily achieve all the health outcome objectives.

The next sections examine more closely the policy environment and policy areas at the time Finland's policy for health for all was formulated.

Steps and timetables

In 1980–1981, the National Board of Health translated the main WHO health for all documents into Finnish and widely circulated copies with the hope of generating awareness and discussion. In 1981–1982, the Board organized three expert seminars to discuss the envisaged broad policy issues. The first seminar included a small group of health sector experts, and the two later meetings included various interest groups outside the health sector.

In 1982 a steering committee was set up to prepare the first draft of Finland's strategy for health for all. The draft was completed in 1984 and circulated widely in Finland. This version included quantified targets related to health outcome or process outcome, which raised a debate: why should some organizations or institutions commit themselves to quantified policy outcomes that may, in reality, lie outside their scope of effect?

To ensure that representatives of other sectors and politicians would read the strategy, a shorter version *(9)* was prepared in 1985 as a Government report to Parliament on health policy. This report used lines of action instead of quantified targets as policy tools. A few quantified targets – mainly related to the use and distribution of public resources – were left in the report. The key strategic lines of this parliamentary report received wide support; there was more debate on such politically controversial issues as food production and nutrition and environmental health hazards.

Finland publishes its strategy for health for all

The final document on Finland's strategy for health for all was published at the end of 1986 *(1)*. The document is a book of about 150 pages published in Finnish, Swedish and English. The book has three chapters: starting-points for health policy; assessment of development of Finnish society and health from 1986 to 2000; and the strategy, including the rationale for the strategy. A total of 34 strategic lines of action were presented.

The first reactions to the publication of the strategy were mixed. The mass media took up the question of whether "promising" health for all in 14 years is reasonable. The hospital sector and specialized medicine were clearly disappointed at the lack of attention they received; only one of 34 lines of action concerned specialized medicine. Health policy-makers used the programme and the political acceptance it received to argue for true intersectoral work. Teachers of public health and health policy rapidly began to use the book in training health professionals.

It was apparently difficult to perceive the new policy document as being very different from the rhetoric that had reverberated throughout the 1970s in Finland. When the document was published in 1986, there was a wide political consensus on the main lines of development in health care. The strategy for health for all was, however, broader than the usual focus on health services. The ideas of intersectoral action met resistance. Good health services and well trained professionals were traditionally conceived as being the best guarantee for good health. Now there were conflicting interests between, for example, food producers and representatives of industry and transport *(10)*.

After the document was published and Parliament discussed the abridged version, the Government proceeded to implement the steps the document had outlined as its tasks. For example, new government funding was allocated for research into socioeconomic differences in health through a special health for all research programme *(11)*. From 1987 to 1991, the health care sector was preoccupied by a shortage of skilled personnel and by new legislation on specialist hospitals and then the new state subsidy system.

Many analysts in Finland think that Finland's policy for health for all constituted an important step at an abstract level, but it did not spark much enthusiasm or lead to much specific action.

Health policy review by a WHO review group

Finland's health sector leaders and the WHO Regional Office for Europe started negotiations that led to an agreement between Finland and WHO in 1988 to conduct a review by a WHO review group in 1990–1991. The health sector leaders were motivated partly by the shared interest with WHO and partly by self-interest in assessing the process and impact of Finland's policy for health for all. WHO was interested in creating from the review a useful model for other European countries.

The method and approaches used by the Organisation for Economic Co-operation and Development in reviewing national policies in such areas as education and the environment were closely studied. A study group of three people and a larger international review group of nine people carried out the review. Three methods of work were used: a review of documentation, on-site interviews and field visits. Three areas were chosen for in-depth study: reorientation of health services, intersectoral action for health (using food and nutrition as an example) and care of elderly people.

The review was published (2). The review aroused considerable interest and debate, perhaps even more than the document on health for all five years earlier. The policy environment at the time of the review had changed. The economy was showing very threatening signs of advancing depression. The health services were still suffering from a lack of trained personnel in 1990, a problem that improved rapidly in late 1991. The service systems were preparing for a major reform of planning and financing to dismantle the traditional detailed state involvement in planning and management. The financing responsibility would be transferred to the 455 municipalities. Many believed that this would constitute a transition to a new era in which the municipalities would become a new kind of power figure, and they would quickly show the hospitals – the big spenders – who is in charge.

The review group was specifically asked to be frank and critical. The review group concluded the following on Finland's process of moving towards health for all.

- The process had been too confined to the health care sector; involvement of other sectors and wider consultation processes might have helped in implementing the policy.
- Although senior experts and policy-makers were committed to the policy, the principles had not received enough visibility in the mass media or at the grassroots level.
- The process had been mostly led by experts and civil servants in a top-down manner; the review group asked why the municipalities were not brought into the process at the initial stage of formulation.
- The WHO policy had been used as a means of legitimizing rather than initiating the national process of formulating policy for health for all.
- The review group gave lengthy but ambivalent argumentation favouring quantified targets instead of just describing the direction of action desired.

- The policy document had referred to the tradition of equity in Finland and to the universal position of equity in the whole society; the review group thought that being more specific in setting objectives and targets for vulnerable groups might have increased the potential for results.
- A small group of civil servants within the health care sector who were busy with their administrative routines had been given responsibility for implementing and monitoring the policy: more human and financial resources should have been used.

Revision of Finland's policy for health for all

In 1989, the Ministry of Social Affairs and Health appointed a steering committee to start revising Finland's policy for health for all. The committee published a revised edition of the original document; the English version *(3)* is abridged.

The revision was based on the committee's own assessment of the outcome and impact of the original policy, the criticism and recommendations of the WHO review group, and a new analysis of the economic situation and policy environment in Finland.

The steering committee outlined seven areas that require action in Finland:

- reducing health differences between population groups;
- maintaining and improving the population's ability to function and to cope;
- achieving wide cooperation in support of preventive health policy;
- improving the effectiveness and efficiency of health services;
- developing human resources in health care;
- prompting management and leadership in health care; and
- enhancing wide public participation.

The new document proposed a very detailed action programme for each area indicating all the institutions, organizations and interest groups that would be expected to take responsibility for action (this was not included in the English edition).

Other results of the policy for health for all and the process of developing it

Numerous developments in Finland can be attributed to the original process of developing the policy for health for all, the WHO review or the revision of the policy. For example, an extensive multidisciplinary research programme for health for all with substantial earmarked funding was launched in the late 1980s. Much of the research was directed towards inequality in health and health promotion.

In 1992–1993, a ministerial committee reviewed the role of national sickness insurance in the financing of health services. The WHO review group had criticized sharply the existence of two parallel collective financing systems in Finland. The ministerial committee produced a political compromise with no major rearrangement, but proposed a number of incremental reforms that would clarify the roles of the two financing systems. Few of these proposals have been implemented.

Active planning for starting a new type of training for health care managers and increasing the volume of training in management, administration, health economics, public health and other relevant subjects started following the criticism of the WHO review group.

Intersectoral action between the health and social sectors has intensified and also found new organizational forms. This is partly a result of the reform of state subsidy policy in 1993, but the Ministry of Social Affairs and Health has also been very active in promoting specific forms of intersectoral action in the municipal primary services. By 1995, 125 of the 455 municipalities had amalgamated the health and social sectors in the municipal administration. Two thirds of the 125 municipalities have integrated their health and social services beyond the mere amalgamation of the municipal agencies. They have joint leadership and joint sectors providing services for elderly people both at home and in local institutions. Although the rearrangement of administrative and financing structures has not necessarily guaranteed active and specific intersectoral action, the most innovative municipalities have made real advances.

A special pilot project called the health for all municipalities project was launched in 1993 in accordance with the 1993 revision of Finland's policy for health for all. Seven medium-sized or larger municipalities are developing their own agendas in accordance with the principles of health for all. This approach is parallel to that of the WHO Healthy Cities project, and some cities in Finland had already become project cities. The focus was municipalities, as the vast majority of Finland's municipalities are far from being cities, both in size and in the types of problems of the residents.

The top priority in the policy of the Ministry of Social Affairs and Health since 1992 has been to reform the service structure of social and health services. This process aims towards structural reform in the care of elderly people, chronically ill people, cognitively handicapped people and people with chronic mental disorders: the gradual reduction of institutional care and transfer of resources to ambulatory services. This is one way of reorienting health services in Finland. The need for such changes was recognized without the process of moving towards health for all, but the process may well have given momentum to this reform.

Equity

Equity is a peculiar theme for health policy-makers in Finland. They commonly believe that the health policy and health care systems are firmly based on equity. At the same time, there is fundamental uncertainty about how such words as equity, equality and other similar concepts should be translated into Finnish.

Finland's 1986 document on policy for health for all does not focus on equity very visibly. It sets the objective of reducing differences in health. It commits Finland to taking special care of the needs of disadvantaged groups in the population. It also states that financial factors should be prevented from hindering the necessary use of health care services.

Why such a low profile for equity? The WHO review group also asked essentially the same question. The answer must be that, at the time Finland's policy for health for all was being built in the mid-1980s, equity was being taken for granted. Socioeconomic and geographical factors that hinder the use of health care services had been successfully removed by either not collecting user fees or keeping hospital fees tolerable. The health promotion approach was progressing on many fronts, especially in areas that would benefit disadvantaged groups. About a decade ago, all major political parties had their own organizations devoted to health and health care policy. There must have been an understanding (an illusion?) that Finland was making progress on equity, and equity therefore did not require a special focus.

The health for all research programme gave equity and socioeconomic differences plenty of attention. Equity concerns have been raised recently in relation to the debates over health care reforms. In addition, the fact that there will soon be as many as 455 different municipal health policies and health care arrangements instead of one national model for policy and services has raised equity concerns.

In the 1993 revision of Finland's policy for health for all, equity is a part of the first area of work: reducing health differences. Equity-related challenges received more precise attention in the detailed proposals, which included:

- developing health education to meet the needs of the population groups with the greatest needs;
- developing the skills of health professionals to address the special needs of these groups;
- orienting information systems and research so that they can detect socioeconomic differences in health as well as differences between the residents of different municipalities; and
- special measures to improve the community environments of disadvantaged groups.

The health differences between socioeconomic groups have continued to widen, mainly because the rapid general reduction in cardiovascular disease morbidity and mortality has been fastest among people of higher socioeconomic status. This trend now poses a very problematic challenge to policy-makers. General social trends, especially the high unemployment rate and reductions in social welfare spending, are counteracting the attempts to reduce differences.

Public participation

Public participation, which is a key principle for achieving health for all, is – surprisingly – missing from Finland's 1986 document on policy for health for all. The WHO review group criticized both the policy process and the policy document for this.

The 1993 revised policy for health for all takes up this issue. The 1993 document humbly admits that public participation, giving patients a voice and similar aspects of Finland's health policy-making and health care have been insufficiently developed.

Why has public participation been underdeveloped? There has been considerable rhetoric in Finland about the Nordic principle of local democratic decision-making, which also includes health issues and services in Finland. All the Nordic countries rely strongly on the democratic autonomy of the local authorities: the municipalities. The municipalities use democratically elected and politically representative governing bodies for multiple purposes, including education, planning the built environment, social services and health. The 1993 reform of the state subsidy system accentuated the role and autonomy of the municipalities. Academic sociological criticism of local democracy has been plentiful in Finland. Does it represent true participation of the ordinary citizens and users of municipal services? The answer has often been negative, although recent developments have tried to clarify the role of local democracy: instead of involvement – often in an unwelcome and unpleasant way – in the everyday operations of municipal health services, the decision-makers should concentrate on policy challenges and on integrating the true needs of the residents. Thus, local democracy, which is sometimes given as an excuse for the absence of participation, might be on its way to turning into a new kind of public participation.

Public participation has also been channelled and institutionalized to take place through large national patients' organizations or public health organizations, in which membership is usually based on the formal requirement of having the specified chronic illness or otherwise through personal interest. Many of these nongovernmental organizations are active at both the national and local levels. It would be very unfair for the work of these organizations to claim that participation does not exist in Finland. The modes of participation, however, have not been oriented towards work with public health policy-making, in the broader sense of participation, until recent years. These nongovernmental organizations vocally defend the benefits and the highly specialized services to which they feel their members are entitled. The voice of the individual may have easily been lost in the large organization, or individual voices are usually expressed within the organizations or in the public relations or fundraising activities of the organizations. In their attempts to influence national policy, these organizations have justifiably demanded clean air for people with chronic pulmonary diseases and healthy food for people with heart problems and for everyone who wishes to eat healthy food.

The health for all municipalities project has given special attention to bringing the public authorities in various sectors and the local nongovernmental activist groups together to promote health. Finland's 1993 policy document on health for all proposed this project and measures:

- to enhance models of local participation between public authorities and nongovernmental organizations;
- to develop skills for health professionals to enable them to work in a more equitable relationship with patients in accordance with a new law (1993) on patients' rights;

- to develop feedback mechanisms to truly use the patient's voice in developing health services;
- to explore the potential of new information technologies, such as in promoting easier access to information and allowing interactive participation;
- to give more power to national nongovernmental organizations in deciding how certain discretionary funds for public health and health promotion are spent.

Intersectoral action

Intersectoral action received central attention in Finland's 1986 policy document on health for all. This was the new feature in health policy compared with various previous policy documents that usually addressed the health care sector only. The Ministry of Social Affairs and Health challenged Parliament to address health with a perspective wider than health care services by presenting the 1986 policy document for health for all to Parliament as part of the policy-formulating process. The text of the 1986 policy document designates two sectors, social services and housing, as necessary partners at the local level in the 34 lines of action.

The WHO review group used food and nutrition policy as a case study on how intersectoral policy and decision-making really work in Finland. Many interesting observations were made. Finland had had a tradition of bringing interested parties in nutrition to the same table by inviting them to participate in state committees and nutrition councils. Representatives of public health interest groups have been involved since the 1960s. Nancy Milio's case study as part of the WHO review *(10)* criticized Finland's traditions of "democratic corporativism"; in the case of nutrition, this might mean that parties with contradictory interests sit in an intersectoral council. They state their views and clash about how to word documents, but all return essentially unchanged to their home bases, with little intersectoral action.

The municipal authorities constitute an exceptional potential for intersectoral action. They arose very slowly. In the 1980s all municipalities were required to establish two local councils. An intersectoral council for health education and health promotion was intended to bring such municipal authorities as those in health care, schools, youth work and sports together with voluntary organizations. A council for rehabilitation issues was oriented towards gathering the different professionals who worked with individuals and families that have health, social, work and other problems to coordinate the professional work instead of passing people around.

The municipalities lacked the budgetary incentive to launch into intersectoral work until the state subsidy system was reformed in 1993. All municipal social and health care services had previously received their earmarked state subsidies, and often little coordination or setting of priorities was needed. The new principle of the state paying subsidies as prospective block grants instead of reimbursing for costs retrospectively has vitalized local intersectoral action. The health care and social sectors now see that they cannot win anything by transferring costs to other sectors. The sectors responsible for housing and for care of elderly people and chronically ill people have learned to work together.

In the health for all municipalities project, the seven municipalities, including central administrators and the popularly elected municipal councils, were asked to list areas in which they would choose to work for health. The following areas were listed by one or more municipalities:

- nutrition
- physical exercise
- teaching plans in schools and health education
- reduction of smoking
- dental health
- aging
- the psychological climate in workplaces
- unemployed people
- children, adolescents and the family
- healthy environment
- health profile or a profile of social problems in the population
- quality development in services
- strategic thinking in health and social matters.

Municipalities are now under increasing pressure to save money and provide more services to populations that are aging rapidly. Intersectoral action is now being truly tested in these circumstances. The idea and visions have been circulated; what will happen remains to be seen.

Health status orientation

Finland has a strong tradition of monitoring health status and the occurrence of illness with various national statistics and registers. The people are also used to responding to population surveys; the response rates are usually very high compared with other countries. It is therefore not surprising that many of the parts of Finland's policy for health for all have been expressed in the form of development objectives for health status, although the use of quantified targets was dropped before the document was finalized.

Health status orientation does not, however, refer only to having a reliable and complete statistical picture. It means moving away from process objectives to ultimate objectives in improving health status. The emphasis in Finland's policy for health for all on common problems that could be either prevented or ameliorated by means other than traditional specialized medicine indicates that health status orientation is the basis of the policy.

What is health status orientation within health care? WHO and the WHO review group use "reorienting health services" instead of "health status orientation". The review group recognized Finland's long and strong tradition of preventive activities in primary health care. The review group asked critical questions about the fact that the preventive work is oriented towards the traditional medical model and about the lack of true teamwork. More work is needed to reorient health professionals in general towards the principles of health for all.

WHO chose Finland to be a pioneer country in health policy-making partly because of the country's success in strengthening primary health care in the 1970s and 1980s. The review group failed to notice that a large proportion of this impressive growth can be explained by the transfer of smaller specialist hospitals to the administrative umbrella of the municipal health centres. Thus, much of the shift from the specialist level to the primary level merely comprised renaming institutions and placing them under new administration. No hospitals needed to be closed until the introduction of a separate programme for reducing the number of inpatient places in specifically psychiatric hospitals.

The review group did foresee a threat that many Finns did not want to take seriously: that specialist medicine would achieve an advantageous position after the reform of the state subsidy, which was in its final phase of preparation at the time of the review. The years 1993–1995 have shown that this concern was well motivated. Primary services have had to bear a disproportionate share of the burden of cutbacks in many municipalities despite the official policy to the contrary.

Finland's revised strategy for health for all of 1993 makes visible the new ideas of orienting health care services to concentrate on the services that produce proven health gain. The strategy emphasizes quality development and allocative efficiency, the essence of Finland's policy line of the 1990s (reform of the service structure). These two approaches have become important policy challenges in the 1990s.

Concluding remarks

The WHO review group scrutinized intensively Finland's process of developing policy for health for all and the documents on strategy for health for all. Many of the group's observations and conclusions were accurate. It repeatedly saw the policy process as being oriented much in accordance with Finland's traditions: mainly within the health care sector, too much command-style process and no clear breakthrough to broader health policy-making shared by broader societal institutions and an active public. The revised strategy tried to address these challenges later.

Even though the 1986 document on policy for health for all restated many familiar themes in health planning and resource allocation, it disseminated the message outside the health care sector. Why did it not kindle much independent action outside the health care sector? The policy must be viewed based on the historical background and tradition of how Finland has operated in the past decades. All power and knowledge was concentrated in the national health care administration, which used resource allocation techniques to effectively reorient grassroots-level actors in accordance with national policies. Substantial human intelligence was used in thinking how to attract state subsidies to good causes in the municipal and regional health services. The heritage of the 1970s – the strong political interest in health and health care issues – was lost somewhere with the fading of the general political radicalism that affected the entire spectrum of political parties.

The present situation in Finland has been shaken up by the realization that the era of asking for more money and human resources seems to be over. The most realistic structure of financial incentives of the new state subsidy system has caused a radical reorientation of thinking. This could constitute an interesting basis for another round of policy-making, which should now somehow grow from the roots to the top, keeping both the people and their nearest health-related authorities, the municipalities, very much in charge.

Recent developments in Finland could offer interesting policy lessons for other countries. Health professionals in many countries view public debate and consciousness about such issues as cost-containment, limits to care, setting priorities and rationing very negatively. In Finland, these issues must be at the top of the agenda. About 15% of all public services, including health services, are financed by the government borrowing more money *(12)*. This is clearly unsustainable. Nevertheless, the representatives of the health care sector in Finland have had many timely and welcome reactions. The new search for efficiency, the most appropriate allocation of diminishing resources and new administrative and organizational arrangements would not have been possible in the spirit of the 1980s, when the only perceived limit to growth in health care was the lack of personnel.

Breaking the link between public financing and public provision of services did not lead to wide privatization. In fact, the net effect has been de-privatization, since the municipal decision-makers have been loyal to municipal staff and they have first cut back privately purchased services. Only in new types of semi-institutional services to elderly people and people with long-term mental disorders have small, often family-based, enterprises won new ground *(13)*.

It has become much more difficult to implement national health policy strategies because of the new autonomy of the municipalities. Policy development could turn out to be difficult to light up and move in coherent directions. Health care professionals now spend much time and attention in contemplating health care reform and in defending the survival of their own institutions. Citizens' initiatives diverge. Some groups are trying to return to the "good old days" when everything was protected by national will and earmarked financing. Others seek solutions from alternative medicine. The most ominous development seems to be the silence of the really disadvantaged groups in the society and the passivity of political decision-makers when they are told that the people in greatest need have been the first to suffer.

References

1. *Health for all by the year 2000 – the Finnish national strategy*. Helsinki, Ministry of Social Affairs and Health, 1987.
2. *Health for all policy in Finland. WHO health policy review*. Copenhagen, WHO Regional Office for Europe, 1991.
3. *Health for All by the year 2000: revised strategy for co-operation*. Helsinki, Ministry of Social Affairs and Health, 1993 (Publications Series 1993:9).

4. PERTTILÄ, K. ET AL. *Seitsemän kuntaa terveyttä edistämässä. Raportti TK 2000 – kuntaohjelman käynnistymisestä.* [Seven municipalities promote health. Report on the beginning of the health for all municipalities project.] Helsinki, STAKES, 1995 (Aiheita 29/1995).

5. KOKKO, S. New developments in the public primary social and health services in Finland. *Dialogi* (English supplement), **1B**:10–13 (1995).

6. PUSKA, P. ET AL. *The North Karelia Project. 20 years of results and experiences.* Helsinki, National Public Health Institute, 1995.

7. KALIMO, E. ET AL. *Terveyspalvelusten tarve, käyttö ja kustannukset 1964–1976.* [Need, utilization and costs of health services in Finland from 1964 to 1976]. Helsinki, National Pension Institute of Finland, 1982 (Kansaneläkelaitoksen julkaisuja A:18).

8. AROMAA, A, ET AL. *Terveys, toimintakyky ja hoidontarve Suomessa. Mini-Suomi-terveystutkimuksen päätulokset.* [Health, functionality and need for health care in Finland: the main findings of the mini-Finland population study]. Helsinki, National Pensions Institute, 1989 (Kansaneläkelaitoksen julkaisuja AL:32).

9. *Health policy report by the Government to Parliament.* Helsinki, Ministry of Social Affairs and Health, 1985.

10. MILIO, N. Food and nutrition policy. *In: Health for all policy in Finland. WHO health policy review.* Copenhagen, WHO Regional Office for Europe, 1991, pp. 153–175.

11. *Programme for research for "health for all by the year 2000".* Helsinki, Finnish Academy of Sciences, Medical Research Board, 1990.

12. HÄKKINEN, U. Terveydenhuollon kokonaismenot [Total spending in health care in Finland]. *In:* Uusitalo, H. et al., ed. *Sosiaali- ja terveydenhuollon palvelukatsaus* [Review of social and health services in Finland]. Jyväskylä, Gummerus Oy, 1995 (Raportti 173).

13. LEHTO, J. Adaptation or a new strategy? Finnish local welfare state in the 1990s. *Kunnallistieteellinen airkakauslehti*, **22**: 303–313 (1995).

Health policy in North Rhine-Westphalia, Germany

Birgit Weihrauch

Introduction

North Rhine-Westphalia is the largest and one of the most densely populated German *Länder* (states) with nearly 18 million inhabitants. It is situated in the heart of Europe and borders Belgium and the Netherlands.

The Ruhr area in North Rhine-Westphalia is one of the most industrialized areas in Germany – and in Europe – but rural areas such as the Sauerland are also typical.

Germany's health care system is pluralistic and self-negotiating, and has substantial autonomy for organizations and institutions such as the health insurance schemes, the associations of physicians and dentists, pharmacists' associations, hospitals, welfare organizations and urban and rural districts. The health care system is derived from the Bismarck model; federal law provides a legal framework for the main structures and financing. This law was modified in 1989, in 1992 and very recently in 1997. Further legislation on health care reform is pending.

The *Länder* have the main responsibility for formulating and implementing health policy. They have legislative authority for most matters related to health. The *Länder* differ considerably in size, geographical structure, political tradition and health policy development (within the framework established by federal law). North Rhine-Westphalia often takes an innovating and initiating role. The Conference of the Ministers of Health of the German *Länder* as an institutionalized organization and its permanent committees on various specific topics regularly meet, discuss and adopt consensus papers on matters of principle and of interest between *Länder*. This guarantees coordination in matters for which each *Land* has the main responsibility.

On the local level, North Rhine-Westphalia's 54 urban and rural districts are also responsible for implementing health policy. The local health authorities (*Gesundheitsämter*) are under the authority of the urban and rural districts.

In North Rhine-Westphalia, the high standard of medical services for the population is ensured by:

- a differentiated hospital system with highly technological and specialized centres, such as 14 heart surgery centres and 16 perinatal centres, and hospitals for regular medical care close to the needs of the population;

- a dense network of large-scale medical equipment available for inpatient as well as outpatient services;
- a highly efficient ambulance system organized by the urban and rural districts that provides emergency services within a very short time (even in rural districts usually within 15 minutes);
- outpatient medical services provided primarily by qualified general practitioners and specialists, supplemented by specialized hospital outpatient services; and
- a differentiated network of supplementary social services and institutions in the outpatient and inpatient sectors.

Progress in medicine and technology, changing social conditions, and legislation on health insurance and nursing insurance that came into force in 1995 are provoking major changes in the health care system. The outpatient sector is being reinforced. Hospital beds are being restructured and the number reduced, medical care by general practitioners is being upgraded, social outpatient services are being differentiated, all services are being linked and integrated better, decentralization is being promoted and the self-negotiating system is being strengthened.

This autonomous, self-negotiating health system involves many partners. North Rhine-Westphalia is an amalgamated *Land* and many institutions and organizations are therefore distinct for the Rhineland and Westphalia.

The development of health policy and of processes and measures described here have to be viewed with this in mind. Cooperation and various new forms of consensus involving all relevant partners from the very beginning of the discussion processes are of central importance and have increasingly been cultivated in recent years. In a way, they have imprinted the approach of North Rhine-Westphalia to health policy, giving government and policy-makers a mainly initiating and steering function in a democratic process. Limited resources make these processes of coordination and cooperation even more necessary.

The activities and programme described here are mostly initiated and coordinated by the Ministry of Employment, Health and Social Affairs. Further initiatives in some defined fields started by institutions or organizations of the self-negotiating health care system are not described. The account includes as many examples as possible, but the measures described here are by no means complete. Further, they were selected according to the aspects required for the case study.

The concepts and guiding principles of health policy in North Rhine-Westphalia are described before details are provided on the principles of the health for all policy. This makes repetition unavoidable and cross-references necessary, but provides an overall impression of the main political directions and demonstrates well that the principles of North Rhine-Westphalia's health policy and its approaches and activities meet again in the individual items of the policy for health for all under very different aspects.

Concepts and guiding principles of health policy

Programmes and health concepts

Health policy in North Rhine-Westphalia has taken special approaches focusing on the needs of its population. It has traditionally taken an interest in health policy issues that are related to social medicine, public health and environmental problems, whereas autonomous, self-negotiating organizations and institutions have taken prime responsibility for questions of individual medical care.

The state programme for North Rhine-Westphalia, which was mostly developed and published in the 1980s, gives an impression of the direction and the differentiation of approaches taken in different health policy topics according to political needs, including previous health policy in North Rhine-Westphalia. For the programmes on AIDS, maternal and child health and drugs developed in the late 1980s, the political need was obvious. AIDS was a new threat for the population and a new infectious disease that caused fear and uncertainty among the population, infant mortality was higher than in most of the other *Länder* and the abuse of illegal drugs was increasing.

The state health conference of North Rhine-Westphalia was first institutionalized in 1992 (see page 45), but expert commissions supported the federal government in developing the programmes.

The AIDS programme

The AIDS programme was published in 1987 (*1*) and has focused on:

* preventing AIDS, including a variety of mass-media and individual communication measures for special target groups and the general public;
* optimizing the health care system for people with AIDS, including inpatient and outpatient care and the medical and psychosocial sectors;
* promoting solidarity with HIV-positive people; and
* information exchange and cooperation, including the establishment of an AIDS Commission in North Rhine-Westphalia involving organizations, institutions and experts.

The programme has successfully been implemented in cooperation with many different partners in the health care system, especially involving AIDS self-help groups; more than 60 youth workers and more than 40 AIDS coordinators are working in the district health departments, and this is still a central element of the approach towards AIDS in North Rhine-Westphalia. The programme is being continually developed to respond to changing needs.

The programme on maternal and child health

The programme on maternal and child health (*2*) was established to reduce perinatal and infant mortality in North Rhine-Westphalia. It has mainly focused on:

- restructuring the obstetrical and neonatal services, now including a network of 16 perinatal centres and 25 obstetrical and neonatal focal points;
- improving services for pregnant women and the newborn in socially disadvantaged areas with particularly high rates of infant mortality;
- reducing sudden infant death syndrome, including obtaining new knowledge on insufficiently known causes and providing psychosocial help to affected families through a cooperative study led by the University of Münster; and
- information exchange and cooperation, including a commission involving various organizations, institutions and experts that critically evaluates the implementation of the programme.

As a result, infant mortality was reduced from 9.5 per 1000 live births in 1987 to 5.9 in 1994. The study on sudden infant death syndrome led to general recommendations on the care of babies. The incidence then declined from 489 cases in 1990 to 252 cases in 1993.

Based on this study, the University of Münster is coordinating a comprehensive multicentre study in Germany as a whole, financed by the Federal Government.

The drug programme
The threat to the general public from illegal drugs and associated criminal activities has drawn political attention for years. The drug programme (published in 1989) has focused mainly on measures to:

- improve information and prevention
- assist drug addicts
- prosecute the illicit drug trade
- promote information exchange and cooperation.

A comprehensive programme on drug addiction has been developed jointly by the expert commission, all partners of the health care and social welfare system (by involving the representative planning board of the North Rhine-Westphalia Health Conferences) and all responsible sectors of the Government of North Rhine-Westphalia.

Other programmes
Special progammes and concepts have been developed in numerous health areas. For example, "Have a heart for your heart", a worksite prevention and health promotion programme, was developed by the former State Health Institute (now the State Institute of Public Health) and the state division of one health insurance scheme.

In addition, North Rhine-Westphalia has developed programmes on:

- environmental health, with a variety of measures in education, information, prevention and medical care;

- supporting self-help activities and thereby involving affected people in the health care sector, focusing on strengthening infrastructure;
- improving social measures for people who are dying, including several measures in social welfare and health care;
- improving psychiatric care, mainly focusing on community-based psychiatric care;
- improving drug safety, including measures ranging from clinical assessment to monitoring therapies; and
- preventing skin cancer, designed in North Rhine-Westphalia in cooperation with German Cancer Aid (a nationwide nongovernmental organization), physicians, health insurance schemes and local health authorities, and implemented locally by the urban and rural districts in cooperation with various partners.

Even if some of these programmes had not explicitly been attributed to the European regional targets for health for all, the specific objectives, the target groups and the comprehensive way of handling health problems clearly show that the principles and targets of the policy for health for all guided their development. The health for all principles of equity, participation, prevention and health promotion as a central strategic orientation, intersectoral action and international cooperation are central to the health policy of North Rhine-Westphalia.

The State Health Conference of North Rhine-Westphalia

The involvement of people who are affected at an early stage of discussion and planning in the development of new concepts and programmes contributes to the success of health policy. This is especially the case for the pluralistic North Rhine-Westphalia health system.

To institutionalize and cultivate the discussion and decision processes, the Government founded the Health Conference of North Rhine-Westphalia in 1992. The system of health information and reporting was being developed, and a functioning committee for consensual decision-making involving all relevant partners of the health and social care system was considered necessary. The 42 members include health insurance schemes, associations of physicians, dentists and pharmacists, the association of hospitals, associations of local governments, welfare organizations and trade unions, and representatives of employers. Yearly conferences are carefully prepared and held on important topics. Consensual decisions and recommendations are published. A representative planning board meets regularly, prepares the annual conferences and decides basic questions.

The yearly conferences have focused on the following topics:

- psychiatric care
- environmental medicine
- health promotion
- the process of health care reform

- ten priority health objectives in North Rhine-Westphalia
- quality assurance in the health care system.

Each conference adopts a consensus paper and resolution formulating tasks for all partners on the specific topic.

Five years of experience have shown that consensual discussion processes can be difficult and may require much time, but are the only way for developmental processes to succeed, especially for difficult health challenges on which different partners have varying opinions. Very often it was felt that the process may already be the objective.

Public health – a challenge for North Rhine-Westphalia

North Rhine-Westphalia had already developed new public health structures based on scientific approaches oriented towards Europe. It is currently working with all relevant partners on further development to respond to new needs. Even before 1990, the Public Health Academy in Düsseldorf was meeting needs in public health training and education for seven *Länder*. Public health initiatives have become more important in several specific areas and for various reasons, including limited financial resources, an increasing emphasis on efficiency and quality, more emphasis on health promotion and prevention, new approaches for disadvantaged social groups and further development of the health information system. For these reasons, more innovation was required for the new public health.

Thus the first faculty of health sciences in Germany was founded at the University of Bielefeld in 1994. Another scientific public health centre is located in Düsseldorf. In addition, there are numerous well reputed public health scientific institutes and academies. One of the five research associations for public health in Germany is based in North Rhine-Westphalia.

In 1995, the State Institute for Public Health (LÖGD) was founded. The former Institute was an important constituent part. LÖGD is a subordinate institute to the Ministry of Employment, Health and Social Affairs and has major tasks such as building up a public health information system. Since 1992 IDIS – now part of LÖGD – has been recognized as a WHO documentation centre.

In 1994, the European Public Health Centre was founded as a nongovernmental association of scientific, practical and political experts with a coordinating office in LÖGD. This centre aims to guarantee information flow between the research, political and practical levels and offers public health cooperation to all member states and institutions. A common understanding of the meaning and the importance of public health (and the new public health agenda) is required to promote joint European efforts to promote European integration.

A reform of the public health service at the district level is being promoted to meet the challenges and needs on the local level, including the current administrative reforms.

The North Rhine-Westphalia courses of study in public health in Bielefeld and Düsseldorf are active members of the Association of Schools of Public Health in the European Region (ASPHER).

Membership in the Regions for Health Network and the implementation of the Network's aims and principles

North Rhine-Westphalia is a founding member of the Regions for Health Network, which was established in November 1992 in Düsseldorf. North Rhine-Westphalia has since then actively promoted the implementation of the aims and principles of the Network and the WHO strategy for health for all in its health policy. This has included setting up explicit health targets for North Rhine-Westphalia that involve all relevant partners, promoting intersectoral action for the development of health policy, using health promotion, participation and decentralization as guiding principles, aiming at an optimum of quality and efficiency and working at optimizing cooperation, coordination and integration of the partners and sectors on the state and especially local level. The experience and knowledge of and cooperation with other (European) regions were considered to be helpful in these efforts. The Regions for Health Network and the link to WHO became well known in North Rhine-Westphalia, and many active partners were found to support the developments described in the following paragraphs, including within the planning board of the State Health Conference and LÖGD.

Targets for health for all

After the Regions for Health Network was founded, North Rhine-Westphalia started a process of discussing target-setting based on developing new public health structures and a health information system involving the North Rhine-Westphalia Health Conference and its planning board.

After almost two years of consensus-finding, a draft document on ten priority health targets for North Rhine-Westphalia was passed at the 1995 State Health Conference. Difficult discussions at the 1995 conference and within its planning board on the specific direction and content of future health policy in these ten areas finally led to the consensus paper being published (4). The ten health targets cover the following topics (the relevant European regional targets for health for all are listed after each target).

1. Reducing cardiovascular disease   target 9
2. Reducing cancer   target 10
3. Settings for health promotion   target 14
4. Tobacco, alcohol and psychoactive drugs   target 17
5. Environmental health management   target 19
6. Primary health care   target 28
7. Hospital care   target 29
8. Community services to meet special needs   target 30
9. Health research and development   target 32
10. Health information support   target 35

The ten topics:

- meet special problems and areas relevant to North Rhine-Westphalia;
- refer to the five areas identified in the 38 targets; and
- tackle health challenges as well as structural challenges.

The target document was an important first step. A workshop on target-setting with international participation was organized in March 1996 in Brussels. It provided more information and knowledge for the further development of the qualitative and quantitative aspects of health targets. A working group of the planning board of the State Health Conference is actively involved in further development.

Healthy North Rhine-Westphalia

The Ministry of Employment, Health and Social Affairs has advertised a competition for the project network Healthy North Rhine-Westphalia, aimed at improving quality, innovation and efficiency in the health care system. All institutions and organizations carrying out projects that are very innovative and of high quality were asked to apply for membership. Several prerequisites have to be fulfilled, one being an orientation towards fulfilling the health targets of North Rhine-Westphalia.

Health prizes are awarded for the best projects. The planning board of the State Health Conference has participated actively in the decision-making process. The first list of outstanding projects has been published, and three projects have been awarded prizes. These projects are excellent examples for other institutions and organizations and are intended to give impetus for further development.

Intersectoral action for health

An important principle of health for all is intersectoral action, as health must be placed on the agenda in many different fields, including research, education, transport, environment, housing and city planning. An interministerial working group within the North Rhine-Westphalia Government was founded to intensify and disseminate the responsibility for health to all sectors in government and administration. Its tasks are:

- to analyse and demonstrate which projects related to health have been carried out in the various sectors; and
- to discuss further intersectoral developments in state policy.

The ministries responsible for education, science and research, environment, city planning and traffic are involved. According to the subject of discussion they are also involved in the discussions of the State Health Conference.

Local coordination – a new approach to meet the need for more coordination and cooperation for health

The traditional sectoral approach no longer meets the requirements of a modern and future-oriented health and social care system at the local level. Strengthening efforts towards more cooperation and coordination is required to improve the quality, effectiveness and efficiency of health and social care.

A pilot project for North Rhine-Westphalia supported by the Ministry of Employment, Health and Social Affairs was initiated in 1995. The project involves 27 of the 54 urban and rural districts. Round tables are being created for the overall assessment and coordination of the health and social care system, and working groups are being set up in turn on such specific topics as health promotion, psychiatric care and linking hospital care and outpatient care to achieve the following aims:

- optimizing the care of people who are ill and need nursing, especially fairness in covering needs, accessibility and open-mindedness with regard to the interests of the citizens; and
- working out efficient models of participation, cooperation, information and coordination.

The project also aims to initiate a new and innovative approach to planning and steering health and social care at the local level. As all of the participating urban and rural districts are choosing their priorities according to their own needs and aims, they are being supported in consensual health planning processes in priority health areas, which may also lead to setting up health targets at the local level. Interest has been expressed in this.

All partners of the health and social care system are involved, including the physicians' association, health insurance schemes, hospitals, nursing institutions and patients' organizations.

For the pilot scheme, the participating counties are centrally supported by:

- project management established at LÖGD;
- data and information management to support the availability of methods and data for analysis and planning;
- a consortium for scientific evaluation, to show whether and how the aims have been achieved;
- the Ministry of Employment, Health and Social Affairs, which is responsible for the overall political steering process; and
- various panels set up to exchange experience between the participating districts, their representatives and those who support the project centrally.

Equity in health – a principal concern of health policy

The principle of equal opportunity has always been of special importance in North Rhine-Westphalia's health and social policy. North Rhine-Westphalia has been governed by the Social Democratic Party for many years and since May 1995 by a coalition government of the Social Democratic Party and the Green Party, and considers itself the social conscience of Germany.

Germany's social insurance system is based on the principle of social solidarity, and the health care system thus provides an excellent basis for realizing the principle of equal opportunity among various social groups. The quality of health care is high, and care is in principle available to all residents in the same way. Very recent changes in federal legislation on the financing of the health insurance system have led to higher co-payments (despite opposition by the majority of the *Länder*, including North Rhine-Westphalia). Effort is required to ensure that the generally equal access for all to health care services is maintained in the future, despite narrowing resources.

In future political discussions about further health care reform, North Rhine-Westphalia will make all political efforts to maintain equal access for all to health care services, while ensuring high-quality care and appropriate financing of the health system.

Despite the formally equal access for all, the principle of equal opportunity is not always fulfilled for some population groups, such as:

- the long-term unemployed, single mothers and the homeless;
- elderly people;
- foreigners and migrants; and
- people with chronic mental disorders, long-term drug addicts, and those with AIDS.

Efforts must be made to ensure that health promotion programmes focus particularly on less affluent socioeconomic groups. For example, the new state programme on drug addiction will especially plan preventive measures for vulnerable target groups. Surveys on lifestyle, alcohol consumption, smoking, participation in health monitoring and disease prevention schemes, and morbidity and mortality data indicate that disparities in health status and in socioeconomic status are closely correlated.

Equity and the principle of creating equal opportunities for health also require considering people's exposure to unhealthy and stressful working conditions. In accordance with the principles of health for all, a further aspect of equal opportunity is the health status in rural versus urban areas and differences between different regions in the country. The state and everyone responsible for public health therefore have to concentrate all their efforts on:

- finding such problems and problem groups by analysis and evaluation within the health reporting; and
- trying to achieve equal opportunity by actively influencing the structures of access, utilization and quality in services for disease prevention and health care.

Equity in health information

Limited resources in the health care system make it even more crucial to set aims and targets and to focus on target groups. Careful monitoring, analysis and assessment of the situation are necessary to identify these groups and to get further information for making political decisions.

North Rhine-Westphalia has therefore developed a public health information system in recent years (see page 58) that includes information on various aspects of the situation of underprivileged groups.

Research
The Ministry of Employment, Health and Social Affairs has led numerous research studies taking a social viewpoint that comprise a basis for analysis and assessment in the health care sector, including the topics:

- disabled people (1993)
- immigrants (1994)
- the social situation of families with many children (1994)
- lifestyles of single mothers or fathers (1993)
- housing shortage and homelessness (1992).

A recently set up ministerial working group, including the social, employment, family and health sectors, is discussing the general effects of such social aspects and the necessity of a common data bank.

Public health reports
A section of a 1995 report as part of the North Rhine-Westphalia public health report series *(5)* deals especially with health status and quality of life and, in this context, with social inequity and health. Further, the 1997 public health report *(6)* deals with the question of equity in various chapters (such as those on smoking, violence against children, violence against women and children's work). Also, the adopted set of health indicators considers various aspects of equity. A new report on the health of immigrants is being prepared.

North Rhine-Westphalia is coordinating the new European Union Health Monitoring Programme for 1997–2001 for the German *Länder*. An application to this programme is planned for a project on social equity, focusing on the health of children and young people.

Infant mortality
In 1993, the Government of North Rhine-Westphalia permitted data from birth certificates to be combined with those from death certificates, enabling statisticians to make conclusions on various social parameters in infant mortality.

More effort is required in monitoring and assessment (see page 59).

Programmes focusing on disadvantaged social groups
The health policy of North Rhine-Westphalia has focused on vulnerable social groups such as mothers and children and drug addicts.

Maternal and child health (see also page 43)
Measures for prevention and early detection of disease are less effective and infant mortality and morbidity are higher among disadvantaged social groups, including those with poor education, very young mothers, migrant families and high unemployment.

A pilot scheme on improving services for pregnant women and newborns in areas with substantial social challenges has been successful. Specially trained midwives working at the local health authorities are paid to look after pregnant women and newborns in their homes, giving them advice and motivating them to take part in the prevention and early detection programme offered. This state-wide service is intended to be established gradually in the whole of North Rhine-Westphalia, involving the health insurance schemes. The limited public resources at the local level have to cover the expenses, at least in part, and this is a problem (see page 53).

Further, North Rhine-Westphalia is working out special approaches to reduce smoking and alcohol consumption in pregnancy and smoking in the living environment of babies (to prevent sudden infant death syndrome). In addition, the reduced hospital stays and increasing outpatient births are prompting a programme for the care and early screening of newborns and young mothers – again, especially in disadvantaged groups. Here a programme is being worked out together with all partners of the North Rhine-Westphalia Commission on Maternal and Child Health.

Drugs (see also page 44)
In addition to a drug prevention programme and the fight against drug dealers, much effort has been made in developing a differentiated help and care system for drug addicts that takes into account the fact that motivation for therapy is often fragile. Care and help services with easy access have been developed that offer support and help to people who are not yet ready and able to take part in a therapy programme aiming at abstinence. The methadone projects in North Rhine-Westphalia are among these services. These efforts have markedly reduced the number of drug addicts dying from drug-related causes in recent years: from 505 deaths in 1991 to 360 in 1995. Special therapy programmes have been developed for addicted women (counselling as well as inpatient therapy institutions).

Other health programmes (see also page 44)
Other health programmes have specifically considered equity, such as "Have a heart for your heart", a special workplace prevention and health promotion programme, and a programme to improve the comfort of dying people.

Because accident insurance is required by law, equity is also guaranteed in principle at the workplace. North Rhine-Westphalia has considered the request for equal conditions in occupational safety and health for all employees in all areas, and for more emphasis on health promotion in the workplace by reorganizing its occupational safety and health administration.

North Rhine-Westphalia is working towards improving the situation of special groups by developing new models of working time to improve the compatibility of family and work, and by developing occupational health examinations for young people.

A status analysis on work and health in North Rhine-Westphalia provides a database to enable policy to be more oriented towards targets and specific population groups.

Equity will be one of the most important guiding principles in future programmes. For example, North Rhine-Westphalia is working on a comprehensive programme to integrate disabled people socially that has an intersectoral approach from the beginning.

Equity in health for the urban and rural populations

Efforts have been made to ensure an equitable distribution of services in urban and rural areas. In 1991 a pilot scheme was adopted in the regular medical care system. Fifteen oncology centres were founded in North Rhine-Westphalia as associations of universities, hospitals and private doctors. The aim is to provide equal, high-quality medical care to everyone with cancer, whether they live in an urban area near oncology specialists or in the countryside. The oncology centres have established a documentation and information system for the treatment and aftercare of people with cancer, involving all partners.

In the 1970s, North Rhine-Westphalia started to develop a decentralized mental health care system for psychiatric patients that especially focuses on community-based psychiatric care with as much outpatient care as possible. A differentiated outpatient care system, more than 90 day clinics and more than 50 psychiatric departments at general hospitals have been established in local communities. This system is being developed further.

North Rhine-Westphalia's programme on environmental protection has contributed to equity in living and health conditions in rural and urban areas. Much has been achieved in the industrialized Ruhr area, where coal mining and other industry caused severe air pollution problems. Projects on environmental medicine in prevention, diagnostics and therapy have been developed in North Rhine-Westphalia after the health conference on this topic in 1993.

Health targets

North Rhine-Westphalia's new target-setting approach is initially focusing on ten targets in accordance with the principles of health for all. The State Health Conference and its planning board discussed equity as a special topic. The Conference decided that equity should not be formulated as a specific target but that it should be regarded as a common theme in all targets. This was explicitly outlined in the preface to the target document *(4)*. The situation for chronically ill and disabled people was also intended to be a common theme.

Importance of public health in the discussion on equity

Public health research, training, education and practice play important roles in the efforts for equity. The special tasks related to social compensation are an important issue in the ongoing discussion on the reform of the public health service at county level in North Rhine-Westphalia. Recent public health development in North Rhine-Westphalia is described above on page 46.

The limited resources of public budgets at the local and state levels in North Rhine-Westphalia are a severe problem, similar to other regions and countries. The 54 urban and rural districts identify the needs and set priorities in social compensation supplementary to the health insurance system. The situation differs substantially according to the size and rural or urban location of the community. Public health policy is challenged to hold its ground in the conflict of interests between the different political sectors.

Public participation in developing and implementing health policy

Health policy cannot be successfully developed and implemented without the participation of all public partners. In the following sections the word involvement is often used instead of participation, because it demonstrates more clearly the intensive nature of practical participation in health policy in North Rhine-Westphalia.

The participation and involvement of different groups at different levels are especially necessary given the specific factors that are important in health policy in North Rhine-Westphalia:

- the federal state (*Land*) with its principle of decentralized structures and with an important role for the local health authorities;
- the health system in North Rhine-Westphalia with relatively autonomous self-negotiating institutions and partners;
- the complexity of health policy processes, which requires the involvement and advice of scientists, professionals and the public; and
- a new understanding of the empowerment of citizens and patients in matters of health and disease, with a new relationship between professionals and patients.

The State Health Conference and local health conferences (see page 45)
The State Health Conference involves partners in discussing the main processes of health policy development.

The pilot scheme on local coordination (see page 48) established local round tables where they did not yet exist. They include institutions and organizations at the local level similar to the State Health Conference. These round tables deal with all relevant challenges related to health.

State commissions and expert panels (see page 43)
Commissions and other expert panels have been founded in North Rhine-Westphalia on specific challenges related to health policy development, such as establishing and implementing, monitoring and evaluating health programmes. Examples include commissions on maternal and child health, AIDS, nursing care, addiction and drugs, and mental health.

These panels involve not only experts and representatives of professional organizations but also lay representatives from the groups affected. As self-help groups and organizations play an important role in nearly all sectors related to disease and health, the groups affected were very willing to participate and the health care system was pleased to involve them.

Public participation in the public health care system

The heads of the local health authorities and the responsible sectors of the Ministry of Employment, Health and Social Affairs meet annually to guarantee information exchange and discussion between the local and central levels on developments and problems in the public health care system.

The European Public Health Centre was founded in 1994 in Düsseldorf and coordinates public health research and education and the flow of information from there to the health care and health promotion workers and distributors at all levels (see page 46).

Participation of politicians

The Government of North Rhine-Westphalia and thereby the Ministry of Employment, Health and Social Affairs have to implement political decisions and to shape the developmental processes; the Diet (Parliament) has legislative and budgetary authority. This requires an intensive exchange between politicians and the administration.

The Diet, and especially the committee responsible for health, regularly discusses topics related to health policy. The Diet is informed of all relevant programmes and activities and discusses many of them intensively. Politicians are regularly involved in important meetings and events oriented towards the future, such as conferences on special subjects organized by the Ministry in which future development issues are discussed. Representatives from all political parties are also regularly invited and have taken part in the annual state health conference.

Empowerment of patients and the general public

The understanding of citizens and patients of their role in health has changed substantially. The increasing importance of health promotion and disease prevention require public involvement and a new partnership between professionals and lay people. Further, increasing rates of chronic disease and long-term treatment require that patients be well informed and become experts in handling their situation optimally. Highly technological medicine and severe long-term diseases require that people receive more information and also psychosocial support.

These changes have led to numerous developments. To support health information and education of the public, various institutions have initiated a variety of programmes ranging from kindergartens and schools to differentiated programmes for adults. In particular, institutions of adult education, health insurance schemes and hospitals are creating diverse programmes.

In addition, a strong self-help movement for health has developed in North Rhine-Westphalia. About 200 000 people have organized in more than 10 000 organizations aiming at better information for people affected by disease and disorders, mutual support for people with similar problems and psychosocial assistance. The Government of North Rhine-Westphalia has been supporting this movement politically and financially in recent years. Contact and information offices in urban and rural districts provide professional support and consultation for the lay groups. The *Land*, the urban and rural districts and the self-help organizations share the financing. Tight public budgets are restricting the further development of this new type of contact and information office as infrastructual support for the self-help movement. It is hoped that the health insurance schemes can be persuaded to increase financing in the future. Further, the *Länder* and local governments are supporting the self-help movement and lay organizations in many other ways.

The further development of consumer consultation and consumer protection in health care (including patients' rights) is a main concern of health policy in North Rhine-Westphalia. An expert workshop took place in 1996. A study on future development in this field involving six interdisciplinary experts is being worked out; a model project on informing patients and consumers started in January 1998. The State Health Conference is considering placing the topic of empowerment and consumer protection in health care on its agenda.

Involving the public

The Ministry of Employment, Health and Social Affairs and its policy-makers have discussed the development of policy in various fields related to health in regular discussion meetings on various health topics open to all professionals and others who are interested. The topics have included mental health, drugs, accompaniment of the dying, AIDS, the self-help movement, hospital planning and financing structures and others. Many meetings had more than 1000 participants.

In addition, several information leaflets and brochures have been printed on different topics with print runs of several thousand. Current public campaigns include prevention of drug abuse and prevention of skin cancer.

International factors

North Rhine-Westphalia is situated in the heart of Europe and is adjacent to Belgium and the Netherlands. Information exchange and cooperation have therefore been important and have influenced health policy for many years, for practical everyday reasons.

Recent international developments have increased the importance of international exchange and cooperation:

- the changes in central and eastern Europe that comprise a challenge and an opportunity for Europe; and
- the development and expansion of the European Union and the Maastricht Treaty, which explicitly made health policy a matter of concern within the Union.

North Rhine-Westphalia has been active in international cooperation and developments related to health policy, especially in recent years. The Ministry of Employment, Health and Social Affairs and many other partners in the health care system have increased their efforts towards international cooperation.

The most important effort is the active involvement of North Rhine-Westphalia as a founding member of the Regions for Health Network. International activities (membership in the steering committee and participation in conferences and workshops) and the active implementation of the aims and principles of the Network in the health policy of North Rhine-Westphalia are consequences of this active membership, and have influenced health policy remarkably within a short time. Another important international effort was the founding of the European Public Health Centre in 1994 to promote joint European efforts in public health among the member states of the European Union and those applying for membership.

Four transboundary European regions ("Euregios", as they are known) involve cities and counties from Belgium and the Netherlands and regions from North Rhine-Westphalia. The Ministry of Employment, Health and Social Affairs has started intensive communication with the Euregios. Optimal efficiency in health care requires especially that unacceptable obstacles to using the health care system on either side of the border be removed. The Euregios have been involved in a comprehensive project to promote local coordination of the health and social care systems.

North Rhine-Westphalia is actively involved in European developments on health information. It also has a leading role among the *Länder* in Germany. In addition, North Rhine-Westphalia has held several meetings and workshops with international participation:

- expert meetings on sudden infant death syndrome in 1991 and 1995;
- a workshop on health information in 1994;
- meetings with the RHINE consortium to prepare proposals on telematics and health information to be submitted to the European Commission to obtain funding;
- a workshop on a minimal set of health indicators for the Regions for Health Network in January 1996; and
- a workshop on setting health targets in March 1996 in Brussels in combination with the official opening of the European Public Health Centre.

Intersectoral action for health to promote efficiency and quality

Many societal sectors influence the health of the population. Improving the health status of the population and the quality and efficiency of the whole health care sector requires intersectoral action at different levels.

The sectors of social affairs, research, school and education, environment, traffic, housing, urban planning and others need to promote health on the state and local levels. Politicians and administrators have to become active, but professionals also have to cooperate to optimize individual care.

Although there are numerous good examples and trends, much has to be done to change current approaches to health. Cooperation does not work without active support; various health care institutions are often still isolated.

Special public health efforts are necessary to change people's general understanding of health, transfer knowledge, establish structures of cooperation and support the development of training and education programmes that consider intersectoral action for health.

Traditional intersectoral activities

Intersectoral cooperation has traditionally been practised in some fields. For example, drug policy has been of great political importance in North Rhine-Westphalia for many years. It is based on preventing drug abuse, helping people who use drugs, and legal repression of illicit drug trafficking. Integrating these requires close cooperation between the Ministries of the Interior, Justice, Schools and Further Education and Labour, Health and Social Affairs. To strengthen cooperation and develop an integrated policy on drugs, an interministerial working group involving all related ministries was established in 1991 and was active for more than one year, led by the Ministry of Labour, Health and Social Affairs. Its task was to work out the future perspectives of integrated drug policy for the Government of North Rhine-Westphalia. A high-level standing committee of the relevant ministries is continuing this work.

Another example is the close cooperation between the ministry responsible for environment and the Ministry of Labour, Health and Social Affairs, which is responsible for environmental medicine, also involving various state institutes and experts. In addition, health care policies and the policies for children, and for elderly and disabled people are coordinated closely.

Some of North Rhine-Westphalia's health targets are closely related to other sectors; the Ministries of Schools and Further Education, Environment, Regional Planning and Agriculture, Science and Research were therefore involved in developing the targets.

New intersectoral activities

New initiatives have aimed at fundamental and long-term structural changes to bring about more intersectoral action. For example, the development of structures for health information is of great importance in promoting intersectoral action.

The courses of study for public health in Bielefeld and Düsseldorf and the public health scientific institutes in North Rhine-Westphalia are important for transferring public health knowledge from research to the political and practical level and for training and education. The new faculty in Bielefeld is interdisciplinary and open to all academic professionals (such as lawyers, economists, pedagogues and physicians) to optimize efforts to promote public health in different sectors and promote intersectoral action for health.

Building a public health information system

In a modern health care system in which public health plays a great role, a public health information system is of special importance for:

- analysing trends in health status and health challenges
- strengthening innovative ability
- increasing the efficiency of resource use
- improving quality assurance
- evaluating health objectives.

How the system is being built

In the past few years, North Rhine-Westphalia has made every effort to build a health information system as part of the very intensive and complex developmental process on public health, taking public health initiatives described previously into consideration. The Ministry of Employment, Health and Social Affairs has charged LÖGD with this task. In addition, numerous regional activities have been developed.

Health indicators related to regional health objectives

North Rhine-Westphalia adopted the set of health indicators passed by the Conference of the German Ministers of Health in 1991, as did the other 15 *Länder*, and joined the health for all database of the WHO Regional Office for Europe, modifying these sets where necessary. An adaptation at the level of the 54 districts in North Rhine-Westphalia is being developed. In addition, ten health targets were adopted at the State Health Conference in 1995 that are related to the indicator set adopted. The other *Länder* are working on implementing this set of indicators with varying progress and intensity.

Health monitoring

Based on the set of health indicators, data are being acquired from various sources to match the proposed indicators. This has been achieved for a substantial part of the entire set. There is a publication series on this. In addition, local information is being obtained from epidemiological cancer registries (Münster) and sentinels are being developed. A special analysis of the national health surveys of 1984–1985, 1988 and 1991–1992 in relation to North Rhine-Westphalia was published in 1995 *(5)*.

Distributed databases and networks

North Rhine-Westphalia participated in the European Nervous System Project coordinated by the WHO Regional Office to Europe to contribute to promoting health information exchange and comparability in Europe. North-Rhine Westphalia has developed two environmental health systems: the Drinking Water Data Entry, Analysis and Presentation System (TEIS) and the Noxious Agents Information System. The Noxious Agents Information System is a computerized index system and data bank for environmental medicine linked with other data banks on health protection, including occupational health and nutrition. It is now in operation throughout North Rhine-Westphalia, comprising another element of the emerging public health literature and information system. The Noxious Agents Information System especially aims at supporting the local level in making comprehensive information available quickly. Other *Länder* have joined the Noxious Agents Information System and TEIS, and the European Union is now funding the project.

Accessibility of public health information and literature
LÖGD, which is the WHO Documentation Centre for Public Health in Germany, produces one of the largest databases on public health literature (almost 300 000 documents on file) called SOMED (social medicine). There are plans for a SOMED database link to other databases produced in Germany and other European countries.

The health information system in North Rhine-Westphalia
North Rhine-Westphalia published the first state health report in 1991 *(6)* and the second in 1995 *(7)*. These health reports, based on expert opinion, report on more than 70 relevant health topics regarding population health and morbidity, health risks, health protection, care institutions, professions and financing. In the meantime, North Rhine-Westphalia has established an information system on health indicators based on a database including tabular presentation of health indicators, indicator definitions and statistical comments, as well as charts and maps illustrating the geographical variation of data. One or two public health reports are published each year, based on the data collected in the health information system. The database, which comprises about 200 indicators, is accessible to the public via the Internet. This enables North Rhine-Westphalia to offer nearly instantaneous access to up-to-date health information as soon as it is produced.

International approaches to health information
International exchange and cooperation in Europe is growing in importance and the development of an integrated European health information system is therefore highly relevant. The WHO health for all database has been an important basis for European health information for years.

The Maastricht Treaty highlights important preliminary considerations and resolutions on the future development of health information in the European Union. A programme of European Community action on health monitoring was adopted in April 1997. It is aimed at building up a comprehensive European health reporting and health information system to collect, monitor and analyse health data. North Rhine-Westphalia coordinates this programme among Germany's *Länder* and has a representative on the European Union committee overseeing the programme.

From 1992, LÖGD began the development of a statistics pilot for hospital data as part of the European Nervous System CARE Project, based on a telematics network for distributed health databases. This work will be continued by the Health Information Exchange and Monitoring System under the European Public Health Information Network funded by the European Union. The System will be part of the Health Monitoring Programme for the years 1997–2001.

The European Union has the political will to bring its policy in accordance with the WHO approach to provide effective cooperation and coordination on these issues in the future Europe.

North Rhine-Westphalia has been actively involved in international activities in this field: an active coordinating role among Germany's *Länder* in the European Union programme on health information;

participation in the European Nervous System CARE project; a leading role in the RHINE consortium, a group of European regions active in the field of health information and telematics; and organizing a Regions for Health Network workshop on a minimal set of indicators for health for all policy development.

Conclusions

North Rhine-Westphalia's health care system has proved to be highly effective. It has been oriented for years towards the principles of health for all and the European regional targets, especially the principles of equity, participation, intersectoral action and prevention and health promotion as a strategic intent.

North Rhine-Westphalia has also reacted with great flexibility to changing conditions and challenges from within and from other *Länder* and countries:

- the changing spectrum of disease towards chronic diseases;
- the increase in the proportion of old people;
- the change in general social conditions, including increasing numbers of single mothers or fathers and increasing numbers of migrants and refugees;
- environmental challenges;
- limited resources and rising challenges for the health care system;
- international changes and developments leading to the further development of structures and new foci in health policy;
- new forms of structures for coordination, cooperation and integration of all partners in the health system;
- development of a new public health system;
- a stronger focus on objectives and a new basis for an improvement in health information and health reporting; and
- intensifying international cooperation with the European Union, WHO and the countries and regions within Europe.

North Rhine-Westphalia now faces further challenges and problems but new opportunities as well. Equal access to services of high quality that are equitably and adequately financed must be ensured despite fewer resources. All opportunities to realize and increase efficiency must be exploited. The State Health Conference adopted a resolution in 1995 advocating competition in a self-negotiating health care system as an important management instrument. This competition must be based on certain general conditions, including solidarity, decentralization, services close to patients, quality assurance, coordination, cooperation, integration and transparency. In addition, the general conditions of medical rehabilitation need to be developed further according to the changed requirements.

Medical and technical progress require a response to ethical challenges as well as intensified efforts to protect users of health services and increase the expertise of citizens and patients.

Given the stagnant or decreasing revenue and corresponding increased need for expenditure in social and health care, the health system will have to compete in the future with other sectors and objectives for resources. Health will only be improved if efficiency and effectiveness are improved and costs are curbed and if, similar to the discussion on the economic situation of North Rhine-Westphalia, health is lobbied for in a more active and differentiated manner. Here, it should be stressed that the health care system does not burden society; on the contrary, it:

- guarantees health-related and social stability as an important component of the welfare state;
- represents one of the most important economic factors in strengthening sales and in stabilizing the job market; and
- it is a driving force for medical and technical innovation.

An active discussion of health as a crucial economic factor should not be reduced to the regional or national level but is of central importance at the European level. In addition to that discussion, health policy issues related to European integration in the context of the European Union, problems of unequal opportunities between east and west Europe and, finally, global questions and challenges of fundamental significance to health policy will constitute great challenges for countries and regions.

The Forty-eighth World Health Assembly decided to renew the strategy for health for all. North Rhine-Westphalia is willing to take part in the future discussion process as an active partner in the Regions for Health Network.

References

1. Landes-Programm AIDS – Aufklärung, Beratung, Betreuung, Behandlung, Pflege [The *Land* AIDS programme – education, counselling, care and treatment]. Düsseldorf. Ministry of Employment, Health and Social Affairs of North Rhine-Westphalia, 1987.
2. Gesundheit von Mutter und Kind – Landesprogramm zur Verringerung der Säuglingssterblichkeit [Maternal and child health – The *Land* programme to reduce infant mortality]. Düsseldorf, Ministry of Employment, Health and Social Affairs of North Rhine-Westphalia, 1987.
3. Landesprogramm Drogen [The *Land* North Rhine Westphalia drug programme]. Düsseldorf, Ministry of Employment, Health and Social Affairs of North Rhine-Westphalia, 1990.
4. Zehn vorrangige Gesundheitsziele für Nordrhein-Westfalen – Grundlagen für die nordrhein-westfälsche Gesundheitspolitik [Ten priority health targets for North Rhine-Westphalia – The basis of North Rhine-Westphalia's health policy]. Düsseldorf, Ministry of Employment, Health and Social Affairs of North Rhine-Westphalia, 1995.
5. BARDEHLE, D. ET AL. ENS CARE health statistics der EU/WHO. Beteiligung des Landes Nordrhein-Westfalen [European Nervous System Care project health statistics of the EU/WHO, Participation by the *Land* of North Rhine-Westphalia]. Bielefeld, North Rhine-Westphalia Public Health Institute, 1995 (Gesundheitsberichterstattung Bund 7/1995).

6. Gesundheitsreport Nordrhein-Westfalen 1990 [North Rhine-Westphalia health report for 1990]. Düsseldorf, Ministry of Employment, Health and Social Affairs of North Rhine-Westphalia, 1991.

7. Gesundheitsreport Nordrhein-Westfalen 1994 [North Rhine-Westphalia health report for 1994]. Düsseldorf, Ministry of Employment, Health and Social Affairs of North Rhine-Westphalia, 1995.

Four variations on one topic: changes in health policy in Hungary (1980–1994)

Peter Makara

Introduction

The challenges that have faced Hungary in developing health policy in the past 15 years have been constant in many respects:

- the deteriorating health status of the population;
- growing inequalities in health status and in access to health care;
- the marginalized situation and inadequate financing of the health care sector;
- the dysfunctional institutional system;
- technical backwardness;
- the significant role played by "gratitude payments" to physicians; and
- the lack of an intersectoral approach.

Many more items could be added to this list. This case study discusses the political responses to these challenges in the 1980s and early 1990s.

The following four periods in health policy can be clearly distinguished:

- Soviet-type socialist health policy, Hungarian style (1970–1985);
- the reform attempts of declining socialism, including the 1987 long-term strategy (1985–1990);
- the health policy experience of the nationalist conservative Government after the political changes and reform of the health care system (1990–1994); and
- the health policy concept of the new 1994 social–liberal coalition.

Despite the continuity in health challenges, Hungary's economy, politics and society have changed fundamentally since 1980. Changes in health policy resulted mainly from alterations in the general political life of Hungary (as clearly suggested by the four stages of health policy development) but international factors, such as WHO health policy initiatives, have played a major role in the these changes and in the move towards a modern health policy.

Today's health policy and health care system have deep historical roots. The concept of health policy and laws and professionals' views worked out under the Austro-Hungarian Empire still affect institutions and their mentality in Hungary, as both positive traditions and sclerotic conservatism. In addition, under-standing the processes of health care requires keeping in mind the larger social, political and economic policy contexts and the characteristics of the political system.

Soviet-type socialist health policy, Hungarian style (1970–1985)

The communist politicians and health decision-makers in Hungary found themselves in a tight and uncomfortable situation when the data on increasing mortality became public. The superiority of socialist health care and health services was one of the basic ideological concepts of the system. The drastic improvement in epidemiological statistics from 1945 to the late 1950s seemed to support this idea. In fact, mortality improved because infectious diseases declined, which resulted from widespread vaccination programmes similar to those in western Europe, and because the social security system was expanded.

The system of health statistics the socialist countries used in the 1960s contained detailed information on successes, but data on problems were almost completely lacking. Such statistics allowed the health policy-makers of the time to pretend that the health situation of Hungary was among the best in the world. This pretence had a characteristic boomerang effect, as it justified cutting back financial support to the health services. Nevertheless, the mortality data would not disappear, nor could they be hidden from the health experts. The first strategies of the Government in response to this situation included secrecy and an off-hand downplaying of the trends. They may have hoped that the increasing mortality was temporary.

A very interesting political and social event occurred in the late 1960s. Facing a decline in population, the socialist Government raised only the question of the birth rate in public and completely ignored mortality, thereby encouraging a rise in nationalism, moralism, anti-consumerism and policies promoting birth and restricting abortion. The Government did not allow the first articles about the deteriorating mortality trends to be published, which effectively suppressed the discussions in the mass media about the high suicide rates in Hungary.

In the late 1970s, it became impossible to keep the lid on the problem that had been apparent for more than a decade. It was no coincidence that the first conference of the newly formed Hungarian Sociological Association in 1978 was entitled Health and Society, thereby signifying that it was talking about basic social problems. Political rhetoric took the stance of blaming the victim and relying on a closed-minded interpretation of risk factors, maintaining that people were responsible for their own health. International comparative analyses and studies, which began to include Hungary and other socialist countries in the 1980s, conclusively ended the myth of the superiority of the socialist health care system and services. In fact, mortality trends were worsening in all the socialist countries but in no other industrialized countries.

Public health and disease prevention had been in a disadvantageous position even within the health care sector. The diminishing financial resources, dysfunctional organizational frameworks, inadequate and unfit personnel, outdated methods and low status of prevention sharply contrasted with the population's deteriorating state of health. Prevention was reduced to a stock phrase, which aggravated the situation. All this induced deep suspicion of any real initiative in health policy. Traditional public health could not respond to the challenges of the new epidemiological era. The existing Soviet-type network was not adequately prepared to take the lead in managing the primary prevention of chronic noncommunicable diseases, whose incidence was growing, and to adopt the ideas of health promotion.

Public health and disease prevention were pushed into the background in the hierarchy of power in the health care sector and professional education, especially in medical education and research. "Gratitude payment" dates back to fee-for-service health care and gained substantial economic significance when health care staff became poorly paid state employees under the national health care system. This contributed to the development of a curative orientation in the medical profession that did not favour the development of policies for health.

The leaders responsible for the health care sector disguised the steadily worsening problems by publishing statistics on successes and disguising the facts. This hindered the effective furthering of public health interests. Even a few years ago in Hungary, it was commonly and frequently voiced that the morbidity and mortality patterns deteriorated parallel to the constantly improving level of health services.

In the spirit of a concept that deviated from reality, health education wasted most of its scarce resources on empty slogans. The network of patient care institutions only sporadically engaged in preventive activities, despite all official declarations. This depended less on the attitudes of health personnel than on the system of interests and values and organizational and material conditions.

Even in 1986, the leadership of the Soviet Union viewed the concept of health promotion with some mistrust and did not favour sending high-level delegates to the first International Conference on Health Promotion held in Ottawa. As a result, Hungary was the only socialist country to send a ministerial level delegation to the Conference.

The attempts of declining socialism to reform health care – the long-term strategy of 1987

By the mid-1980s, the experts and socialist politicians really dedicated to health care recognized that the policy that had been followed could not handle the challenge of health care in crisis, and that current health policy was helpless against the deteriorating health status of the population. In 1988, the Minister of Health and Social Affairs established a health care reform secretariat in the Ministry, under the leadership of Dr András Jávor. He later became the Permanent Secretary of State in the Ministry of Welfare, the highest-ranking civil servant (the current name for the former Ministry of Health and Social Affairs and Ministry of Social Affairs and Health). In the working groups of the reform secretariat, experts who had been sidelined until then developed their ideas about the changes required. The most important reform of this period was the separation of the health insurance fund from the state budget and the transition to an insurance-based system for health care financing.

In December 1987, the Hungarian Government announced by decree a long-term programme for health promotion. This was a unique experiment under socialist conditions in Europe. The programme was to be implemented at the time that basic political reforms took place. Changes that culminated in the collapse of the regime marginalized this initiative, which disappeared along with the old system. Hence this programme cannot be evaluated properly.

The planning and initiation of the long-term health promotion programme in Hungary was made possible by a number of unique circumstances within a regime that was considered "soft" among the other socialist countries. Although Hungary's epidemiological figures were tragic, even by eastern European standards, the health care system developed a good and active relationship with the WHO Regional Office for Europe. The European targets for health for all and the Ottawa Charter for Health Promotion inspired health policy in Hungary. A team of interdisciplinary experts was on hand to plan and implement the programme, and the personal interests of Dr Judith Csehák, the Deputy Prime Minister at that time, were closely tied to the health promotion programme.

Hungary's long-term strategy for health for all was based on a well meant but sometimes naive adaptation of the WHO targets for health for all. The Prime Minister issued a government decree creating the National Council for Health Promotion and the National Health Promotion Fund, which was in charge of securing financing for health promotion. The Council set eight priorities:

- AIDS
- tobacco or health
- drug abuse
- alcohol abuse
- hypertension
- mental health
- the mass media
- accidents.

Action programmes addressed these priorities in 1988–1990.

Next, institutional frameworks were installed: the National Institute for Health Promotion was established and a number of local programmes were developed. The activities of the AIDS and hypertension programmes had positive quantifiable results.

There were, however, signs of difficulty, and only some were linked to the political system. The programme lacked legitimacy. The National Assembly did not debate the population's health and the health for all policy. The medical profession and most other health personnel were hostile to health promotion. The programme failed to implement action that would serve the population's interest directly and obviously: offering services that could have made it popular with and well known to the public in the long term. In the absence of a comprehensive system of societal policy objectives and means, the programme lacked support. Both its supporters and opponents blamed it for problems (ranging from the insensitivity of the taxation system to the issue of commercial supply) that could only be regulated in the framework of a comprehensive policy for health for all.

Even the Ministry of Social Affairs and Health made hardly any effort to harmonize prevention and welfare policy. Health promotion cannot replace the whole of health for all policy. It was a mistake to take responsibility (or to seem to do so) for problems that the programme could not influence, ease or overcome. This led to accusations and scorching criticism and aroused a sense of failure among the programme's supporters. Trapped in the contradiction between the targets set and the real possibilities, the programme was increasingly pushed back within the boundaries of the traditional health care sector.

Despite several positive examples at the local level, no countrywide movement to promote health emerged. Movements and public institutions for health promotion did not cooperate. The National Council for Health Promotion failed to lay the groundwork for a long-term relationship based on common interests with important social movements that had similar objectives, such as the green party and the association of nature lovers.

The programme failed to identify the economic activities and goods with financial interests in health and healthy lifestyles. In addition, the programme did not have sufficient resources to induce comprehensive social effects. During the three years following its formulation, there was no real programme planning or management at an appropriate level to determine targets, strategies, methods, organizational requirements, financing, evaluation and adjustment mechanisms in a coherent system. The whole programme was heuristically regulated and manually controlled.

In the absence of appropriate annual and medium-term programme formulation, there were excessive planning and poor selection processes. Since financial, personnel and organizational resources were hopelessly scarce, plans were over-ambitious and complete subjectivity flourished. In the lack of appropriate programme planning, the National Council for Health Promotion was not accountable for its work. Instead, it swam with the tide and compromised its own conscience by stating that needs were so great that any action taken would have some benefits somewhere. The lack of conditions for fair evaluation made feedback and professionally sound adjustment impossible. Further, there was no research infrastructure to assist the health promotion programme in a comprehensive way.

Although it was considered politically incorrect to admit that one was inheriting policies from one's predecessor from the 1980s, the fact that the major strategies and guidelines for health for all continued into this period permitted substantial elements of continuity in health policy; even in a crisis, this eventually made possible more organic change.

The health policy experience of the nationalist conservative Government – reforms in health care (1990–1994)

Starting in the middle of 1990, the new Government inherited a hard row to hoe from its predecessor: serious problems and health care institutions on the brink of collapse.

The president of the Christian Democratic People's Party, Dr László Surján, became Minister for Public Welfare. A number of talented people active in the socialist period were forced to leave, so the selection of Ministry staff became based even less on merits than previously. Understandably, health policy did not appear to be the main issue during the change in political system, so the problems of the health care sector were marginalized further.

The first document of the new Government *(1)*, outlining a programme of national renewal, was sparing in talking about health and health care and summarized the major themes of health for all in four pages. Virtually nothing has been realized of its well meaning declarations. Health policy centred on certain elements of health care reform in a clear crisis management approach.

A more conservative, medicalized approach to public health emerged. The long-term strategy from 1987 had its own boomerang: health promotion was labelled a "Bolshevik ambition". Nostalgia (idealizing the public health system of the 1930s and viewing it as a model), the centralizing logic of crisis management, bureaucratic reflexes and mistrust of the local authorities led to the formation of the National Public Health Centre and Medical Officer Service (NPHMOS) in April 1991. It was to guide and supervise epidemiology and health protection activities and supervise health care under the direct guidance of the Minister for Public Welfare.

NPHMOS is headed by the chief public health officer. Its central organ is the National Public Health Centre, which consists of national health institutes. The chief public health officer is the director-general of the National Public Health Centre, which controls the local organs of NPHMOS through county and city public health officers. The national health institutes help to fulfil the tasks of NPHMOS. NPHMOS institutes operate in the counties and the capital and in the towns and the districts of the capital. These institutes operate on the basis of the former sanitary-epidemiology stations. This means a homogeneous, decentralized, regimented government-based authority, with seven national institutes and also county and city public health offices.

NPHMOS had the advantage of limited but secure financing from the central budget but was not backed up by clearly formulated plans for health policy, only by quotations from a few outstanding Hungarian public health experts from the nineteenth century and the 1930s.

In the second half of 1992, the Government became interested in quickly producing a strategic document. At first the Secretary of State in the Ministry of Public Welfare wanted to set a two-month deadline, but the Ministry was unable to ensure professional work and clear dedication. After internal discussions, the Chief Public Health Officer secured the right to formulate the health policy document and made it his personal creation.

The Government accepted the document one month before leaving office. Government resolution 1030/1994 (IV.29) on the principles of a long-term health promotion policy states:

With a view to improving and promoting the population's health status, the Government has endorsed the Programme of Public Health Priorities until the Year 2000.

1. According to the Programme, the following five national targets must be attained:

    a. Health should be seen as one of the major values by an increasing proportion of the population. At the same time, efforts will have to be made to ensure that decision-makers attach primary importance to improving the population's health both in legislation and budgeting.

    b. The years of life lived free from disease shall be extended to at least 55 years.

    c. Life expectancy at birth shall be increased to at least 67.0 years for males and 75 years for females.

    d. The difference in life expectancy at birth of population groups in extremely good and extremely poor social situations shall not exceed 3 years.

    e. The difference between the number of deaths and live births shall be reduced considerably, to the advantage of live births.

2. To this end:

    a. Healthy lifestyles that influence the population's health status shall be shaped by means of education, mass media and health education, in the frameworks of which people must be made aware of the harmful effects of unhealthy dietary habits, tobacco and alcohol abuse and sedentary lifestyles. Further, the methods that enhance the adoption of healthy lifestyles shall be disseminated widely. To implement the above, the national core curriculum shall highlight activities related to health education, and the delivery of health care shall include, in addition to medical treatment, counselling tailored to the needs of the individual.

    b. When environmental factors that have a secondary influence on health status are being shaped, due attention shall be paid to reducing pollution of the living environment, especially of the air and waters, to diminishing hazards in the workplace and to shaping the social environment so as to enhance the promotion of the population's health and the prevention of diseases. During these activities, full consideration needs to be given to the regulations that may exist in the countries of the European Union.

c. A priority commitment of the health care delivery system shall be the provision of preventive services to children and young adults. In the middle-aged population, the restoration of health and the prevention of further decline in health shall be ensured by means of early detection of impairment. Acceptable levels of health in the underprivileged and elderly population groups shall be ensured by developing appropriate methods of extended and continuous care.

d. Taking into account the most prevalent disease groups and most frequent causes of death, efforts shall be made to develop the methods of preventing, first of all, diseases of the circulatory system and malignant neoplasms, as well as to establishing an appropriate scheme of screening to ensure their early diagnosis.

3. The Government considers it its duty of high priority to ensure the strengthening of the social recognition of the health care sector, which is indispensable for the attainment of targets set in terms of disease prevention and medical care.

4. Overall responsibility for the implementation of the Programme shall rest with the Minister of Public Welfare, who will submit a progress report to the Government in the fourth quarter of each year. If endorsed, the progress report shall be presented to the National Assembly as well.

Further, the Government calls upon:

a. local governments, as well as the boards of the Social Insurance Administration and their executive bodies, to provide the greatest possible contribution within their jurisdiction to the attainment of the objectives as set out in the Programme;

b. managers and staff of the mass media to take part in making the Programme known and in disseminating information related to the protection and promotion of health;

c. nongovernmental organizations, interest groups and each member of society to contribute, as far as possible, to the attainment of the objectives of the Programme.

This resolution offers an action plan until the year 2000 and 20 useful prevention programmes, but was not discussed or approved by the National Assembly and offered a strategy mainly for the public health network (NPHMOS). The document speaks about a six-year programme: there is no clear long-term strategy, and a government programme is lacking. Priorities are not clearly defined, intersectorality is not sufficiently elaborated and community action and local primary health care are missing. The prerequisites for health, social and economic development are not considered, and there is no clear concern for equity.

The crisis in health care in Hungary, which is now deep and prolonged, evolved over decades as the combined effect of three fundamental processes: the deterioration of the health status of the population, the institutional crisis of the state health care system and the prolonged economic recession. Numerous factors have contributed to this crisis.

The health of the population has been deteriorating for decades; demands are increasing and becoming differentiated, whereas the structure of health care and the quality and quantity of service have not kept up with these changes.

For about a decade, the tension between health care expenditure and the income-generating capability of the economy has been growing. Even already insufficient funding provided for the operation of the existing health care network has constituted an increasing burden on the economy.

Although the possibility of enforcing human rights has improved in a number of areas, no substantial steps have been taken in this regard in health care. The working conditions, opportunities for self-realization and the income of health care personnel – in view of their responsibility and work load – are substantially worse than what should be possible in relation to the level of development of Hungary.

One of the most severe problems of health care is that, in addition to official state health care and yet within its institutional system, a semi-legal sector exists based on gratuities; and the different and frequently contradictory rules and incentives of these sectors influence the operation of the health care system. In a substantial portion of cases, gratuities influence the relationship between health care workers and patients.

Deteriorating living standards, growing poverty, mass unemployment, the aggravation of social tensions, insecurity affecting more and more people and the greater frequency of stressful situations increase the chances that the health status of the population will deteriorate further.

Health care reform measures
Starting in the late 1980s, when the Government openly acknowledged the growing crisis in health and health care, important and radical changes have taken place in the health care sector (see Box 2.1).

Changes in the financing system
Financing of recurrent health expenditures was shifted from the state budget to a compulsory health insurance system. Until 1988, social insurance revenues and expenditures were part of the state budget. In 1988 a separate social insurance fund was created. The social insurance fund then financed pensions, sick pay benefits, family allowances, various forms of maternity benefits and some minor social assistance programmes. In 1990 the social insurance fund took over health care financing from the state budget. The state budget, in turn, took over the family allowance scheme from the social insurance fund. The pension fund and health insurance fund were separated in 1992.

Box 2.1. A chronology of reform measures in health care

1987 Experiment on diagnosis-related groups launched in 26 hospitals. National health promotion programme announced. Reform secretariat set up.

1989 Private health practice independent from the state system authorized.

1990 Starting in January, health care switched from tax-based funding to funding through compulsory insurance under the social insurance system. New Government announces national renewal programme including section on health care reform. Ownership of health facilities transferred to local governments. Ministry of Social Affairs and Health renamed Ministry of Public Welfare. New system of consensus management in hospitals introduced.

1991 Establishment of National Public Health Service (responsibility for local hygiene stations transferred from local governments to national government as part of this Service). Ministry of Public Welfare issues action programme in June to supplement the government national renewal programme. National Assembly adopts resolution defining the strategy for future development of social insurance (including separation into two funds).

1992 Starting in January, the social insurance fund separated into a pension fund and a health insurance fund. The respective share of health and pensions in total social insurance contributions of 54% is 23.5% for health and 30.5% for pension. National Assembly defines terms and conditions for a subgroup of public sector. Employees called public employees, comprising personnel involved in providing services such as health and education and, under a separate act, another subgroup called civil servants comprising personnel in administrative positions, including staff of the Ministry of Public Welfare. National Assembly eliminates universal entitlement of citizens to health care and defines conditions for eligibility. Family physician service created and capitation-based payment introduced.

1993 Voluntary mutual health insurance (supplementary insurance operated by private non-profit institutions) authorized. Act on occupational health protection. First election of members of self-governing social insurance boards with employer and employee representation. Starting in July, outpatient care remuneration based partly on fee for service and hospital care remuneration on a scheme related to diagnosis-related groups; share of family physician remuneration based on capitation increased to about 80% of total.

1994 The Act on the Hungarian Medical Chamber establishes ethical norms and procedures; right of agreement concerning general rules of contracts between health insurance authorities and physicians; and right to participate in defining health policy and legislation.

Government adopts new national health promotion strategy (government resolution 1030/1994 (IV.29)).

In 1991 the Act on the self-government of Social Insurance Boards with representation of the employers and employees was passed. However, the boards were set up in June 1993. The tasks and responsibilities of the Government in the professional, financial, organizational and functional dimensions of social insurance have not yet been clarified adequately.

The Social Insurance Institute continued to pay health care institutions until 1993 in the same way that the state budget did before. Outpatient and inpatient institutions were financed through global budgets set on a historical basis (the last budget was increased by a certain percentage). Doctors were salaried. New systems of remuneration were introduced in 1992 for family physicians and in July 1993 for specialists.

New methods of paying health facilities were introduced based on the following principles: for family physician services, capitation-based pay; for outpatient specialist care, fee for service; for inpatient care, payment based on diagnosis-related groups. Subsidies for retail pharmaceutical sales were also transferred to the health insurance system. Spending caps were built into payment formulas for family physician services, outpatient care and hospital care.

Changes in ownership arrangements
Ownership of public health facilities was transferred from the national Government to local governments, and autonomous private practice, including private health service enterprises, was legalized. Local governments now own the institutions that they operated in the past. One complication that has arisen is that the ownership of a local hospital has been transferred to the town in which the hospital is situated, even if the hospital serves a neighbouring catchment area as well. By law, the owner has to finance the costs of repairing and replacing equipment and investment. Nevertheless, these responsibilities are not factored into the state subsidies to the local governments, and these local governments are unable to support these costs, especially for the very large county hospitals.

Creation of a family physician service
This service consists of the network of (former) district doctors and newly established private family physician practices, with access to the new capitation-based remuneration system. The legal norms allow for privatization by the family physician, who may perform the function of a family physician as a private physician based on a contract reached with the local government and social insurance authorities. Free choice of family physician was instituted. In addition, all non-emergency cases in specialist care (inpatient and outpatient), except for gynaecology, now require written referral from the family physician. The introduction of the family physician system has meant the dismantling of the former integrated service units, which were small outpatient district clinics for most minor medical interventions by specialists.

Recent changes in pharmaceutical subsidies
Before 1989, retail prices for drugs were fixed at a highly subsidized level, with no relation to producer prices (which were also regulated based on production costs). Subsidies were paid directly to producers, and the state

distribution agency, which managed all retail pharmacies, paid producers a price lower than the market price. When the social insurance fund took over payment of drug subsidies in 1989, the method of subsidy was changed. Subsidies were paid at the retail outlet and were set as a percentage of the retail price. Depending on the social or medical value of the drug, the levels of subsidies were 100%, 95%, 80%, 50% or 0%. In 1993, the subsidy structure was adjusted in such a way that, for a certain number of drugs, a fixed subsidy was applied to all drugs with identical ingredients, regardless of price. This change was intended to encourage the use of lower-cost generic drugs. Patients could be exempted from co-payments for either social or medical reasons.

In 1991 import restrictions were lifted, and the drug market expanded significantly. Prices were deregulated, and only a ceiling on commercial profit margins was set. Overnight, a free pharmaceutical market was created. The expansion of the market has had mixed effects: it has promoted drugs of higher quality that are more effective, but it tends to unnecessarily favour the use of expensive drugs.

Issues related to pharmaceutical subsidies
None of the major actors in Hungary – the population, physicians, social insurance authorities and the pharmaceutical industry – were prepared for the radical changes in the pharmaceutical market. The Ministry of Public Welfare and the health insurance fund have been unable to contain expenditure. Actual expenditure has greatly exceeded projected budgets in every year since 1991. Both the subsidies paid by the health insurance fund and government contributions have been decreasing since 1990, whereas consumers' out-of-pocket payments have increased almost fourfold. Although the share of co-payment by the population has been growing considerably, 81% of total drug expenditure is subsidized, which is high by international standards. Nevertheless, some population groups cannot afford to buy necessary drugs. Increases in consumer drug prices are always a highly politicized issue.

Three factors explain the increasing costs of pharmaceutical subsidies:

- increasing prices brought about by the introduction of imported drugs and exacerbated by repeated devaluation of the forint (the prices of drugs made in Hungary are low by international standards, but increases can be expected);
- the subsidy structure, which is insufficiently targeted; and
- patterns of prescription by physicians and patterns of consumption by the population.

The behaviour of physicians and that of consumers are interrelated, and both have been influenced by the aggressive marketing of foreign pharmaceutical companies.

In addition to introducing fixed subsidies for some drugs, the Social Insurance Institute has taken other measures to contain expenditure. It has eliminated subsidies to health care institutions, which have paid the full price for drugs since 1991. It has also introduced a generic drug programme encouraging wider use of generics. These measures have failed to contain expenditure. Further, the pharmaceutical sector suffers from the same problems plaguing other parts of the health care system: lack of professional and financial control. Pharmacies can exploit the subsidy system. There is no professional supervision (or evaluation) of physicians' prescribing patterns.

The conditions for the promotion of health and the transformation of the health care system and of health insurance have deteriorated considerably over the past few years in several respects.

First, the Government's health policy has been undeveloped and contradictory in its practice. The past few years have been characterized by conceptual confusion. There have been no health policy priorities, and decisions have been improvised and made under pressure. In contrast to the election promises, thinking and activity largely narrowed to the required transformation of the system of financing health care. The problem was further aggravated by the fact that certain elements of the financing system were not harmonized with one another. Control, financing and service structure were transformed along different paths, without coordination.

Second, government measures did not even lead to achieving the objectives declared by the Ministry of Public Welfare and created conditions substantially more chaotic than justifiable, giving rise to a high degree of uncertainty. For citizens, the transformation of health care primarily meant the aggravation of uncertainties and a considerably increasing burden in many cases (for instance, the increasing price of medication).

Dissatisfaction with the condition and operation of the health care system grew among patients and the general public, the Government, local state administration and health care employees.

Third, fundamental decisions were essentially made within the Ministry by manual control, without any substantial participation by the other actors (such as the Medical Chamber, the municipalities and representatives of payers of health care contributions). An institutional framework for establishing a consensus among the actors in health care and their decision-making mechanisms was still missing.

The existing institutional structure and political mechanisms were not adequate to implement a successful reform process. That is why society could not develop or accept adequate reform. The existing decision-making system within health care could not rectify itself, which is one of the preconditions for a successful transformation.

Fourth, health care financing was at a critical stage. The position of the health insurance fund had been unfavourably affected by economic recession, inflation and unemployment. Health expenditure per person was exceedingly low because of Hungary's relatively low level of economic development. The real value of health expenditure had decreased since 1991. In 1992 and 1993, the curbing of expenditure and the rapid increase in costs placed health care institutions in a critical situation.

Owing to the prolonged recession, the low income-generating capability of the economy was a basic problem in the 1980s, when welfare expenditure (on social security, health care and welfare benefits) constituted a large proportion of gross domestic product and the national budget. Neverthe-less, expenditure was insufficient to meet needs and social expectations. In the early 1990s, the deepening recession dramatically intensified problems. Funding available to the welfare sector declined, while the demand for welfare benefits and health care increased.

Fifth, the Government did not, in 1990 or afterwards, honestly admit to the public and health care workers that they should not expect more resources and services in the short term and that reduction in access to benefits was probable. The Ministry of Public Welfare failed to make it clear to society that the basic question was to what extent and how the services financed by public funds would be reduced, and how the losers in the process could be compensated.

The health policy of the new social–liberal coalition in 1994

The health status of the population cannot be improved or the health care system transformed during a single government cycle. The Hungarian Socialist Party and the Alliance of Free Democrats therefore wish to implement a health care programme that can achieve a professional consensus as well as a certain degree of political agreement.

Based on objective analysis, the government will have to decide which of the changes taking place since 1990 can be built upon and how to change the processes moving health care in the wrong direction. The interests of both the public and the professional health care workers require that changes in government should not give rise to shocks in health care. This does not mean, however, that Hungarians should miss the opportunity for alleviating or solving problems that may either be new or may have been bequeathed by the past and grown ever since.

The present Government faces a severe legacy and a situation that is more disadvantageous than that in 1990 in several respects. In addition to financial, medical and organizational components, confidence and moral factors have also contributed to the crisis. In the short term, the scope of movement for the reform of health care and health insurance is greatly constrained, and the factors of uncertainty are aggravated by the fact that the transition to a market economy is proceeding with greater difficulty and less speed than expected. The economic crisis continues to deepen, and the social burdens arising from this are growing dramatically. No substantial, spectacular improvement in economic conditions can be expected. The tension between what is economically feasible and what is needed or demanded from the health care sector is expected to increase further.

The present health administration envisages a health care system in which the following objectives could be implemented in the long term:

* the decisions of Government, municipalities, employers and individuals should take account of health promotion, in relation to reducing risks that give rise to common diseases;

- individual users of the health care system should not be passive recipients of health care but partners cooperating with the system on an equal footing;
- citizens should exercise control over the directions of health care development through their voluntary organizations and public participation;
- every Hungarian citizen should have access to basic health care; mandatory insurance should cover everyone and should extend to the services necessary to re-establish health;
- people demanding services of higher standards and with better conditions than those provided by mandatory insurance should be able to buy such services through voluntary insurance schemes;
- social and regional differences in access to health care should be reduced;
- patients' rights, including the free choice of physician, should be enforced;
- situations of conflict or confrontation, both between the population and health professionals and between different groups of health professionals, should be avoided;
- the autonomy of health care institutions and their employees should be guaranteed;
- the organizations representing health care institutions and the groups representing their employees should participate in making decisions on health care development;
- available resources should be utilized more efficiently; and
- the quality of service should improve continually.

These are strategic objectives, not just for a single government period but for the longer term (10–15 years); implementing them requires a multitude of economic, legal, institutional and behavioural changes. These principles should serve as criteria for evaluating short-term, specific decisions. Relative to these principles, the transformation of the financing system or privatization should be regarded only as instruments. The fundamental difficulty inherent in the present situation is that the reactions to short-term pressures should not deviate from the long-term objectives chosen.

During the 1994 election campaign, health and health care were a topic of moderate importance. Public opinion surveys found that, after unemployment and public security, the population considers health care to be the most important social problem. The manifestos of political parties discussed the topic in some detail, paying close attention to the question of health care reform. In November 1993, the Hungarian Socialist Party organized a conference on healthy public policy and invited the main politicians responsible for health from the other parties. The party representatives at the round table had no significant disagreements, suggesting that consensus can be built on a new policy for health for all in Hungary.

The principles of health for all and implementation of health policy in Hungary

Equity
Equity was a basic ideological concept of the socialist system. After the radical political changes, the concept of equity was contaminated by being associated with the socialist system and had a boomerang effect in making equity unpopular after the collapse. Social and economic processes of the transition had a polarizing effect on already existing regional and social inequality similar to that in Latin America.

The social reality in Hungary proved to be much harsher than the predictions of rosy scenarios. Recession and unemployment hit the country very hard. For the people who lost in this transition, it was impossible to understand why the change from communism should be such a painful experience. Living standards declined for many, and poverty, deprivation, social exclusion, unemployment, homelessness, migration and ethnic conflicts increased.

In addition, the shift to a market economy and a decreasing role of a welfare state that was not anchored solidly enough economically and socially have also contributed to increasing inequality.

In these circumstances, the economic and social prerequisites for improving equity in health are lacking.

Hungary's health promotion documents of the early 1990s included statements on equity as a basic value, but an equity-oriented policy for health for all is currently more rhetoric than reality. The health policy has the important features of equity of access and equity in health. The basic health services remain free of charge. Nearly the whole population is covered by social insurance. The Ministry of Public Welfare is coordinating some health and social policies, with clear support measures available in cases of extreme crisis or poverty. In the early 1990s the pioneering and supportive role of nongovernmental organizations and churches increased in working towards promoting equity and reducing deprivation.

In public health, settings approaches such as Healthy Cities and Health Promoting Schools are strongly involved in ensuring equity. There are some special health promotion programmes targeting disadvantaged social groups (gypsies and migrants).

Participation
The whole process of political change, including health policy, was led by the basic values of democracy and resulted in a movement towards participation in political decision-making. The principle of participation is a basic aspect of a pluralistic society.

Hungary has a free press and a parliamentary system, and health issues have been sharply debated in the National Assembly and the mass media.

Hungary's health care services are developing in a pluralistic direction. With many pluralistic actors, determining where health decisions are made can be hard. The roles of the Ministry, the social insurance boards, local government and the Hungarian Medical Chamber are unclear in the decision-making process. Hungary's health policy lacks an institutional framework (board of health), technique and the practice of consensus-building. Skills in dialogue are required to bridge the gaps between different actors. The Ministry of Public Welfare's policy planning system has basically failed to find methods of ensuring public participation for each specific situation. For example, the Government lacks legitimacy in public health, presenting a risk for long-term continuity and sustainability of health strategies.

The role of local communities and public participation in public health has increased significantly. Nongovernmental organizations, community actions and citizens' initiatives are developing and flourishing in Hungary.

It is no accident that, despite promises, not much was done to promote patients' rights. The interest in protecting patients is much weaker than that of the medical profession.

Intersectorality

The economic and social cost of transition in Hungary has been higher than anticipated. Prolonged economic downturn, high levels of unemployment, sharply reduced social security, widening income and health differences, falling health standards and the rise of organized crime do not create an environment stimulating intersectoral action to improve health. In this difficult process of transition, sectoral interests are prevailing and the coordinating mechanisms of intersectorality are weak and fragile.

Public health in Hungary became remedicalized and intersectoral cooperation declined in the early 1990s.

There are some promising examples of good practice even within the Government. One is the high-quality cooperation between the environment and health sectors and the cooperative learning process of the National Environmental Health Programme.

Another example of intersectorality is the Health Promoting Schools project and the cooperation of the Ministry of Public Welfare and the Ministry of Culture and Education in the new school curriculum development.

The government decree creating a National Public Health Committee, co-chaired by the Ministers of Public Welfare and of Culture and Education might be a promising cooperation framework for the future. Intersectorality is much better developed and offers a much more natural form of cooperation in local communities. Good examples include the WHO Healthy Cities Network, the Hungarian Health Promoting Village Association, or the community development project based on a World Bank loan. Despite different fiscal situations, local governments show more and more willingness to cooperate intersectorally for health.

Orientation towards health status

The draft health policy documents in Hungary (not published) have explicit targets for morbidity and mortality and provide potential monitoring and evaluation tools for the health status of the Hungarian population. Mortality statistics and other demographic data are very well developed. There is a regular survey system on health behaviour and lifestyles. The situation is much less favourable for morbidity statistics.

The Hungarian World Bank loan includes a special component for the development of analytical epidemiology, health policy monitoring and evaluation and various training systems for epidemiology.

The policy-making activity of the Ministry of Public Welfare and other actors is guided by the principle of health gain.

The problem is that, although Hungary has high-quality measurement tools, the only thing that can be measured satisfactorily is that Hungary lacks a clearly defined strategic health policy.

Reference

1. *A nemzeti megújhodás programja* [Programme of national revival]. Budapest, Press Office, Prime Minster of Hungary, 1990.

Health policy development in Lithuania[a]

Vilius Grabauskas

Introduction

Unlike some of the countries of the former Soviet Union that have recently regained or achieved independence, Lithuania managed to retain a link to the outside world, and has had long-standing collaboration with WHO, both headquarters and the Regional Office for Europe. This started as early as 1971–1972 with the Community Myocardial Infarction Registry (WHO Regional Office for Europe) and Behavioural Components of Health Intervention Programmes: the Kaunas-Rotterdam Intervention Study (WHO headquarters). This collaboration developed from classical epidemiological studies to community-based programmes in health promotion and disease prevention. Health policy development activities included involvement in the countrywide integrated noncommunicable diseases intervention (CINDI) programme, the Healthy Cities project, the Health Promoting Schools project, the Health Promoting Kindergartens project, the Health Promoting Hospitals project and, from 1992, in the Regions for Health Network in Europe. For many years, especially under the Soviet regime, collaboration with WHO was the only window for continuous international contacts, and Lithuania used it very innovatively. These links also created an atmosphere receptive to the concept and principles of health for all among a critical mass of researchers, public health administrators and politicians *(1,2)*.

The health information collected systematically and the experience accumulated through a number of population-based projects and health intervention programmes had clearly demonstrated that concentrating on the health care sector alone would not substantially improve the health of the Lithuanian population *(3,4)*. Intersectoral action involving the entire structure of the society was considered important. This concerted action requires a comprehensive health policy that is developed and adopted at the highest political level.

This was clearly demonstrated by designing and developing the Lithuanian Integrated Programme for the Prevention and Control of Noncommunicable Diseases, for which implementation started in 1982. Later on, this Programme constituted a part of a CINDI/INTERHEALTH programme coordinated by WHO.

The Soviet regime resulted in a rigid, centrally run, excessively medicalized, hospital-based and physician-centred health care model in Lithuania. Nevertheless, an attempt was made to develop

---

[a] This chapter draws heavily on a paper presented by the author at the European Health Policy Conference: Opportunities for the Future, Copenhagen, 5–9 December 1994 *(5)*.

intersectoral collaboration to implement the Lithuanian CINDI/INTERHEALTH project. The Intersectoral Political Committee for CINDI/INTERHEALTH, which was chaired by the Minister of Health (Dr J. Platukis at that time), was established with the Vice-Ministers of Social Security, Education and Culture, Agriculture, Environment, Commerce and the Interior representing sectors other than health and with representatives of the mass media, the Catholic Church, etc. Nevertheless, this Committee failed because it lacked understanding of the origins of health problems, did not promote community participation and failed to identify the resources in other sectors that could be mobilized for health purposes. This left the health care sector alone, with its limited and modest resources, to try to implement CINDI/INTERHEALTH. The political structure in Lithuania did not support approaches oriented towards health gain, although a few documents pretending to describe the development of a national health programme, while actually describing how to strengthen health care, were prepared as a failed reaction to WHO's initiatives to develop the strategy for health for all.

Process

Following a long and sometimes painful dialogue within the medical community, the Lithuanian Medical Association was re-established in May 1989. These political developments in health care were very clearly part of the overall political fight to regain independence, and Lithuania's declaration of independence on 11 March 1990 considerably added to the enthusiasm and motivation to work on formulating a new concept of health. The Parliamentary Health Commission was created and a new Department of Health Policy and Strategy was established within the Ministry of Health for the first time. This greatly facilitated the organization of the national dialogue on the principles of the new health system that the Lithuanian people would like to have.

A very important resolution adopted by the re-established Lithuanian Medical Association at its congress in 1989, requesting that the health professions develop a new national concept of health for Lithuania, gave a new impetus to health policy development. Kaunas Medical Academy and its Health Research Centre have collaborated with WHO since 1982 as a WHO Collaborating Centre for Training and Research in Chronic Disease Epidemiology and Prevention. The Academy has taken an important leading role in the process of drafting and organizing the national dialogue on the new concept that was developed. The principles of health for all constituted the basis for its development, which means that prerequisites for health, lifestyles conducive to health and a healthy environment were considered equally as important as appropriate health care (1). After intensive national dialogue, this concept was approved by the VII Congress of the Lithuanian Medical Association held in Kaunas and was adopted by Parliament in October 1991. Together with its approval, Parliament requested that a national health policy document and national health programme be prepared, and the Ministry of Health was given the responsibility of coordinating this activity.

The development and adoption of a new national noncept of health for Lithuania (annex to *Lithuanian health report – 1990's (3)*) is a starting-point for a more systematic effort in formulating and implementing national health policy. The concept in itself is valuable, as it contains a number of important principles of health policy development and represents a good framework for its further advancement.

Immediately after the new national concept of health was adopted at the Congress of the Lithuanian Medical Association and submitted to Parliament for approval, the decision was made to ask for international assistance from Finland, which had already undergone the process of formulating a policy for health for all and had experience in defining national health priorities and targeting actions. The support from the WHO Regional Office for Europe and long-standing collaborative contacts between WHO collaborating centres in Kaunas and Helsinki bore fruit: in January 1991, a top-ranking Lithuanian delegation led by the new Minister for Health and comprising representatives of the Parliamentary Health Commission, the Department of Health Policy and Strategy of the Ministry of Health and Kaunas Medical Academy (most of the delegates also represented the Lithuanian Medical Association, being active members) visited Finland on a study mission.

This was a very useful visit, since Finland, assisted by the Regional Office and a team of international experts, was in the process of reviewing their own national policy and programme for health for all (6). The Lithuanian politicians and the new health administration learned many lessons. The most important included the need for a clear political commitment to health; a balance between national, regional and local responsibility for health; equity in health issues; and public involvement in the decision-making process: defining health priorities, targeting actions and mobilizing resources. Of utmost importance was ensuring intersectoral cooperation, especially in health promotion, environmental protection and disease prevention. One of the major determinants of the amount and quality of action at various levels and by various sectors of society is informed public opinion. This is why working with and through the mass media should be an integral component of national health policy development.

Alongside national expertise, another Regional Office initiative contributed considerably to the formulation of national health policy in Lithuania, especially in defining objectives and setting priorities for this process. A Lithuanian delegation was invited to a Regional Office Consultation on Subnational Health Policy Development in September 1991 in Lugano, Switzerland, which subsequently led to the establishment of another initiative: the Regions for Health Network in Europe. Lithuania had been invited to the Consultation before gaining independence to represent health policy development on a subnational level. By the time the delegation attended the meeting, Lithuania had been internationally recognized as an independent country but continued its participation in the establishment of the Network, representing the Baltic region (7).

When the Lugano meeting took place, the Minister for Health (Dr J. Olekas) was representing a country that had just regained its independence. During this meeting of top-level decision-makers, he was exposed to a broad range of experiences from across Europe focusing on the development of policies targeting health gain. The experience of his colleagues in Europe made a strong impression on the new Minister.

At this point, another intergovernmental body entered the picture: the European Union's PHARE (Assistance for Economic Restructuring in the Countries of Central and Eastern Europe) Programme. In the context of the PHARE Programme, Lithuania was asked to prepare a health policy framework, and the Minister and his advisers insisted that such a framework be in accordance with the WHO health for all approach *(1)*. WHO acted as a PHARE consultant and supported the mobilization of over 40 Lithuanian experts, who prepared Lithuania's first public health report *(3)* as the essential background information for the development of a health policy and strategy and the first National Health Policy Conference in 1993. The report was first published in Lithuanian and subsequently translated into English.

A group of national experts representing a very wide range of expertise (the Ministry of Health, academic institutions, professional and voluntary health organizations and the National Health Information Centre) worked together in preparing the National Health Policy Conference, collecting information and critically assessing the Lithuanian health situation in the 1990s *(8)*. The drafts prepared by various groups after consensus was achieved were collated into the *Lithuanian health report – 1990's (3)* by the Health Research Centre of Kaunas Medical Academy. This report served as the principal background document for the Conference itself.

According to the Conference agenda, prepared in consultation and with the support of the Regional Office and the PHARE Programme, case studies on the process of health policy formulation at the national level (Finland, the Netherlands and the United Kingdom) *(6,9,10)* as well as experiences from the Regions for Health Network (Catalonia, Spain and Wales) were presented *(11,12)*. The experiences on models of health care financing presented by WHO and PHARE consultants completed the planned introductory part of the Conference. The *Lithuanian health report – 1990's (3)* had been discussed widely by various institutional and voluntary organizations prior to the meeting, and the report was again critically reviewed at the first National Health Policy Conference, to which a wide representation of various sectors of society was invited. The Conference was opened by the Prime Minister and attended by several members of the Cabinet as well as members of Parliament representing the Parliamentary Committees of Health, Social Security and Labour, Economy and Finance, Education, and Science and Culture.

All major political parties, the State Department for Environmental Protection, all voluntary nongovernmental organizations having even a marginal interest in health, academic and research institutions, regional and municipal health authorities, administrators of national, regional and local health services and the mass media were represented at the Conference and numbered almost 300 delegates from various parts of Lithuania. The active participation of Dr J.E. Asvall, WHO Regional Director for Europe, emphasized the importance of the Conference. Dr Asvall also spoke to Parliament and presented the conclusions of the Conference to the President of the Republic. The close involvement of the President and the Prime Minister alongside the Minister for Health indicates the political interest and commitment at the time.

The resolution adopted by the participants of the first National Health Policy Conference outlined the framework for the priority steps in national health policy formulation and established objectives for action. The priority steps recommended were:

- establishing a National Health Council at the highest political level with consultative authority and function to Parliament;
- preparing intersectoral action plans for health promotion and environment protection;
- working out plans for institutional and public involvement in health matters;
- introducing new curricula for education and training of health professionals at undergraduate and postgraduate levels to meet the new tasks of a health system in transition;
- reorienting the organization of health services to give priority to primary health care structures;
- introducing quality control measures for health care and relating them to the planning and financing levels within and outside the health care system;
- defining mechanisms aimed at ensuring the implementation of the principles of equity in health;
- elaborating schemes for international collaboration in health; and
- updating and developing further the health information system, allowing for proper monitoring and evaluation of health system performance.

The health priorities identified in which immediate actions should be undertaken were:

- maternal and child health
- cardiovascular diseases
- cancer
- accidents
- AIDS
- environmental and occupational health.

The major strategic lines selected for action aimed at introducing healthier lifestyles were:

- reducing tobacco consumption
- reducing alcohol consumption
- promoting healthy nutrition
- increasing physical activity
- conducting sex education
- promoting safe driving.

In developing appropriate health care, the major emphasis was shifting resources to support the development of ambulatory services.

The development of the legislative basis for health was considered as a major and urgent undertaking in shaping a new health system in transition.

Although the national dialogue on health system development as well as the consensus achieved at the first National Health Policy Conference had clearly defined priority areas for action, the day-to-day implementation of the health policy turned out to be more complicated than expected. First of all, the promises of parliamentarians to deal with health legislation as a priority issue were overwhelmed by other problems requiring their urgent attention (such as domestic and foreign policy, the economy and privatization), and the main piece of health-related legislation was thus first adopted by Parliament in July 1994. The rest of the expected health legislation was on a long waiting list.

Unfortunately, the governments changed frequently in Lithuania in this transition period, which also meant changing attitudes towards health system reform. This did not allow a national health programme to be designed and adopted rapidly. However, the Health Reform Management Group established in autumn 1993 took increasingly more leadership in developing a sound basis for health system reform and policies for disease prevention and health promotion. In early 1995, a national task force was established that was charged with preparing a white paper with a health situation analysis for 1995 and an action plan to address major health problems in Lithuania. The Regional Office stimulated the preparation of this document and assisted in preparing the second National Health Policy Conference, originally planned for spring 1996. As an intermediate step in mobilizing political power in Lithuania and enhancing intersectoral collaboration for health, a full-day parliamentary discussion on the health challenges with international participation took place in November 1995. A large number of members of parliament, including four ministers, took part in the six-hour discussion, which was broadcast through the mass media.

As a result of these initiatives, the draft document prepared by the national task force was developed into a national health programme, which was finally approved by the Government in October 1996 after wide discussion in the health care and other sectors. This programme is based on the WHO strategy and principles for health for all, starting with ensuring the prerequisites for health, including equity, promoting lifestyles conducive to health, introducing healthy environments, providing appropriate care and support programmes, developing new public health structures, changing the training of health personnel, and using a newly developed health information system for monitoring and evaluating health outcomes.

Again, as a result of a complete change of government that was expected after the general elections in October 1996, the date for the Second National Health Policy Conference was moved to spring 1997. The major reason for this decision proposed by the national task force and approved by the Ministry of Health was the desire to involve a new government in the process of national health development and a hope that such renewed commitment would have a better chance of success. In the meantime, the health promotion component of the draft health policy had been discussed further during a national dialogue with international participation, and this was reflected in a revised draft of the national health programme.

A nationwide effort to bring together all projects initiated or coordinated by WHO in Lithuania (the CINDI programme, the Healthy Cities project, the Health Promoting Schools project, the Health

Promoting Kindergartens project, the Health Promoting Hospitals project and the Regions for Health Network) was initiated (networking the networks). This contributed considerably to reshaping the national health programme and making it more balanced in terms of health promotion and disease prevention versus health care actions. Among the first decisions of the new Minister of Health was a decision to hold the Second National Health Policy Conference in April 1997 to discuss the draft strategy. The Conference participants suggested a number of changes to the draft and recommended that a revised version be sent to Parliament for approval. They also recommended the development of a policy for food and nutrition within this health for all framework.

Equity in health

Given the wide scope of the policy under development in a country in transition, the equity in health issues are recognized as part of the overall health policy for Lithuania *(13,14)*. The need to promote equity is clearly demonstrated by inequalities in health status that are well documented in Lithuania (see *Lithuanian health report – 1990's (3)*, pp. 12–14). Nevertheless, the equity issue in Lithuania, probably similar to many other post-socialist countries, is not popular for political reasons. The main reason for this is the difficulty in returning to the equity challenge after a long period of declarations under the old regime about equity and solidarity and the experience of "equity in poverty".

This problem is further complicated by the ongoing process of privatization. This is why the present policy framework is addressing equity mainly by providing equal accessibility to health services for the total population with priority given to the most vulnerable groups (mothers and children, disabled people and elderly people). At the same time, some signs indicate that the situation might be improving rapidly, since various nongovernmental organizations and interest groups are already putting considerable pressure on the Government, municipal authorities and health services to take into account the needs of these disadvantaged groups. One example is that the existing legislation provides a good basis for requesting actions; for example, the law on integrating disabled people into society provides good opportunities to put considerable pressure on national, regional and local authorities. To support the scientific evidence for taking issues of inequalities in health seriously, the research group from Kaunas Medical Academy is carrying out a research project designed to study health inequalities in Lithuania in more depth. The issues of lifestyles, environment and accessibility to health care are being taken into account.

Participation

Lithuania has the privilege of having a solid database that combines the health statistics collected routinely at the national, regional and local levels with the data from research projects carried out on representative population samples. The national health data extend back to the 1930s, and some data from the research projects are available for at least the last two decades. Paradoxically, this has not influenced the development of health policy or enabled informed participation in decision-making. One explanation for this might be that, until the Soviet regime collapsed, substantial health or health-related information (especially at the national level) was not accessible to researchers, health administrators or the public. This did not allow the long-term trends in health status in Lithuania to be assessed properly, discussed openly or compared with similar health indicators and their trends in western European countries.

As mentioned earlier, the development of a new national concept of health for Lithuania, which was adopted by Parliament in October 1991, is a starting-point for national health policy formulation. The health professions initiated the development of this concept, and representatives from all levels (national, regional and local) have participated actively in initiating this process. After a task force formed by the Lithuanian Medical Association and chaired by representatives of Kaunas Medical Academy prepared the first draft, a national dialogue started, with the full text of the concept being published in *Atgimimas*, a very popular weekly newspaper at that time.

A special effort was made to involve all health professional associations in this consultation process as well as non-health government and nongovernmental organizations and interest groups, such as other ministries, municipalities, charitable organizations, sports and leisure organizations and clubs, health clubs, the Catholic Church and the mass media. This process was greatly facilitated by the active role of the Parliamentary Health Commission, which assisted in organizing the dialogue nationwide. Nevertheless, national politicians and experts had the major responsibility and accountability for the final version of the document.

One of the most serious problems in formulating the major principles of the new national concept of health was the apparent intention of the medical profession to limit the concept itself and the related dialogue mainly to the functions of the medical profession and health care structures. This arises from a restricted medicalized perception of health and consequently concentrates on more or less medical approaches to solving health problems. As might be expected, the involvement of sectors other than health care in the national dialogue on health policy and strategy was a decisive component of moving towards a much broader concept of health and the approaches to dealing with this. The group of professionals that was most opposed to and obstructive of health policy development was the newly established Association of Privately Practising Physicians.

The general public traditionally has had limited interest in health policy issues, as this has been considered the responsibility of the politicians. Fortunately, this attitude is changing; one way is the growing numbers of nongovernmental organizations.

The Parliamentary Health Commission played a decisive role in a parliamentary health discussion day in November 1995 in collaboration with WHO. A large number of members of parliament took part in discussing the main health challenges, and the public galleries were packed with representatives of nongovernmental organizations, municipalities and other local groups. The whole discussion was broadcast on radio, and excerpts were shown on television.

Many political parties participated both in the first National Health Policy Conference and in the parliamentary discussion. This willingness to engage in open dialogue and a search for a degree of consensus on health issues has been an important feature of the post-socialist era.

International opinion, standards and expertise have played a very important role in helping to achieve acceptance of the broader concepts of health both among the health professions, as well as in the public at large. WHO has played a decisive role in this. Lithuania started to formulate health policy as a subnational entity under the Soviet regime. Later, the first National Health Policy Conference was organized in 1993 and the first Lithuanian health report was published under the stimulating role of the Regional Office for Europe and with its considerable help.

Lithuania is now serving as a test case for the formulation of a comprehensive health policy extending to 2005 by collaborating with WHO to network the networks. Those involved in the WHO Regions for Health Network, Healthy Cities project, Health Promoting Schools project, Health Promoting Kindergartens project, Health Promoting Hospitals project, Baby Friendly Hospitals project and CINDI programme are collaborating in formulating the draft policy document and are discussing their potential role in implementing the policy. Thus, not only strong synergy is expected as the various networks collaborate but also wider participation, ownership and commitment from many more groups and prospective partners.

Intersectoral policy

Fortunately, the new national concept of health clearly spelled out the major principles of a policy for health for all. This gave numerous opportunities to initiate health policy implementation parallel to parliamentary discussion on health legislation. Joint action plans have been elaborated by the Ministries of Health and of Education and Science on a national programme for healthy schools; by the Ministries of Health and of Environment on a national programme for environmental health protection; by the Ministries of Health and of Social Security and Labour on a national programme for the integration of disabled people in society; and by the Ministries of Health and of the Interior on a national programme for preventing traffic accidents. National action programmes with intersectoral involvement have also been prepared, discussed and approved by various authorities on tobacco or health, hypertension control, healthy nutrition, prevention of AIDS and prevention and control of cardiovascular diseases.

Although these programmes have clearly defined objectives and targets as well as mechanisms for implementation, the planned implementation suffers considerably because of lack of resources. Another obstacle is the resistance of old structures to planned changes. A narrow and excessively medicalized, hospital-based and physician-centred model of health care services often continues to be the focus of attention. This means that further efforts are needed to keep forthcoming changes in the Lithuanian health system closer to the health for all principles and approach. Enhancing the health promotion and disease prevention activities in health services will rely heavily on the experience accumulated in the CINDI programme *(15)*.

The reality is that intersectoral collaboration for health still remains a delicate issue in Lithuania. Regardless of the general acceptance that other sectors of society are important for the health of the population, no effective mechanisms to implement this intersectoral collaboration have been in place until recently. Many of the limited-scale activities referred to previously have occurred at the local level and have been based on the enthusiasm of certain individuals or interest groups.

A somewhat more systematic approach was developed in the CINDI experimental areas and more recently in Kaunas within the Healthy Cities Project, which is now developing a healthy cities network in Lithuania.

The research teams, mainly from Kaunas Medical Academy, disseminated information. The Academy was also involved in health intervention projects that helped to publicize the concepts of intersectoral collaboration for health. The ongoing process of developing new legislation in Lithuania has considerably helped to involve other sectors in setting common objectives for health. The Law of the Health System, adopted by Parliament in 1994, has considerably strengthened the potential for intersectoral collaboration for health. For example, this Law stipulates that a National Board of Health reporting to Parliament is to be established on which all sectors of society should be represented. At the level of government, an Intersectoral Executive Committee for Health is to be established, supported by similar structures at the municipal level. The adopted laws on alcohol control, tobacco control and consumers' rights, which were either guided or drafted by those involved in health policy formulation (such as the group from Kaunas Medical Academy), provide a good legislative basis to move more aggressively towards intersectoral collaboration for health. During the 1995 parliamentary health discussion, a number of ministers other than the Minister for Health took part and showed clearly that they recognize their responsibility for health.

Putting health on the agenda of other sectors is still not easy. For example, a multinational tobacco corporation (Philip Morris, which entered Lithuania in 1993) was the major obstacle to the adoption of the Tobacco Control Law, which gives priority to the health needs of the people.

The Public Health Faculty at Kaunas Medical Academy was established in 1994. This is an important factor that is already contributing to strengthening the process of developing intersectoral policies for health and is planned to contribute much more in the future. The faculty will conduct bachelor degree undergraduate training programmes covering such important areas as health planning, health system development, health education and environmental health. The postgraduate School of Public Health, which all those having a university degree will be eligible to enter, is planned to be organized as a consortium of universities, academies and institutes in Kaunas. It is hoped that this structure can provide information and research support to find further evidence of the role of various risk factors on the level of health of the population. It will assess the effectiveness of interventions and will, therefore, strengthen the development and implementation of intersectoral policies for health.

Orientation towards health status

Lithuania has a well developed health information system. In addition to the routinely collected health indicators such as morbidity, disability, mortality, health service operations and financing, a solid database exists on the determinants of ill health, including lifestyle and behaviour and biological, environmental and social factors, which are systematically collected from representative samples of the Lithuanian population. A research team from Kaunas Medical Academy has collected these data since 1972.

This database enables baseline assessment of the health situation, with a wide range of choices for starting-points for assessment or monitoring. An example of this type of exercise is the health situation assessment for the 1990s published in the *Lithuanian health report – 1990's (3)*. The selection of this baseline point in time has special significance for Lithuania, as it represents the drastic changes in the political, social and economic life of the people after regaining independence. The monitoring process will represent the natural trend of national efforts to improve the health situation of the population.

It is, perhaps, also natural that health objectives and targets as well as the monitoring process will be related to WHO European targets and indicators for health for all, given the long-standing contact with WHO and its support for national health policy development. In fact, the health status orientation of the existing database, as well as experience accumulated by research groups of Kaunas Medical Academy, also contributes to international efforts for health policy formulation promoted by the Regional Office.

Kaunas Medical Academy has organized, since 1994, three Baltic training seminars on epidemiological foundations for health policy formulation at the regional and local levels for experts from Estonia, Latvia and Lithuania as part of the activities of the WHO Regions for Health Network in Europe and Lithuania's commitment on behalf of the Baltic region. This has led to the joint preparation of public health reports for the Baltic region and has greatly increased collaboration between the statistical services of the Baltic countries. These reports and the *Lithuanian health report – 1990's (3)* emphasize some of the differences in health status between all the countries around the Baltic Sea.

Summary and conclusions

The process of formulating a national health policy in Lithuania, a country in transition, has undergone several stages. Despite the existence of a national critical mass of professionals who understand the major principles of health policy development and who have a solid database to scientifically back the suggested decisions, and despite general acceptance by the public of the broader dimensions of health, the actual process of developing health policy is still facing considerable difficulty. Many factors obstruct this process, such as the inflexibility and resistance of the medical profession, traditions from the previous health service model and an extremely difficult economic situation. Nevertheless, one of the most important factors is the frequent change of government and, subsequently, of ministers of health, which makes continuity difficult. Fortunately, however, in contrast to the political level, the health professionals involved in health policy development and implementation assure at least one level of this necessary continuity. As a result of continuous efforts by the Health Reform Management Group and research and education institutions, and with the constant support of WHO, a policy and strategy for health for all continues to be developed, and the groundwork is being laid for improved dialogue and participation.

References

1. *Health for all targets. The health policy for Europe*. Copenhagen, WHO Regional Office for Europe, 1993 (European Health for All Series, No. 4).
2. *Priority research for health for all*. Copenhagen, WHO Regional Office for Europe, 1988 (European Health for All Series, No. 3).
3. *Lithuanian health report – 1990's*. Kaunas, Medical Academy Press, 1994.
4. *Demographic data for health situation assessment and projections*. Geneva, World Health Organization, 1993 (document WHO/HSF/GSP/93.2).
5. GRABAUSKAS, V. Health policy development in Lithuania: experience and lessons. *In*: Harrington, P. & Ritsatakis, A., ed. *European Health Policy Conference: opportunities for the future, 5–9 December 1994. Volume V: Health challenges for countries of central and eastern Europe and the newly independent States*. Copenhagen, WHO Regional Office for Europe, 1995, pp. 141–150 (document EUR/ICP/HFAP 94 01/CNO1(V)).
6. *Health for all policy in Finland: WHO health policy review*. Copenhagen, WHO Regional Office for Europe, 1991.
7. *The process of health policy development*: report of a WHO Working Group. Copenhagen, WHO Regional Office for Europe, 1992 (document EUR/ICP/HSC 418).
8. *Health statistics of Lithuania 1993*. Vilnius, National Health Information Centre, 1994.
9. *A strategy for health: Netherlands health policy document 1992*. Rijswijk, Ministry of Health, Welfare and Cultural Affairs, 1992.
10. *The health of the nation: a strategy for health in England*. London, H.M. Stationery Office, 1992.
11. *Health plan for Catalonia for 1993–1995*. Barcelona, Generalitat de Catalunya, Departament de Sanitat I Seguretat Social, 1993.
12. *Investment in health gain*. Cardiff, NHS Directorate, Welsh Health Planning Forum, 1991.
13. WHITEHEAD, M. *The concepts and principles of equity and health*. Copenhagen, WHO Regional Office for Europe, 1990 (document EUR/ICP/RPD 414).
14. DAHLGREN, G. & WHITEHEAD, M. *Policies and strategies to promote equity in health*. Copenhagen, WHO Regional Office for Europe, 1992 (document EUR/ICP/RPD 414(2)).
15. *Protocol and guidelines: Countrywide Integrated Noncommunicable Diseases Intervention (CINDI) programme*. Copenhagen, WHO Regional Office for Europe, 1996 (document EUR/ICP/CIND 94 02/PB04).

Health policy development in Malta

Ray G. Xerri

The birth of a national health policy

In 1984, Malta's House of Representation endorsed the WHO European strategy for health for all. A year later the Health Division undertook the task of developing a national health policy in a joint project with the WHO Regional Office for Europe. Although no formal policy document was produced at that stage, the published document *Health services development plan for Malta, 1986–1990 (1)*, incorporated many aspects of this newly developing policy for health for all.

Since the 1980s, the health sector has undergone major reforms, expanded existing services and created new ones. Changing patterns of demography, disease and risk factors, a spurt in new sophisticated technology, greater numbers of highly skilled health care personnel, overspecialization and escalating costs have been superimposed on a rapidly rising standard of living and higher expectations of the Maltese people.

In the early 1990s, the need for an explicitly formulated national health policy was increasingly felt. It became evident that a five-year plan was not sufficient to adequately address the present challenges:

- improving the healthy life expectancy of the Maltese people;
- reorienting policies towards health rather than health care;
- improving allocative and technical efficiency; and
- responding to the Government's commitment to WHO.

To effectively address the current and future constraints on the health care sector, the Health Division needed to reorient its role and functions and to formulate a vision for rational and sustainable development in health care based on priority criteria and value for money. The Department of Health Policy and Planning, set up in 1993, was mandated to develop this vision and to draw up a national health policy on the basis of this vision.

In December 1995, Malta published its first national health policy as a consultative document entitled *Health vision 2000 (2)*. This policy was formulated after wide consultation with all key actors, including both political parties. The inclusion of all key actors ensured political consensus and commitment to the implementation of the policy. Based on this broad political endorsement, the change in Government following the October 1996 elections has not affected the strategic planning for the implementation of the policy.

Following the launch of the consultative document, comments were invited from all key actors to ascertain that the policy formulated was acceptable to them. Based on this later consultation, the policy was revised and asthma was included as an additional priority area to the ones already identified.

Method used to formulate policy

A multidisciplinary steering committee was appointed to formulate the national policy, and chaired by the Director of the Department of Health Policy and Planning. A consultant adviser, Dr Paul Abela Hyzler, was contracted by the Department to act as project manager. A technical working group was also set up to carry out the research required to prepare the policy.

Wide consultation was used throughout the whole process of policy formulation, and such an approach is also planned for the next phases of implementation and monitoring and evaluation. Liaison with the WHO Regional Office for Europe was fostered from the inception through personal communication and correspondence. It continued throughout the drawing up of the policy document, during which drafts were disseminated for comments and recommendations.

Stages in policy formulation

Situation analysis
The health status of the Maltese people and the trends and projections in patterns of illness and risk factors of disease were analysed in detail. Then the organization, structures, services and new developments in the health sector were reviewed. This enabled existing problems and deficiencies to be identified.

Setting priorities
In the second stage, a wide process of consultation was used to broaden the ownership of the policy among the different stakeholders. Personal discussions or interviews were held with key stakeholders, and numerous senior health care workers, heads of departments and representatives of political parties, professional organizations, institutions, commissions, agencies, unions, other nongovernmental organizations and some client groups were contacted by letter and invited to submit their views on local key health and health service areas that warranted targeting to improve health status. The WHO Regional Office for Europe was also consulted at this stage.

By a process of consensus, the steering committee defined the criteria for the selection of key areas for priority action. Each area should be an actual or potential cause of premature death, avoidable ill health or health-related psychosocial problems. Effective intervention should be possible, offering scope for:

- health gains or avoiding further deterioration in health status;
- improving the delivery of health services; and
- cost–effectiveness.

The area chosen should enable objectives and targets to be set and progress towards achievement to be monitored through indicators. Areas should not be exclusively limited to health status gain but may also include appropriate management objectives linked to health status.

The steering committee decided that, to avoid duplicating effort, wasting resources and promoting undue conflict, it would not select areas for action for which the Health Division did not have the main responsibility.

All submissions from the key stakeholders were then scrutinized. Suggested key areas were ranked in order according to the number of times they were proposed overall. The committee considered all submissions, even those ranked lower. Nevertheless, since the committee strove towards wide ownership of areas for selection, the top-ranking areas were rigorously scored against the selected criteria. Mean scores were computed, and the higher-scoring areas were selected and grouped under three main categories: diseases and other entities, risk factors and health and supportive services.

The diseases and other entities chosen include coronary artery disease and stroke, lung cancer, breast cancer among women, diabetes, traffic accidents, mental illness and asthma.

The risk factors selected include smoking, elevated blood pressure, unhealthy diet, obesity and elevated serum cholesterol levels, and substance abuse.

The health and supportive services in focus are primary health care, including general practice and community services, communication, research, human resource development, management, setting and maintaining standards, and disseminating information.

Setting objectives and targets
For each key area selected in the first two categories, the committee proceeded to set objectives and targets, using the WHO policy for health for all as a guideline. Objectives and targets were not proposed for health and supportive services, as the committee felt that these should be formulated at the operational or unit level in accordance with the policy of decentralization and subsidiarity being adopted in the reform of the management structures within the health care sector.

Mechanisms for achieving the targets were then broadly stated, highlighting an intersectoral approach and spanning the whole spectrum of health and health-related interventions, from health promotion and disease prevention to cure and rehabilitation.

Futures workshop
A futures workshop was organized under the auspices of WHO with a number of leading academics and economic planners. The aim of the workshop was to forecast future changes in demography, social values, cultural, scientific and technological advances, educational patterns and economic

trends. The workshop was useful, as it helped in considering the future changes that may affect health status and to take such considerations into account during the drafting of the policy document.

Equity in health

Scope of the policy
The scope of Malta's national health policy is to maximize health gains by reorienting health care and health services to meet epidemiological and service priorities through a rational planning cycle and a multisectoral approach. The policy will form the cornerstone for all the reforms envisaged within the health care sector. A reform model has been devised for this purpose.

The concept of equity is incorporated within the policy and is explicitly documented. Malta's national health policy is guided by WHO principles as reasserted in the Ljubljana Charter. Further, the policy builds on the existing health care delivery system, which is a publicly provided health care system, encompassing the whole range of health care interventions: health promotion, disease prevention, treatment and rehabilitation. Different care groups are appropriately targeted to avoid vulnerable groups and inequities.

Equity issues were considered in the process of selecting the key areas. The objectives and targets chosen, as well as the action programmes outlined, gave due importance to gender and age differences as well as to other relevant vulnerable groups.

Vulnerable groups
The situation analysis carried out before policy formulation started undertook to identify inequities and vulnerable groups. Similar to other western European countries, some differences were noted between men and women, women faring better in most instances, except for some chronic conditions such as arthritis and in certain specific cancers such as breast cancer.

Although some regional variation in morbidity was identified between the northern and southern parts of the island, this was not statistically significant except for blood pressure differences. There were no statistically significant regional differences in the use of private general practitioners, health centre physicians, specialists and hospitals.

Variation in self-reported morbidity was noted among different socioeconomic groups: asthma and hay fever were highest in groups A and B (professionals and managers) (19%) and lowest in group E (unskilled workers and people depending on transfer payments) (3%); arthritis was highest in group E (35%) and lowest in group A (8%); and high blood pressure was highest in group E (25%) but lowest in group D (semi-skilled workers) (6%) (1992 survey data; socioeconomic groups were determined according to the activity of the head of the household).

Various special programmes and specific government departments or organizations cater for a number of vulnerable groups. Some of these are outside the umbrella of the Health Division, which nevertheless provides its support as needed. Such groups include elderly people, physically disabled people, substance abusers (drugs and alcohol), single mothers and battered wives. Where necessary, intersectoral and joint action programmes are formulated.

The Department of Health Policy and Planning has formulated and published a separate policy document on mental health entitled *National policy on mental health services* (*3*). The document encompasses the new philosophy needed to radically reform this sector. Its principal parameters and objectives are:

- to enhance mental health within Malta by fostering conditions for healthy environments in family, school, workplace and community;
- to provide a range of appropriate services to empower people to cope better with mental health issues, thus maximizing their productive and social life;
- to attain a shift from the traditional patterns of mental health care to modern comprehensive and diversified services for the prevention, treatment and rehabilitation of mental illness;
- to coordinate and converge services provided by the public, private and voluntary sectors within a national strategy to prevent duplication of resources and ensure synergy towards national objectives; and
- to introduce efficient and effective management systems to manage the hospital and community mental health care services.

Equal access

Health care
Access to a comprehensive public health care system in Malta and Gozo is universal since health care is free of charge at the point of contact. Public health care is financed through central taxation. Primary health care centres are regionally distributed around the island so that distances are not a significant barrier. Twenty-four-hour domiciliary services by general practitioners and community nurses and midwives are also available. Pharmaceuticals are free of charge for outpatients provided that the client is suffering from a chronic condition scheduled under the Social Security Act or is entitled for free medicine based on a means test. If treatment is not available locally, clients are referred abroad for such care at Government expense.

Healthy lifestyles
Health promotion and education are integrated in all school curricula, from kindergarten to secondary schools. As school is compulsory between the ages of 5 and 16, this ensures that the upcoming generation receives basic health promotion and social skills to enable a choice of healthy lifestyles.

Although health promotion literature is freely distributed, most is provided in English. This may be a barrier to some people. Nevertheless, the mass media, and especially the audio and video media, is full of health promotion messages and advice, and the whole population therefore has access to such information.

Specific vulnerable groups may have problems that may prevent them from adopting healthy lifestyles. Specific programmes by various government departments or voluntary organizations cater for such groups.

Healthy environment

Similar to other European countries, Malta has had to face complex environmental problems brought about by growing industrialization, the increasing use of chemicals, more intensive agricultural practices, increasing motor traffic and an explosion in tourism, with its overload effect on waste and sewage disposal, food outlets and noise pollution. These problems, superimposed on a very small country with a high population density, may place residents of certain parts of the island at more risk of environmental pollution than others. Unfortunately, some of this inequity may be difficult to redress, but both the Department of Public Health and the Department of the Environment (under the Health Division) strive to address any ensuing problems. Collaboration between the two departments facilitates better forward planning of environmental policies, which may have potential public health implications.

Equity policy

Malta has no formal equity policy and no structures in place to support equity. Further studies of small-area variation in health care and more refined disaggregation techniques are needed to identify possible inequity that may not be apparent now. There are no plans for commissioning research on the subject or any specific training on equity issues, given that equity is not considered an area of concern.

Participation

National, regional and local groups

Given Malta's geographical size and culture, regional and local groups are not very evident. Since 1993, elected local councils have been set up covering all towns and villages. However, these councils were not consulted in policy formulation since they were still finding their feet and the steering committee believed that it would be futile to consult them at that time.

Key stakeholders, government departments and agencies, political parties, professional organizations, institutions, commissions, trade unions and other nongovernmental organizations were widely consulted during the initial stages of policy formulation. The process of wide consultation is one of the strongest factors behind Malta's new health policy. The sense of ownership of a policy is absolutely essential for successful implementation. Another strong point is the explicitness and transparency of the selection process in priority-setting. This enhances the disposition for wider acceptance of the policy.

Interest groups

Some specific disease or client groups were consulted in the initial stages of policy formulation, but the list was not exhaustive. It is envisaged that such groups will be involved directly in drafting strategies for each key area for action.

Certain client groups, such as the Hospice Movement and the Commission for the Advancement of Women, consulted widely among their members before presenting their recommendations to the Department of Health Policy and Planning. The Commission organized a well attended seminar for women and translated the recommendations for action identified by the participants into a policy paper and forwarded it to the steering committee for its consideration.

The method used in the final selection of priority areas and the explicit description of the process in the policy document seemed to be the best manner of resolving conflicting interests.

Communication with the public

There were no specific attempts to obtain the public's views during the policy formulation stage. Considering the special characteristics of Malta, it was felt that such a step would have hindered or slowed down the efforts to formulate an effective and unbiased health policy. At the same time, the steering committee, throughout all its deliberations, took into account the current local concepts, views, values and expectations of health and health care. Despite the lack of direct consultation with the public, it is not envisaged that implementing the policy will be a major problem. In fact, the strategic plan for preventing accidents has been finalized and has received very favourable comments from the public and the mass media as a specific action plan to reduce such accidents. When the policy document was drafted, great effort was made to write the document in a friendly style that makes it easily understood.

Following the publication of the health policy document (2), a few articles appeared in the local printed mass media, and health policy is also occasionally referred to on the broadcast media. Nevertheless, health for all has not yet really become a public domain. Once specific strategic plans are formulated on each key area, the public response to and awareness of the national health policy is expected to increase. This is already becoming evident from the concern expressed and feedback received from the general public and the mass media, urging the Department of Health Policy and Planning to expedite the implementation of the strategic plan on road traffic accidents.

International factors

Malta has a good working relationship with WHO. The Regional Office for Europe has played a key advisory role throughout the whole policy formulation process. The Regional Office sponsored and coordinated the futures workshop mentioned previously. It also contributed financially towards printing the policy document.

Malta was also honoured by the presence of Dr Jo Asvall, Regional Director for Europe, who visited to officially launch the policy document. Dr Asvall highlighted the contribution that Malta can offer to other

European countries in health policy, epidemiological research and analysis of health service operations. He opined that Malta should take a more proactive lead in international health fora, especially in health issues pertaining to the Mediterranean basin.

Malta places a high value on international cooperation in health. Only through such cooperation can countries learn from each other and confer the necessary help and support. At the WHO Conference on European Health Care Reforms held in Ljubljana, Malta proposed that the Regional Office become a clearinghouse for research on health service operations. The Conference adopted this idea.

The collaboration with the Regional Office will be maintained throughout the implementation of the national policy, and it is envisaged that the Regional Office will be represented on the monitoring and evaluation committee once this is set up.

Intersectoral policy

Health-related policies in other sectors
An essential consideration in the drafting of Malta's national health policy was that *(2)*:

Improving a country's health does not depend on the efforts of the health sector alone. Intersectoral participation is needed to ensure the prevention and control of disease, the promotion and maintenance of health, the ensuring of a healthy and health conducive economic and social environment, and the provision of health services appropriate to people's needs. Such action implies cooperation among government departments, agencies, voluntary organizations, and other sectors such as business and industry, labour unions, local councils and professional groups.

During the deliberations on the drafting of the national health policy, the steering committee had considered the serious health and social challenges associated with substance abuse, disabled people, single-parent families, home and occupational accidents, AIDS and the environment. It had, however, noted that the Health Division was not responsible for remedial action for these areas, which fell under the umbrella of specific government departments, agencies, commissions and nongovernmental organizations. Since all these constituted bodies are mandated to formulate policies and implement action programmes within their respective areas, the steering committee explicitly decided from the start that these areas would not be considered for inclusion in the national health policy, although *(2)*:

> alliances are being, and will continue to be formed … with a view to adopting an intersectoral approach to their solution.

Similarly, the committee had felt that the Secretariat for the Care of the Elderly was satisfactorily addressing the problems of elderly people. This care group therefore was also excluded as a priority for action.

Mechanisms

Mechanisms that strive to ensure that health is put onto the wider public agenda include the system of adopting wide consultation, seeking political commitment to the policy by all political parties, and the use of all forms of mass media to increase public awareness of the vision and content of the policy document.

Intersectoral collaboration has been foreseen for the implementation stage of the national health policy. A strategic plan will be drawn up for each key area identified. The Department of Health Policy and Planning is responsible for formulating such plans. It will set up a multisectoral planning team and direct it to carry out this task. Each strategic plan will then be presented for approval to an interministerial committee that, in turn, will appoint an intersectoral task force. The task force will implement the strategic plan. The intersectoral collaboration envisaged at the strategic and implementation phases is absolutely vital to the success of the policy.

Alliances and partnerships

An explicit commitment was made to strengthen the old alliances with other bodies primarily accountable for a number of health-related issues. New alliances will be formed through the intersectoral collaboration described above. In fact, this has already occurred, since a multisectoral committee has almost finalized the first strategic plan for the first area chosen for priority action, road traffic accidents. The effect of using this approach has proved to be a very positive and enriching experience. The end result is much better than the Health Division could have achieved working in isolation. Further, the feeling of ownership of the strategic plan will be a positive factor in promoting implementation.

Specific examples of national intersectoral policy action

Alcohol and drugs

The Commission against drug and alcohol abuse acts as the main policy-formulating body that brings together experts and operators from government departments, professions and voluntary organizations to discuss policy issues, make recommendations and oversee the quality of services related to substance abuse. There are three advisory boards focusing on preventing disease, treatment and rehabilitation and illicit drug trafficking.

A government-funded agency has been founded specifically to coordinate, develop and manage the various government prevention and care services. It further actively collaborates with and supports other government departments and nongovernmental organizations working in this sector. This consolidates effort and makes more efficient use of resources.

Food and nutrition

In 1988, the Government endorsed a food and nutrition policy for Malta formulated by the Nutrition Branch of the Health Promotion Department. By its endorsement, the Government declared its intention to improve the nutritional wellbeing of the Maltese people, by empowering the public to adopt healthy eating patterns and by promoting health considerations in the provision and production of food. This policy, the extensive health promotion campaigns and the strong alliances fostered and sustained by the Nutrition Branch of the Health Promotion Department with the Departments of Trade, Agriculture and Industry have had notable achievements. For example, more healthy food choices are now available at reasonable prices. All foods are labelled nutritionally and are marked with a date by which they are to be used, a best before date or an expiry date. In addition, consumers have become more informed, and attitudes towards healthy food have improved. Public demand for healthier food is therefore rising.

The success of Malta's nutrition policy illustrates how intersectoral and multidisciplinary cooperation at a national level can change a population's attitudes and behaviour favourably.

Specific examples of local intersectoral policy action

With the establishment of elected local councils in 1993, many councils are undertaking initiatives to improve the local environment. These include promoting effective means of waste disposal, developing gardens and children's playing areas, traffic-calming measures to ensure pedestrian safety and the introduction of child care centres and day centres for elderly people.

Several local councils are participating with the Health Promotion Department in a joint community-based action programme. The participating local councils have identified a health promotion need in their community and planned a specific action programme to address that need, and are expected to implement it and then to evaluate the effectiveness of both process and outcome in terms of behavioural change. This programme has been planned by the Health Promotion Department in association with the Department of Health Policy and Planning, the Commission for the Advancement of Women and representatives of the local councils. The programme included a series of public discussions, activity programmes within schools and a series of television programmes aimed at explaining the concepts of the health policy formulated and at mobilizing the public to take up health issues.

Local councils are also represented on the first strategic planning committee, which is formulating the strategic plan of action on road traffic accidents.

Health status orientation

Monitoring

The Department of Health Information issues annual reports on mortality, cancer and hospital activity analysis. Besides giving disaggregated statistics according to age and sex, these reports attempt to analyse and evaluate trends. Notifiable infectious diseases are monitored and reported monthly.

The *Yearly demographic review* published by the Central Office of Statistics breaks down deaths by age, sex and socioeconomic groups.

The Health Promotion Department monitors attitudes and lifestyles. The Department of Public Health regularly carries out limited environmental monitoring, such as drinking-water and sea-water quality. The Food Safety Branch of this Department monitors the quality of all imported and locally produced food items.

Malta has no formal mechanism for monitoring morbidity on a regular basis. The national health policy has emphasized such a gap, and proposals have been put forward to remedy this situation. This information is a prerequisite to monitoring and evaluating the success of the strategic plans implemented based on the national health policy.

Quantitative targets

The Health Division reviews biannually its success in achieving the European targets for health for all and reports to WHO. In some instances Malta has bettered these targets, but in others more progress is still needed.

Health vision 2000 (2), sets quantitative targets for each area selected for priority action. These targets have been inspired by the European targets for health for all, and have been adapted to the local situation in Malta.

Quality issues

Quality has always been an implicit criterion for the Health Division. The ultimate objective of Malta's national health policy is to improve the healthy life expectancy of the Maltese people. This requires improving the quality of life through intersectoral action programmes. Such programmes strive to achieve the highest affordable quality in their implementation.

The Department of Health Policy and Planning is currently embarking on a total quality management project that aims to improve the quality of health care at all levels.

Evaluation

Health vision 2000 (2) recommends a permanent committee to periodically monitor, evaluate and report on the progress made in achieving the targets set under each key area. The Department of Health Policy and Planning would then be able to revise targets as appropriate. As targets have been devised to show changes in health status, this mechanism would monitor and evaluate the progress in improving health status.

This monitoring and evaluation committee will also report on the action being taken to implement national health policy. This would be necessary to relate the association between successful or unsuccessful policy implementation and the resultant changes in health outcome, which will enable the policy to be revised appropriately.

Feedback mechanisms (Fig. 2.1)

The policy document highlights the various feedback mechanisms necessary to ensure that the strategic plans implemented based on the national health policy are attaining their targets and objectives.

Fig. 2.1. Feedback mechanisms in national health policy

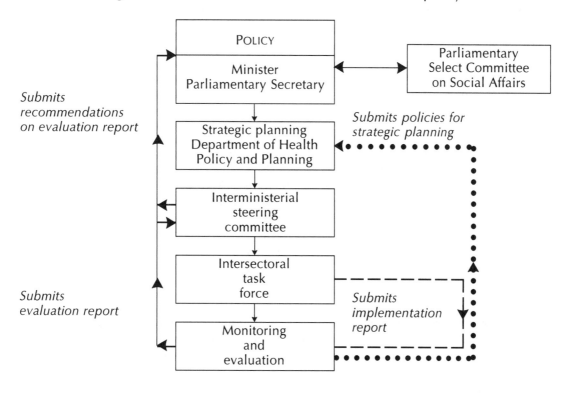

The intersectoral task forces, which implement the strategic plans, will regularly submit implementation reports to the monitoring and evaluation committee. The monitoring and evaluation committee will analyse such reports and submit evaluation reports to the interministerial committee and the Department of Health Policy and Planning. These evaluation reports will analyse critically the achievements in health gain and will identify any remedial action needed if targets, objectives or time frames are not achieved.

Based on the evaluation report, the interministerial committee will submit its recommendations to the minister responsible for health (the Minister for Social Development) to either revise the national health policy or suggest remedial action to resolve the problems highlighted in the evaluation report. The Department of Health Policy and Planning will revise the national health policy or the strategic plans.

The evaluation report submitted to the Department of Health Policy and Planning will elaborate new key areas and indicators of progress and allow targets and strategic plans to be revised as appropriate.

The interministerial committee will give the intersectoral taskforces feedback on their performance and inform them of any remedial action needed to attain the desired targets, time frames and objectives.

Summary and conclusions

Strong points in Malta's policy development included political commitment, wide consultation, intersectoral and international collaborating and the formulation of explicit criteria for the selection of key areas for action.

Strong political commitment

A strong political commitment was acquired from the very beginning, prior to the initiation of the planning phase. The efforts of the health sector alone are insufficient to improve a country's health. Therefore, unless government actively supports health policy, health would never be at the top of the political agenda. Government commitment is crucial in ensuring interministerial and intersectoral collaboration and the adequate mobilization of resources. Political interest must be sustained throughout all the phases of policy development and, equally important, must be transmitted to the public. A point was therefore specifically made to have the national health policy endorsed by the Government and other political parties and to promote mass media coverage of its launch.

Methods used to keep the Minister briefed on policy development included frequent personal discussions, monthly memoranda highlighting progress, copies of the minutes of steering committee meetings, and other relevant communications. Early cooperation with the parliamentary opposition was also promoted. This was done by personal communication with the shadow Minister responsible for health, as well as through correspondence. The response was very favourable.

Wide consultation

Wide consultation was absolutely crucial to producing commitment to implementation. The various stakeholders were included in the planning stages of policy development. Policy must be shared and owned to bring forth positive results. Consultation in the strategic planning phase facilitates implementation and paves the way for true intersectoral collaboration.

Intersectoral collaboration

The intersectoral collaboration adopted in the strategic planning phase has been a rich experience to all concerned, and the alliances built give great hope for the success of the implementation phase.

International collaboration

International collaboration must be mutually beneficial to all partners concerned. Malta has benefited from close collaboration with the WHO Regional Office for Europe in all stages of policy development and it is hoped that the Regional Office has also obtained an enriching experience from such collaboration. Malta has also perused other countries' experiences, which were a rich source of learning and guidance.

Formulating explicit criteria for selecting key areas for action

Another strength of the process was that explicit criteria were formulated for the key areas for action, as some suggestions that emerged from the consultations had to be excluded. Contributors whose suggestions were excluded would have otherwise become potential sources of noncompliance and could also become potentially damaging to further policy development. The predefined explicit criteria were therefore a tool that aided the selection of the key areas by the steering committee, but also served as a justifiable yardstick for those who had contributed ideas.

Possible weaknesses included the method of evaluating recommendations for key areas of action as well as insufficiently wide collaboration.

Method of evaluating recommendations for key areas for action

One deficiency arose from the fact that, although the steering committee considered all submissions, only the areas recommended most frequently were objectively scored against the criteria. This could have biased selection in favour of numbers and away from disadvantaged groups or areas.

Insufficiently wide collaboration

Despite all our efforts, in retrospect we feel that we have not been exhaustive enough. All stakeholders must be included. Time must be spent on situation analysis in policy development to assess the relative contributions of different sectors, government departments, trade unions, political parties, institutions, professional organizations, commissions, interest groups and other nongovernmental organizations, key individuals and the general public in the development and impact of health policy and to analyse the strengths, weaknesses, opportunities and threats involved and how best to handle them.

The future

The national policy document presents a vision for the health gains that can be attained in the next decade by optimizing the use of resources to address priority health and health service areas through an intersectoral approach. This will remain a mere vision unless detailed strategic plans with time frames are formulated. Rational planning demands regular monitoring and evaluation to measure progress and correct any problems encountered.

Strategic plans

For each key area identified in *Health vision 2000 (2)*, the Department of Health Policy and Planning will formulate a detailed strategic plan for action through the joint collaboration of a multidisciplinary and multisectoral planning team (Fig. 2.1). This plan will be presented for approval to the interministerial committee, composed of the permanent secretaries within the various ministries who are the final arbiters in the decision-making process and who can allocate the necessary resources to implement such plans. This committee will in turn appoint intersectoral task forces to implement such strategic plans.

Monitoring and evaluation

A monitoring and evaluation committee (it is hoped to include a WHO external assessor) will be set up to report periodically on the progress made in achieving the objectives and targets and in the process of implementation. This information will be necessary to adjust and refine the initial strategic plan appropriately to complete the policy development cycle.

The national policy and health care sector reforms

Given the current and future constraints on the health care market, the public health care sector needs to be reformed to ensure appropriate development in the years to come. Various health care sector reforms in other countries have failed to achieve their objectives in terms of quality indicators, equity issues, cost containment and health gains. Such failures are often attributable to a lack of understanding of the intrinsic characteristics and market weaknesses inherent in the health care sector. Health care reforms cannot be based solely on economic criteria.

Health care sector reforms must have as their cornerstone a health policy based on a priority ranking of health problems that addresses adequately the issues of equity and high-quality and affordable health care.

Thus, the Department of Health Policy and Planning has developed a philosophy to guide all reform action programmes: the Malta model (Fig. 2.2). Briefly, this philosophy contemplates that any reform within a health care sector must have three dimensions:

Fig. 2.2. The Malta model of developing health policy

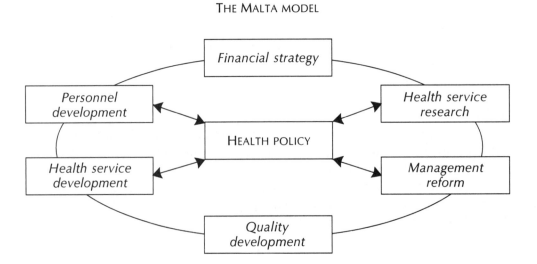

THE MALTA MODEL

- an internal dimension to enhance the operational efficiency and the effectiveness and quality of the services provided by each individual health care unit;
- an external dimension by which each health care unit identifies its new role and functions to attain the targets laid down in the national policy; and
- a horizontal dimension by which each health care unit identifies how it can collaborate with other health care units to facilitate attaining the targets of the national health policy.

References

1. *Health services development plan for Malta, 1986–1990.* Valletta, Department of Health, 1986.
2. *Health vision 2000.* Valletta, Department of Health Policy and Planning, 1995.
3. National policy on mental health services. Valletta, Department of Health Policy and Planning, 1995.

Health policy in the Netherlands: description and analysis of ten years of national health policy development emphasizing the health for all strategy

Evert Dekker

Introduction

Definition and frame of reference

In this study, policy is defined as a set of objectives, priorities and strategies for future action. Policy development is the process that gives the actual form to the policy-making; it is characterized by the merging of content and structure (Fig. 2.3). Health policy is defined as any explicit government policy related to health status and health care intended to promote the principles of or attain the goals set by the health for all strategy of WHO, taking into account the structural conditions in a given political and administrative environment (Fig. 2.3).

During the session of the WHO Regional Committee for Europe held in September 1984, the Netherlands and the other European Member States endorsed this policy for Europe. Since then the policy has been formulated and implemented in various ways in the Netherlands.

General characteristics of the Netherlands

The Netherlands is located in northwestern Europe and covers an area of 41 864 km^2; almost 20% of this is inland water. The capital is Amsterdam and the seat of government is The Hague.

The Netherlands has a developed market economy based largely on financial services, light and heavy industries and trade. The Netherlands has one of the largest reserves of natural gas in western Europe, providing more than half the domestic energy used. The agricultural sector accounts for less than 5% of the gross domestic product and employs a similar percentage of the workforce. The long growing season and excellent grazing lands on the polders, however, put the Netherlands among the top exporters of cheese, butter and eggs.

General characteristics of the population

The Netherlands has a population of over 15 million and is one of the most densely populated countries in the world (Appendix 1).

Fig. 2.3. The Y model for health policy development

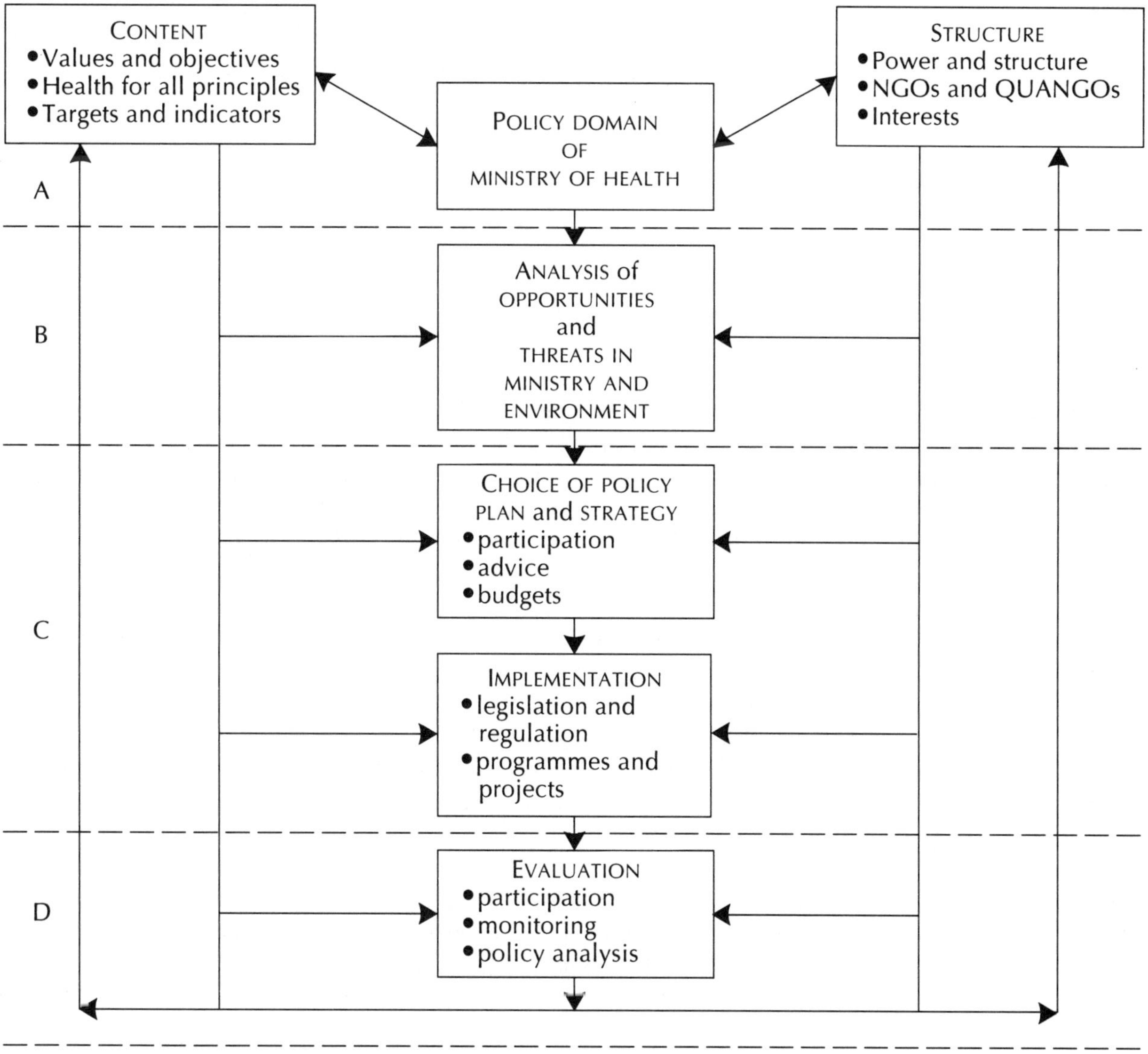

CONTENT		STRUCTURE
•Values and objectives	POLICY DOMAIN OF MINISTRY OF HEALTH	•Power and structure
•Health for all principles		•NGOs and QUANGOs
•Targets and indicators		•Interests

A

B — ANALYSIS of OPPORTUNITIES and THREATS IN MINISTRY AND ENVIRONMENT

C — CHOICE OF POLICY PLAN and STRATEGY
•participation
•advice
•budgets

IMPLEMENTATION
•legislation and regulation
•programmes and projects

D — EVALUATION
•participation
•monitoring
•policy analysis

This model combines not only the confrontation of content and structure but also the policy cycle (stages A, B, C, and D) and the SWOT model (strong-weak opportunities and threats).

NGOs: nongovernmental organizations; QUANGOS: quasi-autonomous nongovernmental organizations.

Source: Unpublished paper by Bosboom & Hegoner (1979).

The ethnic composition is 90% Dutch with a considerable proportion of Turks, Moroccans and Germans. Current immigration exceeds emigration and is mostly from Turkey, Morocco, the United Kingdom and Surinam, a former Dutch colony.

Mortality figures are relatively favourable. The average age at death and life expectancy at birth are increasing gradually (Appendix 2).

The long-term demographic trends show not only population growth but also an increasing proportion of older people. This has tremendous consequences for health policy.

General characteristics of health status

The life expectancy in 2010 is projected to be 1–1.5 years longer than in 1990, but only part of this gain in life span will consist of healthy years.

Trends in life expectancy (mortality) are largely determined by a limited number of important causes of death. In 1990 the most important causes of premature death in rank order were: coronary heart disease, stroke, lung cancer, breast cancer, chronic obstructive pulmonary disease (including asthma), road accidents, colorectal cancer, suicide, diabetes mellitus and stomach cancer. These ten causes are responsible for about 48% of the total potential years of life lost through all causes of death.

Trends in health expectancy are largely determined by a limited number of important diseases and disorders, most of which are different from those that determine life expectancy (mortality). Health expectancy is calculated based on data about poor health experienced, long- and short-term functional disability and stays in institutions. Calculated this way, health expectancy is largely determined by the occurrence of chronic diseases and disorders but also by ones of short duration. About 80–85% of those who describe their health as "less good" have had one or more chronic diseases, compared with 30–35% of those describing their health as "good".

By 2010, the total number of people with diseases and disorders, especially the chronic ones occurring mostly in old age, is expected to increase by 25–40% above the level in 1990. This increase is especially associated with the growth in and aging of the population and has considerable consequences for health care.

Changes in lifestyle may lead to considerable health gains, especially as regards the reduction of premature death. Smoking makes the biggest demonstrable contribution to total mortality in the Netherlands (calculated at about one quarter), posing numerous challenges for prevention (1).

Increasing the healthy life expectancy and quality of life will also be a challenge. This especially applies to chronically ill people, including those with mental disorders.

The political system

The Constitution from 1814 vests legislative power in a bicameral Parliament, the Staten-Generaal, with a 75-member First Chamber and a 150-member Second Chamber. The members of the First Chamber are elected to six-year terms by members of provincial councils; members of the Second Chamber, which has greater authority, are directly elected to four-year terms. Executive power is exercised by an appointed Cabinet under the leadership of the Prime Minister. The judiciary is headed by the High Court.

Governments after the Second World War comprised Roman Catholic and Labour Party coalitions. From the late 1950s until the early 1970s, the Christian Democratic Party, a reorganized Catholic Party that included Protestants, controlled the Government. That control was lost in 1973 to the Labour Party, followed by a succession of various coalitions from 1977 on. Since 1994 the Government has comprised the Labour Party, the People's Party for Freedom and Democracy (a right-wing liberal party) and the Democrats '66 (left-wing liberal democrats).

Policy environment

The Netherlands has a pluralistic health system *(2)*. Such systems have long been common in continental western Europe. The pluralistic system in the Netherlands combines two types of decentralization: functional and geographical (Fig. 2.4). The functional type of decentralization covers cure, care and some preventive aspects of the health system and is therefore a dominant characteristic of the health system.

The pluralistic health system in the Netherlands has a historically embedded liberal tradition combined with the social responsibility of private organizations, especially those with a religious background, thus reducing a potential strong role of government. Government and social actors share responsibility for formulating and implementing policy.

Social insurance is the main source of health care financing. This separates the health and social welfare systems administratively, as social welfare is financed by tax revenues. The social insurance, historically originating from sickness funds and the labour movement, traditionally focuses strongly on protecting the most vulnerable people.

In addition to government administration, the social actors or nongovernmental organizations join forces in quasi-autonomous nongovernmental organizations. This represents the functional type of decentralization (Fig. 2.4). They play a major role in regulating the actual provision of health services. The actors in these quasi-autonomous nongovernmental organizations are care providers, insurers (sickness funds and private insurers), consumer organizations and, in one case, organizations of employers and employees. This characteristic accounts for a relatively strong tradition of consultation and negotiation between all actors, including the Government.

One of the consequences of this structure is that the agenda for national health policy is mainly dominated by planning, financing and organizing health services and less by health status, equity and intersectoral

Fig. 2.4. Types of decentralization of the health system in the Netherlands

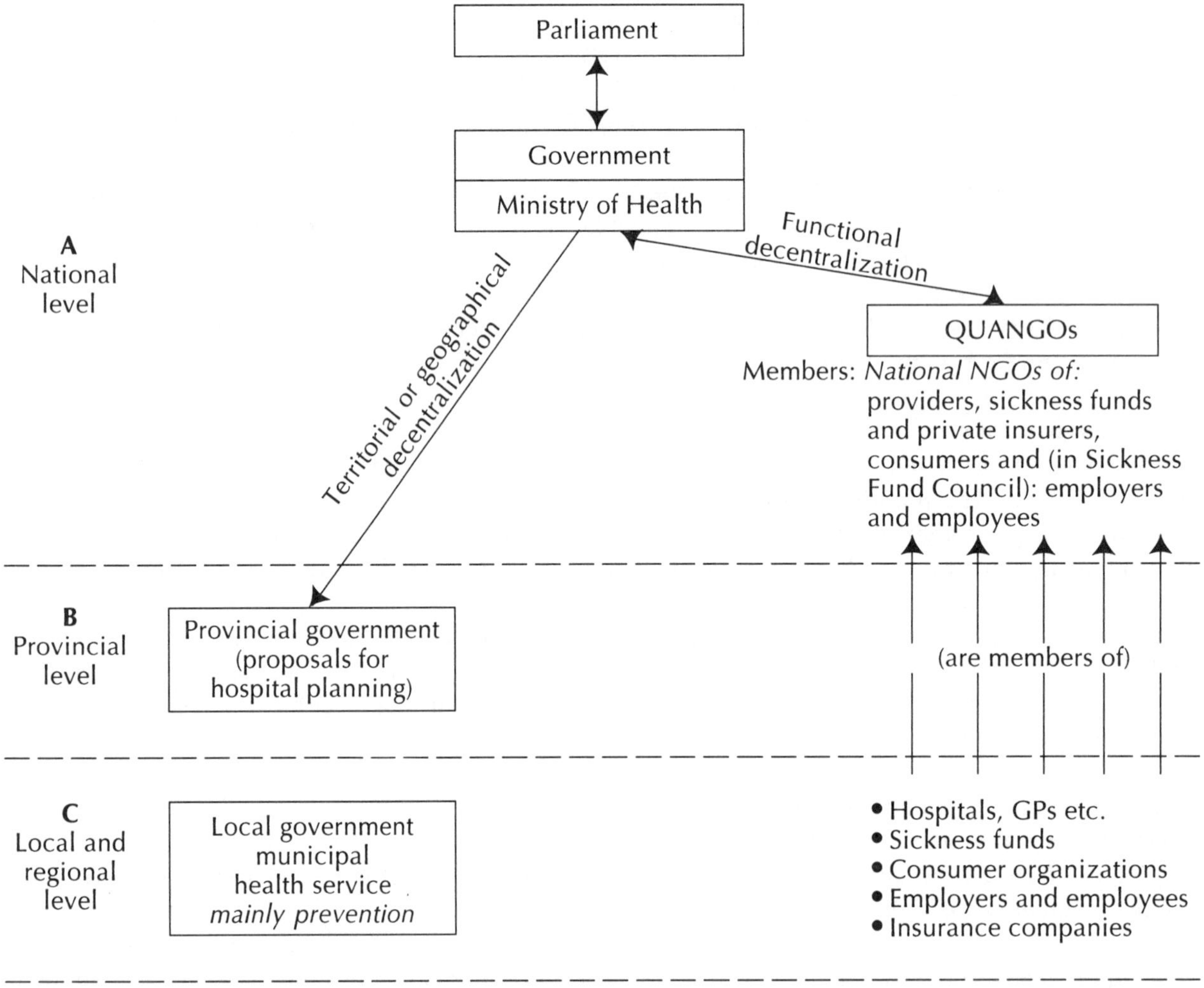

	Parliament

A
National
level

Government
Ministry of Health

Functional decentralization

Territorial or geographical decentralization

QUANGOs

Members: *National NGOs of:* providers, sickness funds and private insurers, consumers and (in Sickness Fund Council): employers and employees

B
Provincial
level

Provincial government (proposals for hospital planning)

(are members of)

C
Local and
regional
level

Local government municipal health service *mainly prevention*

- Hospitals, GPs etc.
- Sickness funds
- Consumer organizations
- Employers and employees
- Insurance companies

QUANGOs (Quasi-autonomous nongovernmental organizations)
1. Sickness Fund Council   } *advise and regulate*
2. Central Council for Health Care
3. Hospital Facilities Council
4. National Council for Health Care   } *advise*
5. Health Council

action. Despite these structural features of the system, the Government of the Netherlands has always endorsed the WHO regional strategy for health for all.

A second characteristic of the policy environment influencing the health for all strategy in the Netherlands is the ongoing debate since 1986 on health care reform *(3)*. These reforms were described as "balancing corporatism, etatism and market mechanisms" *(4,5)*. Proposals by the Dekker Committee *(6)* and subsequent government actions have dominated the policy agenda since then. The social and political debate emanating from restructuring and financing the health care system has mainly focused on cost containment and its financial consequences for the population, especially the most vulnerable groups.

Both pluralism or (neo-)corporatism and care reforms have largely determined the opportunities for developing a health policy leading to health for all *(7,8*, E. Dekker, personal communication, 1993).

Start of the process

The Netherlands has a relatively long history of health policy development. In 1983, a first step was taken by the establishment of the Steering Committee on Future Health Scenarios. Scenario analysis is a means of forecasting, formulating strategy and allocating resources that has developed in response to the problems of making decisions in complex and rapidly changing societies. It integrates traditional discipline-specific forecasting methods within a multidisciplinary framework and adds qualitative methods that project assumptions about the future. It also integrates plans and future intentions with projections derived from past trends and causes *(9)*.

This step appeared to be of strategic importance, as information on the future of health status and its determinants (including health care) has formed the basis of health policy documents since then. Moreover, Parliament showed great interest in the health scenarios from the start, thus facilitating the introduction of health policy on the basis of health for all.

The scenarios, together with the launching of the European regional strategy for health for all by WHO, were the main sources of inspiration for the first health policy document in the Netherlands, the *Health 2000 memorandum (10)*. The document was prepared by the staff responsible for health policy development using informal consultation with experts. The document mainly described the health status of the population, the policy component being very modest. The Government only committed itself to start changing in the direction of health policy, but did not implement the health for all principles with a visible reorientation of the existing policy towards care-oriented health.

Main stages of the health policy process

In 1987, Parliament debated the *Health 2000 memorandum*. The Parliamentary Commission on Health endorsed the policy commitment to develop health policy, but expressed disappointment about the content of the memorandum, suggesting that it should be more oriented towards policy. In the same year, the Dekker Committee published its proposals for restructuring the financing and organization of health services (see below).

In response to this criticism, the Ministry of Welfare, Health and Cultural Affairs prepared a new health policy document in 1989, the *Target document on health policy (11)*. This included quantitative targets on cancer, cardiovascular disease, accidents and the use of alcohol and tobacco. This policy approach was strongly supported by new scientific studies *(12)* quantifying the health gain of possible health policy measures. Specific measures were designed to meet the targets, but budget proposals were not included. Soon after a draft version of the document was issued, the Government fell and the new Government did not continue the proposed health policy.

As the *Target document on health policy* did not acquire the status of a policy document, a third national health policy document was prepared in 1991: *A strategy for health (13)*. This document represented a more modest approach and appeared to be more in line with the existing health care policy. It also contained some new priorities for intersectoral policy relating to people's incapacity for work.

Parliament debated *A strategy for health* in 1992. Although the Parliamentary Commission on Health expressed disappointment about the modest scope of the policy proposals, the Parliament approved the document as it was and it became accepted policy. In the same year, the Dunning Committee published *Choices in health care (14)*, thus starting a national debate on criteria for setting priorities in health care.

The health status orientation of health policy was strengthened by a new document: *Public health status and forecasts (1)*. This document integrated all available information on the health status of the population, its determinants and on socioeconomic differences in health, thus forming an adequate basis for new health policy proposals.

A new Government used this document to formulate a comprehensive framework for health policy in 1995, embracing a broad health policy agenda for the current Cabinet period (1994–1998). The latest health policy document, *Healthy and sound (15)*, used the new data on health status to introduce general health objectives such as extending healthy life expectancy, and covered such traditional issues as pricing policy for pharmaceuticals.

Criteria used in defining the policies, objectives and targets
The criteria used in defining the content of the health policy have shifted over the last decade. The first two (draft) policy documents focused on preventing premature death, and measures to prevent the main causes of death – cardiovascular disease, cancer and accidents – were prominent policy measures. As statistics on mortality caused by these diseases and the underlying determinants (such as nutrition and alcohol and tobacco use) were readily available and the documents did not have a real political impact, quantitative health targets (like the European regional targets for health for all) could be used.

At a later stage, the emphasis shifted from "adding years to life" to "adding life to years". This new approach was based on the increasingly favourable health status of the population; consequently, chronic diseases, mental and psychosocial disorders and the health problems of elderly people require more attention.

The criterion of extending healthy life expectancy clearly scored higher than avoiding premature death in multi-criteria analysis. In this process the most important policy-makers of the ministry were asked to rate, based on epidemiological data, the most urgent priorities of health policy, using general objectives and criteria. The interactive nature of the process (computerized scores shown on a central display and subsequent discussion) greatly enhanced the quality of this method of preparing policy.

The latest health policy document, *Healthy and sound (15)* describes the Government's general health policy objectives as:

- increasing healthy life expectancy
- preventing avoidable deaths
- increasing the quality of life.

This case study describes the implementation of the principles of health for all in the Netherlands, except for the principle of reorientation to primary health care, because there are no striking changes. The health system already emphasizes primary health care.

Equity

General principles

Equity in health and equal access to health care play an important role in health policy. Equal access to health care services is a traditional cornerstone of the neo-corporatist health system. Sickness funds play a major role in such systems. With their tradition of solidarity, they greatly contribute to the principle of equal access. Private insurers are required by law to follow this principle, although during the last few years both types of health insurance have tended to offer all kind of extras to the consumer on an unregulated basis.

Equity, in the sense of equal opportunities for health for different socioeconomic, regional and ethnic categories of the population, did not play a role in health policy for a long time. Awareness of existing differences in health started to increase in the 1980s and was especially promoted by the launching of the WHO strategy for health for all.

Equity programme

The *Health 2000 memorandum (10)* described extensively the known socioeconomic differences in health. The following year the Scientific Council for Government Policy organized a national conference. Actors within and outside the health system attended. This conference, initiated by the Ministry of Welfare, Health and Cultural Affairs, ensured a favourable political and social context for the subsequent programme. The main conclusion was that there is enough evidence about socioeconomic differences to justify a specific effort by government and social actors to reduce these differences. A special programme committee was set up, and a five-year research programme started in 1989. The broad political support for equity in health was shown, for example, in the fact that the chairperson of the programme committee was a well known member of a right-wing political party. Part of the programme was (and still is) a long-term research project together with several smaller projects concerning, for example, lifestyle factors and socioeconomic position and health. Within the programme a special documentation centre (which evolved into a WHO collaborating centre) was set up, and a series of research reports drew national and international interest.

In 1991 the Scientific Council for Government Policy organized a second national conference. The original actors from the first conference were now invited to report on the progress made in putting equity on the agenda and on the specific measures taken in various sectors. The research programme ended with an international conference in 1994, but it had become clear that equity should remain a policy priority. Thus, a second equity programme started, now focusing on implementation of the research results, particularly in distressed areas in large cities.

A strategy for health (13) recognized vulnerable groups: people incapable of working, homeless people and, to a lesser extent, ethnic minorities. Special measures were taken, such as intersectoral action to protect the position of those incapable of working and support for local initiatives, including subsidizing local support groups and taking national action to prevent the exclusion from work of people with physical or mental disabilities or chronic illness.

In conclusion, the equity programme is a successful spin-off of health policy. Awareness of existing inequities has increased; for example, this now plays a role in the debate on reforming the law on sick leave. Protecting the position of people with chronic illness and mental disorders is at stake. Nevertheless, the equity issue has clearly shown the limitations of health policy relative to other policy domains. First, economic interests are often more dominant in the political debate. Second, health policy in the Netherlands, because of the policy environment, does not have a strong tradition of intersectoral policy aimed at improving social conditions outside the health care sector.

Participation

Participation in policy preparation
The pluralistic nature of the health system includes a strong tradition of involving social groups in preparing government policy. After the *Health 2000 memorandum (10)* was issued, five national conferences were organized to discuss the strengths and weaknesses of the proposed new policy approach. These conferences focused on sectors of health care, such as primary care (general practitioners and health centres), mental health, hospitals and administration. These conferences showed strong support for the empirical underpinning of the document but mostly scepticism towards the feasibility of the new policy, especially in dealing with the strong vested interests of hospital organizations, medical specialists and health insurance organizations. As explained previously, the policy environment is dominated by care suppliers and insurance organizations and therefore tends to focus on health care services instead of improving health status.

In the following stages of policy development, this pattern of responses appeared to continue. The draft *Target document on health policy (11)* was discussed informally with about 80 organizations, clustered according to the subject, and later about 100 formal written responses were sent to the Government.

No special participatory processes were organized for the third and fourth draft health policy documents, but special national meetings were organized to focus on the quality of care, preventive policy, local health policy, health impact assessment and, as mentioned, equity.

At the local level, the WHO Healthy Cities project has enhanced participation by the population. About 20 municipalities have entered the Netherlands National Network of Healthy Cities. Since 1995, the Netherlands Union of Local Authorities has formally recognized and supported the Network *(16)*. Participation is promoted on a wide range of issues, often broader than health care services; for example, the general living conditions in neighbourhoods. Projects to increase the self-determination of elderly people and self-care of people with mental disorders and their relatives, as well as self-help groups for those who are incapable of working, have enhanced participation *(17)*.

Interest groups

The position of patients' organizations was enhanced during the 1960s and 1970s as part of a general democratization process in society. Sickness funds and the cross organizations providing extramural care, both associations consisting of members, have traditionally claimed to represent health care consumers. Nevertheless, this increasingly proved to be too theoretical.

The quasi-autonomous nongovernmental organizations are interest groups with a dual function: public regulation of health care within a legal framework and representing the interests of a special category, such as medical specialists (Fig. 2.4). Patients' organizations have acquired an increasingly important but still modest role in these nongovernmental organizations. Nevertheless, creating a federation of all patients' organizations at the national level has strengthened the consumers' voice considerably.

Patients' organizations have strengthened their position as an advocate for special problems and as platforms for mutual support often with government support. Given the epidemiological transition from infectious to chronic diseases, the establishment in 1991 of an official National Commission on Chronic Illness marked the recognition of the increasing importance of this category of consumer. This Commission actively defends the rights of people with long-term health problems in the debate about reforming the law on sick leave and the accumulation of co-payments (users' fees).

Communication with the public

Only the first health policy document, the *Health 2000 memorandum*, was issued in both a technical and a popular version. The Netherlands has not had a special mass campaign related to overall health policy. Nevertheless, intensive campaigns have been carried out on, for example, alcohol abuse, traffic accidents and AIDS. In addition, to follow up the Dunning report *(14)* on making choices in health care, a campaign was launched via various mass media, including television and leaflets, to make the public aware of the financial and ethical limits of health care and the need to make choices. The television shows especially aroused intensive debates by asking an audience to choose how limited health care money should be spent; for example, on an old person versus a young alcoholic, both with the same medical problems.

This last example represents a case of two-way communication; all the other types are one way. The public's views are normally taken into account via patient or consumer organizations.

International factors

The European regional strategy for health for all is one of the main roots of Netherlands health policy. During the first stages of this policy, *Targets for health for all (18)* was an explicit reference book for national policy. In later stages when it became clear that the European strategy for health for all as a whole would not be attained by the year 2000, the emphasis of cooperation with WHO shifted to parts of the strategy such as equity and Healthy Cities. During the last few years, the Netherlands' attitude towards the health for all strategy has become slightly critical because of a growing discrepancy between the actual policy agenda in many countries, notably the ongoing debate on health care reform and the fact that WHO is holding on to the (partly revised) targets for health for all.

Since the Maastricht Treaty came into force on 1 November 1993, public health policy within the European Union is becoming more prominent. A framework for action in the field of public health *(19)* embraces several action programmes, most of them disease-oriented. The Netherlands has proposed that the framework be reformed and based more consistently on WHO's principles for health for all.

Intersectoral action

New initiatives

Intersectoral action in the sense of interdepartmental cooperation concerning mutual activities exists as long as a separate policy unit for health exists, be it an agency or a ministry. This applies to policy on tobacco and alcohol, nutrition, health care pricing and labour conditions in the care sector, and education and training. Nevertheless, the launching of the strategy for health for all has given rise to new initiatives, including:

- social security: efforts to protect the position of chronically ill people and people with mental disorders;
- health policy and health services for asylum seekers and refugees;
- strengthening the tobacco and alcohol policy: regulating advertising;
- strengthening nutrition policy: reducing fat consumption;
- improving instruments for accident prevention, especially traffic accidents; and
- encouraging physical activity by subsidizing research and education campaigns.

New alliances and strategies for intersectoral action

In implementing intersectoral health policy, policy-makers become aware of their policy domain in relation to those of other social or political interests. Each policy domain, such as government finance or labour, has its own policy agenda and sociopolitical network. Knowing these agendas and networks is a prerequisite for successful intersectoral policy and a starting-point for choosing an adequate strategy for cooperation. An important step in recognizing these mechanisms was a workshop on Making Partners: Intersectoral Action for Health, organized by the WHO Regional Office for Europe in cooperation with the Ministry of Welfare, Health and Cultural Affairs *(20)*. By developing specific proposals and practical checklists, this workshop proved to be a crucial step in developing intersectoral action for health.

Policy domains can have conflicting and parallel policy agendas. For example, the interests of a ministry of health conflict with those of a ministry of finance concerning alcohol and tobacco policy. In contrast, the interests of a ministry of labour coincide with those of a health ministry in matters of labour protection and preventive policy at the workplace. Experience with intersectoral health policy in the Netherlands shows that different strategies should be used according to the interests, policy agenda and sociopolitical network of the other actors. A cooperative strategy, using negotiation as the main method, was used in getting the Ministry of Transport and Public Works to strengthen road safety policy. A disruptive strategy can be necessary for an opposing and powerful actor such as the Ministry of Finance. Disruption can be achieved by encircling tactics such as supporting and subsidizing the anti-tobacco lobby or continually publishing data on the harmful consequences of smoking and alcohol abuse, thus influencing public opinion *(21)*.

Most of these strategic phenomena were tested in two studies on the dynamics of intersectoral decision-making. In these studies, analysing the relative power position of other actors reliably predicted the chances of success of a ban on tobacco advertising and of a new health care reform. Both issues required considerable collaboration with other ministries. This method has been described extensively *(22–24)*.

To conclude, successful intersectoral health policy requires analysing different aspects of the policy domain of other political actors. Second, the pluralistic nature of the health care system in the Netherlands, combined with the high priority given to health care reform, diminishes the opportunities for successful intersectoral health policy *(25)*. The pluralistic character of the health care system makes it fragmented, especially its administrative and financial structure. This impedes strong collaboration between the health and social systems and the labour sector.

Intersectoral policy at a local level

At the local level, the lines of communication are shorter, which enhances the making of new alliances. The establishment of a Healthy Cities network with a national focal point has stimulated new projects with various objectives. Depending on the subject, cooperation has been established on social and cultural work in neighbourhoods (health promotion for elderly people), the local police (social safety) and the public works sector (road safety). In general, small projects are the most successful *(17)*.

Health status orientation

Monitoring
Monitoring as part of health policy covers aspects of health status, use of health services and the structure and financing of health care. The following agencies are responsible for monitoring:

- the Central Bureau of Statistics (mortality and health surveys);
- the Foundation for Information on Health Care (use of health services);
- various national institutes, oriented towards sectors or categories such as primary health care (general practitioners and health centres), mental health and handicapped people; and
- quasi-autonomous nongovernmental organizations in health insurance and tariffs.

Most of the data gathered by these actors have been compiled in a national integrated document called *Public health status and forecasts (1)*. This was the first epidemiological document (after the *Health 2000 memorandum*) with such a broad approach, bringing together all available data on health status and its determinants. The results of this document were then used inside the Ministry for a multicriterion analysis. In this process all responsible directors expressed their preferences (via a linked computer system) on the basis of the summarized data on health status.

In the future, such a document will be issued every four years. It is envisaged that the next document will also contain data on the effects of diseases, including disability or loss of quality of life, and data on use of health services. A commitment to issue such a report regularly is an invaluable precondition for developing health policy on a permanent basis.

A programme of health impact assessment has been started. The first step in the programme was an expert report *(26)* followed by an intensive workshop attended by scientists and policy-makers experienced in other forms of impact assessment, such as environmental impact assessment. Following this first step, the strengths and weaknesses of several kinds of policy impact assessment (such as the environment, road safety and criminality) were analysed to create a framework for health impact assessment *(27)*. The report of this analysis was sent to Parliament.

Health status orientation and making choices
Abel-Smith et al. *(28)* suggest that the first criterion to be used in setting priorities should be "the extent and seriousness of the problem". This implies focusing on health status as a starting point in the process of making choices in health care, a problem facing an increasing number of countries all over the world. The same criterion, albeit formulated in another way, is followed by *Choices in health care (14)* and in

the Swedish report *Priorities in health care (29)*. Quantitative and qualitative health status should remain the cornerstone of the health for all principles.

Summary and conclusions

Developing health policy guided by the health for all principles takes much time and effort. Whether this policy is successful depends on the historical, political and administrative context Fig. 2.3 and 2.4). It seems to be crucial to analyse well these contextual factors to avoid a too idealistic approach, which will fail in the end.

Essential factors in the Netherlands are the pluralistic character of the health system, with its emphasis on health services policy, and the fact that the policy agenda was dominated by health care reforms for many years. This situation changed when the new Cabinet came into power in 1994. Cost containment is now the first priority. In previous years it had been proven that the pluralistic, neo-corporatist structure of the health system resisted radical reform *(5)*, showing that the Netherlands is no exception to the rule in Europe *(30)*.

Given these contextual factors, especially the pluralistic or neo-corporatist structure of the health system and the dominant position of health care reform on the policy agenda, health policy (in the sense used in this study of policy oriented towards improving health status) has not become the leading policy model. The focus is still on the supply side and not on the demand side (the core of public health and health for all). Nevertheless, introducing the health for all strategy influenced the acceptance (again) of an approach focusing on health instead of just health care and has certainly led to interesting and encouraging spin-offs, such as:

* the equity programmes;
* a revitalization of public health at the local level;
* more attention for vulnerable groups such as chronically ill people and people with mental disorders;
* strengthening preventive policy;
* using innovative approaches in intersectoral action;
* strengthening epidemiology in general and an approach focusing on health status in particular; and
* the establishment of the Netherlands School of Public Health.

Health policy oriented towards health for all allowed new concepts and principles to be introduced into the overall health policy, such as the epidemiological transition to chronic diseases, the decompression of morbidity and the competing causes of morbidity and death. These illustrate a health status orientation and, as such, an adequate mechanism of underpinning the need to make critical choices in health care.

Soon after the strategy for health for all was introduced, two independent policy lines developed: health care reform, which has dominated the political agenda ever since, and policy oriented towards health for all. Health care reform scarcely took health criteria or improvement in health into account, whereas health policy oriented towards health for all missed the link to health care reform. The latest policy document *Healthy and sound (15)* has a more balanced approach. Nevertheless, the translation of such health-oriented policy objectives as extending healthy life expectancy into specific structural and financial policy measures remains a challenge for the future.

Most countries encounter difficulties in strengthening their intersectoral policy for health because of the relatively weak political position of the health sector compared with, for example, government finances. Nevertheless, the specific administrative conditions of the health system in the Netherlands (Fig. 2.4), together with a focus on care reforms, creates a certain introversion that hinders an active policy integrated intersectorally in the system as a whole. Some new initiatives have been taken, however: intersectoral policy in the new legislation for sick leave, better living conditions for elderly people (housing, home care and social security) and the use of new methods such as health impact assessment and analysis of intersectoral decision-making.

The Netherlands thus shows that political support, together with a determined and astute attitude, shape the opportunity to implement health policy based on the principles of health for all.

A decade of experience may provide general lessons. WHO launched the health for all strategy in Europe shortly before a wave of health care reforms arose in many countries *(30–33)*. This explains in part the obstacles to the health for all strategy becoming the leading model in the health policy of European countries. In addition, the enormous ambition of the strategy as a whole and the rather formal structure of the 38 targets in particular may have marginalized the strategy in the course of the last decade. It is hoped that a drastic renewal of the strategy for the twenty-first century will address these problems while preserving the health for all principles as guidelines for a policy oriented towards public health. Such a policy should not only include monitoring of health status but also focus on analysing the administrative aspects of the system and how they can best serve health policy, and on the strategies for implementation.

This renewal will have to take into account the integration of content and structure (Fig. 2.3): integrating the implementation of the public health approach into the existing political and administrative environment while changing this environment. All current health care reforms should be assessed for how they contribute to public health.

More specifically, the main supportive factors for such health policy in a pluralistic or corporatist context are:

- the distinction between providers and purchasers, which could become such a factor (as it has in Sweden and the United Kingdom) because, in principle, it allows improvement in health status to be included in contracts;
- analysis of the relative power position of the health system in the intersectoral environment, together with consonant strategies;

- building support systems and strengthening the relationships with existing systems, such as the public health sector, and research institutes on health promotion, epidemiology and health impact assessment;
- organizing publicity on health status, risk factors and the options at stake in making critical choices; and
- exploring the possibilities of integrating policy oriented towards health services with policy oriented towards outcome, by introducing such concepts as healthy life expectancy and quality of life and by developing health impact assessment as a tool in health policy.

It is to be hoped that the lessons from the Netherlands support the present WHO intentions of renewing the strategy for health for all. The key factors in such a policy seem to be: maintaining the public health approach (also as a sound basis for the increasing problem of making choices in health policy and health care) and integrating content and structure; that is, placing the principles of health for all in a proper political and administrative environment, which should also be transformed.

The renewal of the strategy for health for all requires much closer collaboration between WHO, the European Union (on the basis of Article 129 of the Maastricht Treaty *(28)*) and the World Bank *(34)*.

References

1. RUWAARD, ET AL., ED. *Public health status and forecasts: the health status of the Dutch population over the period 1950–2010. Summary of a report in Dutch.* The Hague, SDU Publishers, 1994.
2. DEKKER, E. & VAN DER WERFF, A., ED. *Policies for health in European countries with pluralistic systems.* Houten, Bohn Staflen Van Loghum, 1990.
3. OKMA, K.G.H. Restructuring health care in the Netherlands. *In*: Williams, R., ed. *International developments in health care: 1990s.* London, Royal College of Physicians, 1995, pp. 95–102.
4. MORONE, J.A. ET AL. European health policies: welfare states in a market era. *Journal of health politics, policy and law*, **20** (special issue): 557–785 (1995).
5. SCHUT, F.T. Health care reform in the Netherlands: balancing corporatism, etatism, and market mechanisms. *Journal of health politics, policy and law*, **20**: 615– 652 (1995).
6. *Bereidheid tot verandering* [Willingness to change]. The Hague, State Publishers, 1987.
7. DEKKER, E. *Pluralistic structures and processes of health policy development.* Copenhagen, WHO Regional Office for Europe, 1991 (document ICP/HSC 417/5).
8. DEKKER, E. Health care reforms and public health. *European journal of public health*, **4**: 281–286 (1994).
9. BRENNER, M.H. Scenarios, decision making and strategic planning: a framework. In: Brouwer, J.J. & Scheuder, R.F., ed. *Scenarios and other methods to support long term health planning.* Rijswijk, Steering Committee on Future Health Scenarios, 1986.
10. *Nota 2000* [Health 2000 memorandum]. The Hague, Ministry of Welfare, Health and Cultural Affairs, (1986). Abridged English version: *Health as a focal point. An abridged version of the*

memorandum Health 2000, the Netherlands. The Hague, Ministry of Welfare, Health and Cultural Affairs, 1987.

11. *Ontwerp-kerndocument gezondheidsbeleid* [Target document on health policy]. The Hague, Ministry of Welfare, Health and Cultural Affairs, 1989.

12. GUNNING-SCHEPERS, L. *The health benefits of prevention.* Dissertation, Erasmus University, Rotterdam, 1988.

13. *A strategy for health.* Rijswijk, Ministry of Welfare, Health and Cultural Affairs, 1992.

14. *Choices in health care.* Zoetermeer, Government Committee on Choices in Health Care, 1992.

15. *Healthy and sound. Framework for health policy in the Netherlands 1995–1998.* Rijswijk, Ministry of Health, Welfare and Sport, 1996.

16. KOORNSTRA, A. Putting public health on the Dutch municipal policy agenda. *Research for Healthy Cities, newsletter,* **7**:1 (1995).

17. SAAN, A. ET AL. *Intersectorale actie; voor grensbewoners is smokkelen normaal* [Intersectoral action: for inhabitants of the border zone, smuggling is normal]. Assen, Van Gorcum, 1994.

18. *Targets for health for all.* Copenhagen, WHO Regional Office for Europe, 1985 (European Health for All Series, No. 4).

19. *Communication of the Commission on the framework for action in the field of public health.* Brussels, European Commission, 1993 (COM(93)559 def).

20. TAKET, A.R., ED. *Making partners. Intersectoral action for health.* Copenhagen, WHO Regional Office for Europe and Rijswijk, Ministry of Welfare, Health and Cultural Affairs, 1990.

21. BENSON, J.K. The interorganizational network as a political economy. *Administrative science quarterly,* **20**: 229–249 (1975).

22. STOKMAN, F.N. & VAN DEN BOS, J.M.M. A two-stage model of policy making with an empirical test in the US energy policy domain. *In*: Moore, G. & Whitt, J.A., ed. *The political consequences of social networks,* Vol. 4. *Research and society.* Greenwich, CT, JAI Press, 1992, pp. 219–258.

23. STOKMAN, F.N. & VAN OOSTEN, R. The exchange of voting positions: an object-oriented model of policy networks. *In:* Bueno de Mesquita, B. & Stokman, F.N., ed. *Twelve into one: models of policy making in the European Community.* New Haven, CT, Yale University Press, 1994, pp. 105–127.

24. STOKMAN, F.N. Modelling conflict and exchange in collective decision making. *Bulletin de méthodologie sociologique,* **49** (December): (1995).

25. DEKKER, E. & VAN DER GRINTEN, T.E.D. Tien jaar facetbeleid; terugblik en perspectief [Ten years of intersectoral health policy in the Netherlands]. *Tijdschrift sociale gezondheidszorg,* **73**: 484–492 (1995).

26. ROSCAM ABBING, E.W. ET AL. *Gezondheidseffectscreening: een verkenning* [Health impact assessment: an introduction]. Nijmegen, Catholic University, 1993.

27. PUTTERS, K. *Gezondheidseffectscreening; rationele modellen in hun bestuurlijke context* [Health impact assessment; rational models in an administrative context.] Rijswijk, Ministry of Health, Welfare and Sport, 1996.

28. ABEL-SMITH, B. ET AL. *Choices in health policy: an agenda for the European Union.* London, London School of Economics and Political Science, 1995.

29. *Priorities in health care: ethics, economy, implementation.* Stockholm, Ministry of Health and Social Affairs, 1995.
30. *Four Country Conference (1995) on Health Care Reforms and Health Care Policies in the United States, Canada, Germany and the Netherlands. Conference report.* Rijswijk, Ministry of Health, Welfare and Sport, 1995.
31. HAM, C. & BROMMELS, M. Health care reforms in the Netherlands, Sweden and the United Kingdom. *Health affairs*, **13**: 106–119 (1994).
32. *Health care systems in transition. The search for efficiency.* Paris, Organisation for Economic Co-operation and Development, 1990.
33. *The reform of health care systems. A review of seventeen OECD countries.* Paris, Organisation for Economic Co-operation and Development, 1994.
34. WORLD BANK. *World development report 1993. Investing in health.* Oxford, Oxford University Press, 1993.

Appendix 1. Size and sex distribution of the population of the Netherlands, 1992–1994 and projections for 2000 and 2010

Population	1992	1993	1994	2000	2010
Male	7 480 422	7 535 268	7 585 887	7 984 491	8 450 707
Female	7 648 728	7 703 914	7 755 666	8 094 766	8 492 023
Total	15 129 150	15 239 182	15 341 553	16 079 256	16 942 730
Non-Dutch citizens as a percentage of the total population	4.8	5.0	5.1		
Population density per km^2	446	449	452	474	499

Source: Statistical yearbook of the Netherlands 1995. The Hague, SDU Publishers, 1995.

Appendix 2. Vital statistics for the Netherlands, 1991–1993 and projections for 2000 and 2010

Mortality	1991	1992	1993	2000	2010
Deaths					
Total	129 958	129 887	137 795	139 876	158 774
Male	66 679	66 264	69 884	70 182	80 898
Per 1000	8.6	8.6	9.0	8.7	9.4
Standardized death rate per 1000					
Male	8.2	8.1	8.4	8.1	7.7
Female	6.7	6.6	6.9	7.0	6.8
Total	7.5	7.3	7.7	7.5	6.4
Average age at death					
Male	70.9	70.9	71.3	71.9	73.0
Female	77.1	77.2	77.7	78.5	79.3
Life expectancy at birth					
Male	74.1	74.3	74.0	75.4	76.0
Female	80.2	80.3	80.0	81.0	81.5

Source: Statistical yearbook of the Netherlands 1995. The Hague, SDU Publishers, 1995.

Development of a policy for health for all in Catalonia

Ricard Tresserras, Conxa Castell & Lluís Salleras

Introduction

Catalonia is a region in the north-east of the Iberian Peninsula. It has 6 million inhabitants and two official languages: Catalan and Spanish. The region also has a history, a culture and an idiosyncrasy that distinguish it completely from the bordering regions. Since 1979 Catalonia has had its own government and has been able to organize itself within the framework of the Spanish State and the European Union. The Autonomous Government of Catalonia is convinced that Europe should be operationally organized based on regional policies, and therefore supports all initiatives by the Spanish state and the European Union that encourage regional policies in any area, including health.

Political structure
In 1985, the Spanish Government passed the General Health Act (GHA) which, under the protection of the Spanish Constitution, clearly encouraged the decentralization of the health services, given that it foresaw a pluralistic system in which each Autonomous Community (the term employed for the regions) had to establish its own health service. This service comprises all the public health centres, services and establishments within the Autonomous Community. All these activities have been carried out in a politically stable democratic environment, both in Catalonia and in Spain.

Structure of the health care system
To implement the mandate of the General Health Act, the Catalan Parliament passed the Reorganization of the Health Services in Catalonia Act, which created the Catalan Health Service. The Catalan health system comprises three major components: the health care providers (public and private), the Catalan Health Service as the public financing agent, and the Department of Health as the main instrument in planning.

The process of developing policy for health for all
The first stage in the process of developing a new health policy in Catalonia based on the principles of health for all was the preparation of a framework document *(1)* to elaborate a health plan for Catalonia. The document was elaborated through a centralized interdepartmental process based mainly on epidemiological data. This document analysed the situation in 1989–1990, selected the health problems and priority interventions, and set the targets for general health improvement and risk reduction for the year 2000 in accordance with the WHO European strategy for health for all.

The document was written by the professionals of the central health administration services in collaboration with external experts, and was published and launched in 1991 during a health policy conference held in Barcelona with the participation of representatives of the WHO Regional Office for Europe. Professionals working in decentralized health services, including district health authorities and primary health care, then analysed the framework document in depth with a view towards putting the document into operation, and with the final objective of producing the first health plan for Catalonia. A draft for a model local health plan was prepared with the contributions of all these local partners. This decentralized process included the participation of health professionals working in multidisciplinary teams, and community involvement was guaranteed through the participation of the municipalities, local and district authorities, trade unions, consumers' associations and other community partners.

Role and content of the health plan

The health plan for Catalonia *(2,3)* is the fundamental instrument for the health policy of the Autonomous Government of Catalonia. This plan sets the targets, the guidelines and the action the Catalonian Health Service needs to carry out to implement the right to health protection guaranteed by the Spanish Constitution. Convergence and Union, a Catalan nationalist party in the Autonomous Government of Catalonia, had a general political alliance with the Spanish Workers' Socialist Party at that time. Although the party in the Autonomous Government had a majority in the Catalan Parliament, many health and non-health policies had been adopted based on agreements reached among the different political parties. The health plan is one of the main aspects of the health policy reform, which the Autonomous Government approved and then presented to the Catalan Parliament for its general support.

The fundamental objective of the new policy embodied in the health plan is to improve life expectancy in good health and the positive health of Catalonia's population.

Public health in Catalonia

Life expectancy at birth in Catalonia is one of the highest in the world. In 1986, a man born in Catalonia had a life expectancy of 74 years. A woman born in the same year could expect to live on average for 80 years. The overall life expectancy was 77 years. Nevertheless, not all the potential years lived by Catalonians are lived in good health. The data for mortality and the data for morbidity, disability and institutional inpatients show that a large proportion of years lived are lived in poor health, with some sort of temporary or permanent disability of varying severity. In 1986, only 63.9 years of a total life expectancy of 77.4 were lived in good health. It is logical, therefore, to emphasize improving life in good health by adding life to years and not just increasing total life expectancy by adding years to life. This is the approach adopted by Catalonia and many European countries based on the WHO European strategy for health for all. To be specific, assessment of the potential increase in life expectancy in good health was one of the main criteria used in setting priorities among various types of intervention in health policy in Catalonia until the year 2000.

Selecting health problems and priority interventions

Health problems had to be selected and priority interventions determined when the first health plan was formulated.

First, the extent (mortality and morbidity) and severity (including the potential years of life lost, temporary or permanent disability, loss of working days, institution inpatients and health and social costs) of the various health problems were analysed to assess how reducing or eliminating the problems would improve the life expectancy in good health of the population of Catalonia. The prevalence and population-attributable risk of risk factors for chronic illness such as an unbalanced diet, smoking, hypertension, physical inactivity, alcohol abuse, hepatitis B and C virus infections, exposure to harmful substances in the workplace and in the environment were analysed to assess the potential reduction of health problems and improvement in the population's life expectancy in good health.

Second, the sensitivity of the health problem or risk factor to preventive or curative intervention (the effectiveness and efficiency of the intervention or the instrument used to solve the problem or control the risk factor) was assessed.

Third, the feasibility of the intervention aimed at solving the problem or controlling the risk factor was assessed economically, politically and organizationally.

This was the first time explicit criteria had been used in Catalonia for selecting priority problems and strategies. Based on these criteria, 19 priority health problems to be dealt with were selected (Table 2.1), as were the interventions that need to be implemented by 2000 to improve the life expectancy in good health and positive health of the population of Catalonia (Table 2.2).

Table 2.1. Priority health challenges selected in Catalonia's health plan for 1993–1995

Diseases of the circulatory system	Occupational health problems
Cancer	Tuberculosis
Diseases of the respiratory system	Nosocomial infections
Accidents, poisoning and external causes of injuries	Dental health problems
Diseases of the digestive system	Mental health problems
Alcoholism and other types of drug dependence	Diabetes mellitus
AIDS	Osteoarticular pathologies
Infectious diseases that can be prevented by routine and non-routine immunization	Environmental and food hygiene related diseases
	Maternal and infant health problems
Sexually transmitted diseases	Health problems of foreigners

Source: Department of Health and Social Security *(2)*.

Table 2.2. Priority interventions selected in Catalonia's health plan for 1993–1995

Detecting and controlling arterial hypertension	Preventing and controlling sexually transmitted diseases
Preventing and controlling smoking	
Improving dietary habits and nutrition	Preventing occupational health problems
Detecting and controlling hypercholesterolaemia	Preventing and controlling tuberculosis
Promoting physical activity	Preventing and controlling nosocomial infections
Reducing obesity	Preventing and controlling dental caries
Creating a healthy environment	Promoting interventions aimed at reducing mental health problems
Improving food hygiene	
Screening for cervical and breast cancer	Encouraging interventions aimed at reducing osteoarticular pathologies
Preventing accidents	
Preventing and controlling alcoholism and other types of drug dependence	Preventing and controlling maternal and infant health problems
Preventing and controlling AIDS	Promoting interventions aimed at foreigners' health problems
Performing routine and non-routine immunizations	

Source: Department of Health and Social Security (2).

Setting targets

The European regional targets for health for all set in 1984 were taken into account in deciding what Catalonia could achieve by 2000 for each health target. The WHO targets for the problems and interventions covered were taken as a minimum, and the levels proposed by the European targets were generally accepted for Catalonia. There were some special situations. Some European targets, such as life expectancy at birth, had already been achieved in Catalonia when the health plan was formulated. In other cases, such as infant mortality and maternal mortality, the WHO targets were considered to be too low and more ambitious targets were set for Catalonia.

Health problems or interventions for which WHO had not set specific targets were given their own targets and levels specific to Catalonia, bearing in mind the experience of countries at a similar socioeconomic level. An example is targets for serum cholesterol levels in the population.

Health plan targets were set up according to epidemiological information, taking into account the principles of equity and strengthening primary health care, health promotion and disease prevention.

Health system organization

The Catalan Health Service plans, evaluates, finances, guarantees community involvement and has direct contact with users but it does not manage. Services are administered and provided by various suppliers, public and private, through service contracts that aim to create a certain degree of competition between them.

One of the major changes stemming from the new organization of the health care system is based on this separation of financing of services and their provision. A system has therefore been established that distinguishes between the service contractor – the Catalan Health Service – and the health care service providers. This was the organizational environment in which the health plan was developed. Otherwise the public provider had no competition to force it to accomplish the objectives.

The contracts define the general framework of the relationship and principles that characterize the service supply: equity, access to services, quality of activities, priorities, coordination between the various care levels and user satisfaction.

One of the most important issues is that the contract allowed preventive activities related to the priority health problems defined in the health plan to be included. Further, the contract has become a positive and dynamic factor in orienting the work of health professionals based on Catalonia's targets for health for all and the introduction of an evaluative culture at every level of the Catalan health organization.

Emphasizing prevention

In Catalonia, as in other countries in western Europe, the main health problems are chronic disease and accidents; immediate life-threatening environmental pollution (water, air and food) is now largely under control. Improving the population's life expectancy in good health therefore fundamentally requires measures in health promotion and disease prevention. These preventive activities can relate to people collectively, by such means as information and health education campaigns for the population, immunization campaigns and mass screening, or individually, including personal vaccinations, case finding and health advice in health care delivery.

In fact, the preventive activities that health professionals can apply in their day-to-day work have the greatest potential for improving the life expectancy in good health of the population of Catalonia. The approach to the strategy for health for all in Catalonia is mainly based on the health care sector, although some activities were considered from an intersectoral viewpoint.

Even if all experts are convinced that preventive activities need to be integrated into health care (health advice, preventive immunization and screening), the reality in medical care is that most physicians and medical care teams apply preventive medicine very little in their day-to-day work. Most of the effort and the time spent are dedicated to diagnosing and treating diseases and very little is dedicated to preventing them. This has several causes: the main ones are lack of time, lack of knowledge about the preventive measures to apply (because protocols are lacking and because different sources make different recommendations), scepticism about the effectiveness of some of the preventive measures and, finally, the fear that the risks exceed the benefits (including medicalization, false-positive and false-negative results in screening and labelling), as many minor complications and side effects with which ill people would cope reasonably well are generally poorly accepted by asymptomatic people.

To achieve objectives in improving health and reducing risk and by common agreement, health experts of the Department of Health and Social Security of Catalonia, representatives of the Catalan Society of

Family and Community Medicine, representatives of the General Medicine Society and the Catalan Society of Nursing and other health administration bodies and institutions have reached a consensus on a package of preventive interventions that can be applied gradually to asymptomatic adults targeted according to age and sex. Only interventions with proven effectiveness and efficacy (or for which these are likely to be proven, such as some types of advice) according to groups of experts from Canada and the United States over the last 15 years have been included. This consensus was published in the document *White paper: basis for the integration of prevention into health care practice (4)* (Fig. 2.5).

During 1994 and 1995, the white paper was broadly disseminated all around Catalonia through its publication in several documents and journals and a process of training the trainers among the primary health care professionals (physicians and nurses).

Fig. 2.5. Development of a health plan in Catalonia

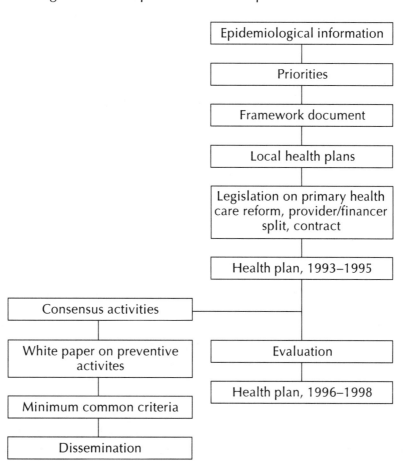

Nevertheless, the adoption of an individual-oriented strategy for preventive activities does not mean that the population strategies were abandoned, especially health promotion activities (including health information and education for the population through the media and restrictive and supportive legislative measures). This refers especially to nutrition, alcohol, smoking, physical activity and accidents.

Equity

The Catalan Health Service considers the user – as an individual – the main target of its actions. It also considers the staff working in the health system as the backbone of that system in implementing the changes the Health Service wants, and in formulating and applying the new health policy included in the health plan for Catalonia.

The Catalan Health Service has to provide health coverage for the whole population of Catalonia, enduring that all residents have access to quality health services. The principles inspiring the Health Service include the consideration of health as a public service, the integral conception of the system, and the efficacy and efficiency of the organization.

The Catalan Health Service came into being with the explicit mandate to take the health services closer to the people, both for primary health care and for hospital care. Further, the Catalan Health Service also provides preventive care, social health services and mental health care, which traditionally have not been part of the public health services provided in Catalonia.

One of the main principles that inspired health policy was equity: equal access and opportunities to obtain quality health services (preventive, curative and rehabilitative) free of charge and for the whole population. The health plan explicitly recognized the objective of equity. Nevertheless, housing and socioeconomic factors do not have specific targets in the health plan. These topics are taken into account by other departments in Catalonia such as that responsible for social welfare.

Equity in targets and in its development through corresponding activities was enhanced by the establishment of a local health plan for each of the eight health districts in Catalonia (Fig. 2.5) in accordance with the guidelines of the health plan for Catalonia. For example, some areas have a substantial immigrant population from developing countries, which can have special problems, whereas other places do not. Each local health plan takes these differences into consideration. The local health plans are drawn up based on the targets for health and risk reduction of the health plan for Catalonia, but special operational targets are adapted to the local needs. The resources to implement the health plans are allocated to each health district.

Healthy lifestyles are promoted through general activities using mass media resources targeting the general population, and specific preventive activities in primary health care targeting the attending population. Because it is known that media campaigns are more successful in reaching people of higher socioeconomic status, special activity programmes target groups of lower socioeconomic status. Such people of low socioeconomic status need special attention for diseases that have a high prevalence (AIDS, tuberculosis and sexually transmitted diseases). The groups are selected for special attention according to the frequency of the health problem.

In recent years, a special programme has been developed aiming at integrating health promotion and disease prevention in primary health care. Equal access to a healthy environment is promoted through legislative measures. A new Ministry for Environmental Affairs was created in Catalonia. Equal access to health care is guaranteed by an equal territorial distribution of primary health care centres and hospital resources. Each resident of Catalonia has a primary health care centre in his or her neighbourhood and a hospital no further than 30 minutes from home by car. An assessment of the progress in equity of services is a part of the assessment of the health plan. This is especially considered in the operational targets of the local health plans.

Participation

The elaboration of the health plan was a dynamic process, both because of the people involved in it and the dimensions of each of the phases: analysing the situation, formulating targets and interventions, and assessing the feasibility of the interventions.

Elaboration was based on two structures exclusively devoted to this activity: a territorial team consisting of a coordinator and an epidemiologist in each of the eight health districts, and a central technical team from the Catalan Health Service.

The territorial teams of the health districts collected and analysed information and identified the health and service problems using the comments of professional health staff. Based on the framework document for the formulation of the health plan for Catalonia *(1)* they drew up the operational targets and the interventions for the preliminary health plan projects for each health district or area. The district manager managed the whole development process, and much of the work was carried out in cooperation with professionals of the health care system.

Both the territorial team and the central team received technical and methodological support from the various units of the Department of Health and Social Security of Catalonia and the Catalan Health Service and from other multidisciplinary work teams including epidemiologists, planners, health managers, economists and health care professionals. This ensures that consistent criteria are used to elaborate the preliminary health plan projects for the health districts.

To ensure that the community is involved in elaborating the local health plans, health committees have been established for each district or local area with representatives of municipal and local councils, trade unions, businesses, professional organizations and user associations. These local health committees were informed about the preliminary plans and expressed their opinions and contributed to them. The

Executive Council of the Catalan Health Service approved the local health plans first, and the Autonomous Government of Catalonia gave the final approval.

One of the basic instruments necessary to analyse the situation in local areas was the definition of a set of basic indicators common to all health areas. During this phase, it became clear that the various sources of information available on health have to be classified and standardized. Some new sources also have to be created, including the Catalan Health Survey during the current health plan. This survey includes as major areas of interest socioeconomic and demographic characteristics, health status, utilization of health services, lifestyles and risk factors, and user satisfaction.

The problems identified in each health area were subjected to professional consultation with the following objectives: to determine the professional staff's opinions and perceptions of the problems identified; to include these opinions in preliminary health plan projects for each health district; and to provide an opportunity for professional staff in the health areas to take part in the elaboration process.

The operational targets were formulated bearing in mind their feasibility. Thus, the following aspects were considered: acceptability of the measures, intersectoral implications, organizational repercussions, expenditure repercussions, and existence of the necessary conditions for its application such as human, material and legal resources.

The health plan was disseminated all around Catalonia, including to all health professionals. It was also submitted to the Catalan Parliament for consideration and published through scientific journals and public mass media. The Department of Health and Social Security is thus committed to the residents of Catalonia through Parliament.

The public participated in developing policy through public organizations, including consumer associations and the association of users of the public health services.

International collaboration

Catalonia's involvement in the health-related projects and activities of WHO and the European Union has also been important. The WHO Regional Office for Europe was consulted in the process of elaborating both the framework document and the health plan for Catalonia. In fact, Catalonia adopted the European targets for health for all as its targets. The health plan draft was discussed by a WHO working group on the development of subnational policies for health.

International cooperation has been very important as a trigger for the development of new activities and as a source of learning from the experience of other countries.

The health plan very clearly states that international cooperation is necessary, not only in the planning stage but also in implementation.

On such challenges as controlling the use of illegal drugs, cooperation is absolutely essential. The solution to this problem depends largely on controlling the trafficking and consumption of such products on an international scale. For other health challenges, participation in projects and international networks allows information and experience to be exchanged, enriching and thus positively influencing new health policy implementation.

The Catalan Department of Health and Social Security has been involved in the WHO MONICA (monitoring trends and determinants in cardiovascular diseases) programme since 1983. This is an international applied research programme in which many European and non-European countries are cooperating. The objective of the research is to monitor the incidence of and mortality from cardiovascular diseases. In 1989 it joined the European Union EURODIAB project for the study of the incidence of insulin-dependent diabetes mellitus in children under the age of 15. In addition, it is a founding member of the WHO European Regions for Health Network, created in 1992 within the framework of the WHO Regional Office for Europe. Since 1993, it has been a member of WHO's countrywide integrated noncommunicable disease intervention (CINDI) programme, aimed at preventing chronic diseases. Some Catalan hospitals are involved in the European Health Promoting Hospitals project.

The involvement of Catalonia in all these WHO programmes has benefited the region in several ways. Catalonia has undertaken new projects based on its specific background. It has learned about other experiences and drawn lessons from this. Catalonia's participation in international projects has helped to consolidate local groups working in the same field. In addition, new initiatives have been launched with the support of the WHO Regional Office for Europe.

The Department of Health and Social Security is involved in projects coordinated by the European Union on health information (influenza monitoring) and smoking (a programme disseminating information on smoking and promoting quitting among health professionals).

The Catalan AIDS Programme is involved in several international activities. Among the research projects, the programme is collaborating with Columbia University and the University of California at Berkeley (USA) on research on the vertical transmission HIV. The programme is also the team leader of the European Union BIOMED Project on cancer and AIDS. During the last three years, the AIDS programme has been providing technical support to the WHO Regional Office for Europe to train epidemiologists in central and eastern Europe and the newly independent states of the former Soviet Union.

Through the Institute of Health Studies, the Department of Health and Social Security is collaborating with the European Union in such programmes as Europe against Cancer and the European Concerted Action EDUCTRA. The Institute is also a collaborating centre of the WHO Regional Office for Europe.

In 1993, the Department of Health and Social Security and the Pan-American Health Office signed a collaborative agreement to exchange information and experience in health promotion with Latin American countries.

Finally, the Department of Health and Social Security is actively involved in the Victoria Declaration Implementation Group. As a result, the 2nd International Heart Health Conference was organized in Barcelona in 1995. Its main product was The Catalonia Declaration on investing in heart health.

Intersectoral policy

The health plan recognizes that protection from environmental risks and the reduction of behavioural risk factors largely depend on the decisions and actions taken in sectors other than health (such as environment, agriculture, industry, government, employment, social security, transport, economy and taxation). Accidents, occupational health problems and environmental problems are examples of health problems that require intersectoral cooperation, as the health sector cannot solve them alone. Smoking, alcohol and drugs are other risk factors requiring intersectoral cooperation.

The Autonomous Government of Catalonia has authority over many of the intersectoral cooperation actions that could contribute to health protection and promotion of the population of Catalonia. This is the case, for example, for environmental control activities, health education at school and legislative actions aimed at restricting cigarette and alcohol advertising and reducing the consumption of tobacco and alcohol in public places.

For some actions, the Autonomous Government of Catalonia shares authority and responsibility with the Government of Spain (such as food production policy, safety of industrial products, health and safety at work, road safety and government actions against illegal drug trafficking).

The Government of Spain has sole authority and responsibility for such actions as tax policy on tobacco and alcohol, legislation concerning the trafficking and consumption of illegal drugs and social security policy.

The district (district councils) and local (municipal councils) bodies also have an important role in intersectoral cooperation: protection from environmental risks, health information and education for the population, and promotion of facilities for physical exercise, such as sports facilities and walking and cycling paths. These bodies are very close to the citizens and are fully aware of their problems and can help to find solutions. In fact, community involvement is fundamentally channelled through these formally established institutions.

Industry, commerce, the mass media and private volunteer workers also have an important role in protecting and promoting the health of the population. Much of industry is producing products that are increasingly healthy and safe. They do not simply comply with the legal minimum; they go much further by adapting their production to the health needs of the consumer. The food-processing industry is a clear example of this, producing food with less saturated fat and more vitamins, minerals and fibre. It seems that industry considers it benefits by manufacturing products in accordance with official and/or international recommendations. Official organizations should therefore state the minimum criteria for the production of any kind of products related to health.

Private volunteer workers also have a role to play in dealing with many health problems, especially alcohol abuse, smoking, drug use and AIDS.

In order to coordinate action and join forces, an Intersectoral Involvement Advisory Committee was created with representatives of all the departments and organizations of the Autonomous Government of Catalonia that can contribute to and collaborate in improving the health of the population. The Committee is not currently active, however, as intersectoral cooperation could be accomplished without it.

Several mechanisms at the central level in Catalonia ensure intersectoral action: interprofessional committees, advisory boards, monitoring commissions and task forces. All these mechanisms are in agreement with the health plan targets. Working groups, commissions and task forces can be created to solve specific problems for several targets established in the health plan for Catalonia. These groups mainly comprise health professionals, including physicians, nurses and pharmacists, but patients and teachers also participate. The group composition depends on the specific problem.

Permanent intersectoral collaboration has been established in programmes such as health education in schools, occupational health and road safety.

Health status orientation

The implementation of the new health policy is expected to produce a detectable improvement in services and health indicators. Evaluation is a fundamental stage of the planning and implementation process of the new health policy for Catalonia and is essential to determining progress on targets. The system that has been designed evaluates the results, the service structure and the process of developing the activities of the suppliers.

Evaluation is especially necessary for planning and decision-making when new social, demographic and health phenomena are shaping complex scenarios in constant change. The health system as a whole must respond flexibly and appropriately to these phenomena in social, health and financial terms.

Evaluation must be used to determine whether the health care system can adapt to these changes and incorporate the results into the planning, management and redistribution of resources in a setting of limited resources. Evaluation therefore needs to be incorporated into all levels of the health care system.

Since the framework document was published in 1991, and especially since the 1993–1995 health plan was approved and published, the Catalan health system and the related non-health sectors have oriented their actions in accordance with the strategies contained in both documents. Thus, Catalonia is in the full policy implementation stage. The monitoring and evaluation stage is also fully under way.

The structure (existence of suitable resources among the suppliers) and the process (their proper use in the form of activities appropriate in number and quality in accordance with the operational targets set in the health plan) are evaluated through the process of contracting out services to providers.

The health plan for Catalonia set process targets related to activities that should be carried out to achieve the risk reduction and health targets. These activities included the production of specific health education material (leaflets, protocols and guidelines) at the central level in Catalonia and specific health care activities (curative as well as preventive) at the most peripheral level.

The results (achieving the health and risk reduction targets) are evaluated, however, by analysing epidemiological data obtained from permanent and one-off information sources.

The service suppliers must provide the Catalan Health Service with information about the human and material resources of the centres and the services forming part of the contract, in order to evaluate their sufficiency and quality. The suppliers, both public and private, usually carry out simple, administrative self-evaluation at least once each year.

Evaluating the process is, however, more complex. The contracts force the suppliers to provide information to the Catalan Health Service (or allow it to get the information directly) about the quality and quantity of activities carried out in the services to which the contract refers, in order to evaluate their suitability and coverage in relation to the targets set in the health plan. Quantitative evaluation is complex but feasible if the methods and the information the suppliers have to provide to the Catalan Health Service are well defined. The qualitative assessment of the health services provided has two main components. The first is the ordinary information the health care system usually provides (such as waiting lists). The second is the evaluation of the health plan targets, which requires a more complex approach such as the involvement of the professionals themselves, including peer review, clinical record auditing, and even surveys about the activities carried out by the professionals or user surveys about the preventive or curative interventions carried out by the professionals.

Evaluation of the results of the interventions – the attainment of the health and risk reduction targets set in the health plan – is eminently epidemiological. It is based on monitoring indicators of effectiveness calculated from data obtained from permanent sources (such as mortality statistics, hospital morbidity statistics, morbidity registers, the compulsory reporting of some diseases and compulsory microbiological reporting) or non-permanent sources (such as general health surveys, specific surveys on the prevalence of smoking, alcohol, drugs, food habits and physical activity, and sero-epidemiological surveys about diseases for which there are immunization programmes).

An important effort was made to set up quantitative targets for the year 2000. Although some targets in the health plan merely indicate the direction of desired change, most quantify the change desired. General health targets are usually related to mortality or morbidity and are quantitative. Mortality by causes is monitored year by year, whereas morbidity is planned to be monitored by periodic health surveys and health examination studies every four years.

The policy implementation process is monitored by peer review carried out through discussion groups composed of professionals working at different levels in the health system. These groups assess, for example, whether activities have been carried out and/or whether the expected resources have been invested in the predetermined points. One important aspect is to analyse legislative developments as well as implementation.

In Catalonia as a whole, the feedback from evaluative mechanisms is received by the managers and technicians at central and local level. These professionals also assess the evaluation of each health area. Furthermore, technicians working in the health areas are responsible for disseminating the evaluation results among the professionals of their own health area.

Differences in process and outcome indicators, both among and between areas, are critical to order to adopt new strategies and readdress the old ones. Catalonia is currently in the process of formulating the health plan for the next three years. The analysis of the most recent indicators is the base used to set up the new operational targets. The general health and risk reduction targets are based on the year 2000 (Tables 2.3 and 2.4).

Conclusion

The development and implementation of the new health policy would have been impossible without a democratic political environment and a supportive legislative framework.

Drawing up the health plan for Catalonia was a critical point. It is the basic instrument for planning and the backbone of all the policy developments in health care and health services. A high degree of participation was attained, although wider involvement is still necessary.

Considerable effort was expended in compiling epidemiological information to determine the main health problems and the interventions to be given priority. In some cases there were not enough epidemiological data, and then it was crucial to know about the experience of other countries and to bear in mind the 38 European targets for health for all.

Table 2.3. Some operational targets related to hypertension

Indicator	Target quantification for 1995	Evaluation of health plan for Catalonia, 1993–1995	Evaluation procedure
Percentage of doctors having a mercury sphygmomanometer	Desirable 100%	94%	Inspection services contract evaluation
Percentage of primary health care settings with hypertension management protocol	Desirable 100%	98%	Services contract evaluation
Percentage of clinical records with blood pressure data (>15 years)	60%[a]	58%	Audit

[a] For the health plan for 1996–1998, the proposed target is 70%.

Promoting the participation and involvement of professionals working in the health care system and other sectors was difficult. Substantial time and effort was required to reach an agreement among all people participating in the elaboration of the health plan, mainly because this was a new, time-consuming way of working based on targets and consensus. Adopting and adapting all contributions from local plans and fitting them into the health plan was often difficult, especially since Catalonia's eight health districts have vast socioeconomic and geographical differences.

Achieving equity in health is a long-term process that requires a permanent system for readdressing the interventions and policies. This is also the case for achieving true community involvement in policy-making. In both cases, much progress is needed. The empowerment of the community in achieving better knowledge of its rights and duties, identifying health-related needs and demanding them requires further development that is highly related to the difficulty of achieving intersectoral collaboration.

A very crucial point in the dissemination of the health plan was the accountability of the Ministry of Health to the Catalan Parliament and thus to the population for the health plan of Catalonia. In this sense, the Minister officially approved the targets and accepted the commitment to achieve them.

Although lifestyles and the environment are very important determinants of health, and health promotion and disease prevention policies are recognized theoretically as being relevant, great effort is still needed to disseminate this idea among health care and health-related professionals and also the health administration, so that they reallocate and invest more resources in implementing these practices and policies while focusing on improving the efficacy and efficiency of the health care system and the satisfaction of users.

Table 2.4. Risk reduction and general health targets related to hypertension

Indicator	Objective	Baseline (1990)	Results of health plan evaluation for 1993–1995	Targets for 2000 quantification	Evaluation procedure
Percentage of the population with hypertension:	To increase				Epidemiological studies
who are aware that they have hypertension		60%	75%	75%	
who are being treated for hypertension		40%	47%	60%	
who are controlling their hypertension		20%	30%	35%	
Cardiovascular mortality in those < 65 years	To reduce	47 per 100 000 population	40 per 100 000 population	40 per 100 000 population	Mortality trends
Stroke mortality	To reduce	121 per 100 000 population	90 per 100 000 population	97 per 100 000 population	Mortality trends

Note: These targets are not modified in the health plan for 1996–1998.

Achieving all these changes requires not only adopting central measures such as legislative support, but also disseminating these policies among all partners and their active involvement in the process. In our current environment, we think that this is still an important challenge.

A permanent, well structured evaluation system is difficult to achieve. It should be simple and cost-effective, and its usefulness in policy-making should be constantly demonstrated and highlighted. Both health managers and practitioners should be persuaded that evaluation is necessary and useful. This trend is just beginning, but most sectors consider the initial results of the evaluation to be useful. These results have been used to modify the targets, when necessary, of the health plan for the period 1996–1998.

References

1. *Framework document for the elaboration of the health plan for Catalonia.* Barcelona, Department of Health and Social Security, 1991.
2. *Health plan for Catalonia 1993–1995.* Barcelona, Department of Health and Social Security, 1992.
3. *Health plan for Catalonia 1996–1998.* Barcelona, Department of Health and Social Security, 1997.
4. *White paper: basis for the integration of prevention into health care practice.* Barcelona, Department of Health and Social Security, 1993.

Health policy development in Sweden: action at three levels

Bosse Pettersson

Introduction

In Sweden, three autonomous political and administrative levels – national, regional and local – have different roles to play in all aspects of public policy, including health.

Consequently, the case studies from Sweden (see also pages 161 and 185) are based on a national overview complemented by a case study on Östergötland County and another on the city of Gothenburg. These case studies indicate how policies based on the health for all approach have been developed at the regional and local levels in Sweden. This first section describes in detail the overall move in Sweden towards a more equity-based health policy and how international health policy development has interacted with the trends in Sweden.

The national level

At the national level, the Ministry of Health and Social Affairs has the main responsibility for formulating policy, initiating the parliamentary process and undertaking discussions with standing committees. The main policy instruments applied at the ministerial level are legislation, financing and strategic planning, which includes setting priorities for national agencies funded by the state. The role of the state in public health is:

- to formulate national policy, establish legislative requirements (such as the delegation of responsibility to the county councils for disease prevention and equal access to care) and issue overall policy guidelines such as those on promoting equity in health;
- to take responsibility for research by, for example, funding research institutions at universities or other research bodies;
- to facilitate and coordinate intersectoral action at the national level;
- to promote the development of public health initiatives at all levels of society; and
- to be responsible for specific challenges that, at certain stages, are best taken care of by national agencies, such as HIV and AIDS and parts of the prevention programmes related to drugs and alcohol.

National agencies such as the National Institute of Public Health and the National Board of Health and Welfare are responsible for administering various health matters at the national level. Largely self-governing, tax-funded bodies, their main task is to monitor common standards for all citizens and in all parts of Sweden, for example in relation to equal access to health care and delivery of health services. On policy issues and related priorities, however, the national agencies are largely bound by ministerial priorities.

Semi-public organizations at the national level, such as the Federation of County Councils and the Swedish Association of Local Authorities, represent Sweden's 26 county councils and 288 municipalities. These organizations play an important role in formulating health policy, as do the professional organizations of nurses and physicians, which have formulated explicit policies based on the European targets for health for all [1,2]. Other organizations that influence policy are the associations for social medicine, occupational health, public health and community medicine, epidemiology, and health systems research.

The regional level

The county councils are ultimately responsible for delivering health care, except for home care for elderly people. Health care comprises about 80% of overall expenditure. Public health or community medicine units have been set up in nearly all county councils [3]. Many activities initiated by public health units take an intersectoral approach. Most county councils have developed comprehensive public health plans and/or programmes and public health reports based on data from national and regional registers, surveys and other data. The reports generally present results for the county in a comparative perspective with other Swedish counties and at the municipal level to compare the municipalities in the same county. Equity is strongly emphasized both in the programmes and plans and in the reports as the overall strategy for health for all. This can be explained mainly by the following factors.

- The European targets for health for all were strongly promoted at an early stage by: translating the targets into Swedish; establishing consultation processes and conferences; and disseminating related documents in the mid-1980s coinciding with the work of the Commission for Health Services for the 1990s [4] and the production of the first national public health report in 1987 and every third year since [5–8].
- The state provided 48 kronor per person per year to the county councils to reinforce disease prevention and health promotion from 1984 to the early 1990s [9,10].
- Given that Sweden has no national health targets, the European targets for health for all [11,12] offered an opportunity for health promoters and educators to advocate for specific issues and to produce a structured programme or plan. The credibility of WHO, both by being the leading international health agency and by virtue of the targets themselves, was especially important at the time.

Despite the existence of health policy programmes and plans that focus on equity and other principles of health for all, the link to focused action and implementation is weak.

Sweden and many other countries have not generally emphasized the preventive dimension of hospital care. An organized exception since the mid-1990s is the WHO Health Promoting Hospitals network.

Linköping University Hospital represents Sweden in the network. A national network began to be established in 1997 and will include ten hospitals in the first phase.

The Swedish case study on Östergötland County Council (see page 161) presents in more detail how a county council can operate in public health.

The local level

The county councils also operate locally. Local action is largely centred around primary health care. There is an idea that the primary health care centres should be the vehicle for health promotion on the local level. Nevertheless, curative responsibilities seem to dominate to such an extent that little or no time is left for primary prevention, with the exception of maternal and child care, health in schools and dental care for young people. Surveys among physicians in Sweden have revealed that they are generally sceptical towards disease prevention (except in relation to tobacco and alcohol consumption), the contribution they can make and their skills in health promotion. Physicians also feel that, in view of other more pressing health matters, disease prevention cannot be given priority. In Sweden, the occupational health services are organized separately and are linked to the labour market.

More apparent and proactive developments in local health promotion have taken place at the municipal level during the 1990s. In particular, most county councils have local health planners, and they have had an important role. Intersectoral local public health committees have also been established in 60% of the municipalities *(13)*. A national network modelled on the WHO Healthy Cities project involves about 80 cities. In addition, three separate networks have been established: one involving Sweden's three largest cities, Stockholm, Gothenburg and Malmö; one involving seven cities with more than 100 000 inhabitants; and one involving cities with between 50 000 and 100 000 inhabitants. Since the municipalities are ultimately responsible for the welfare of individuals, the focus of public health is gradually shifting from a medical to a social approach and to major structural determinants of health such as economics, unemployment, education, demography (including home care for elderly people), the environment and sustainable development. The process of developing local Agenda 21 plans has linked public health and environmental issues and also some aspects of equity and social welfare *(14)*.

Fig. 2.6 shows how public health is organized at the national, regional and local levels in Sweden and the division of roles in public health.

Moving towards an equity-based policy

Health – a universal value
The United Nations Universal Declaration of Human Rights lays down that "enjoyment of the highest possible standard of health is a fundamental right of everyone without distinction according to race,

Fig. 2.6. Organization of public health in Sweden

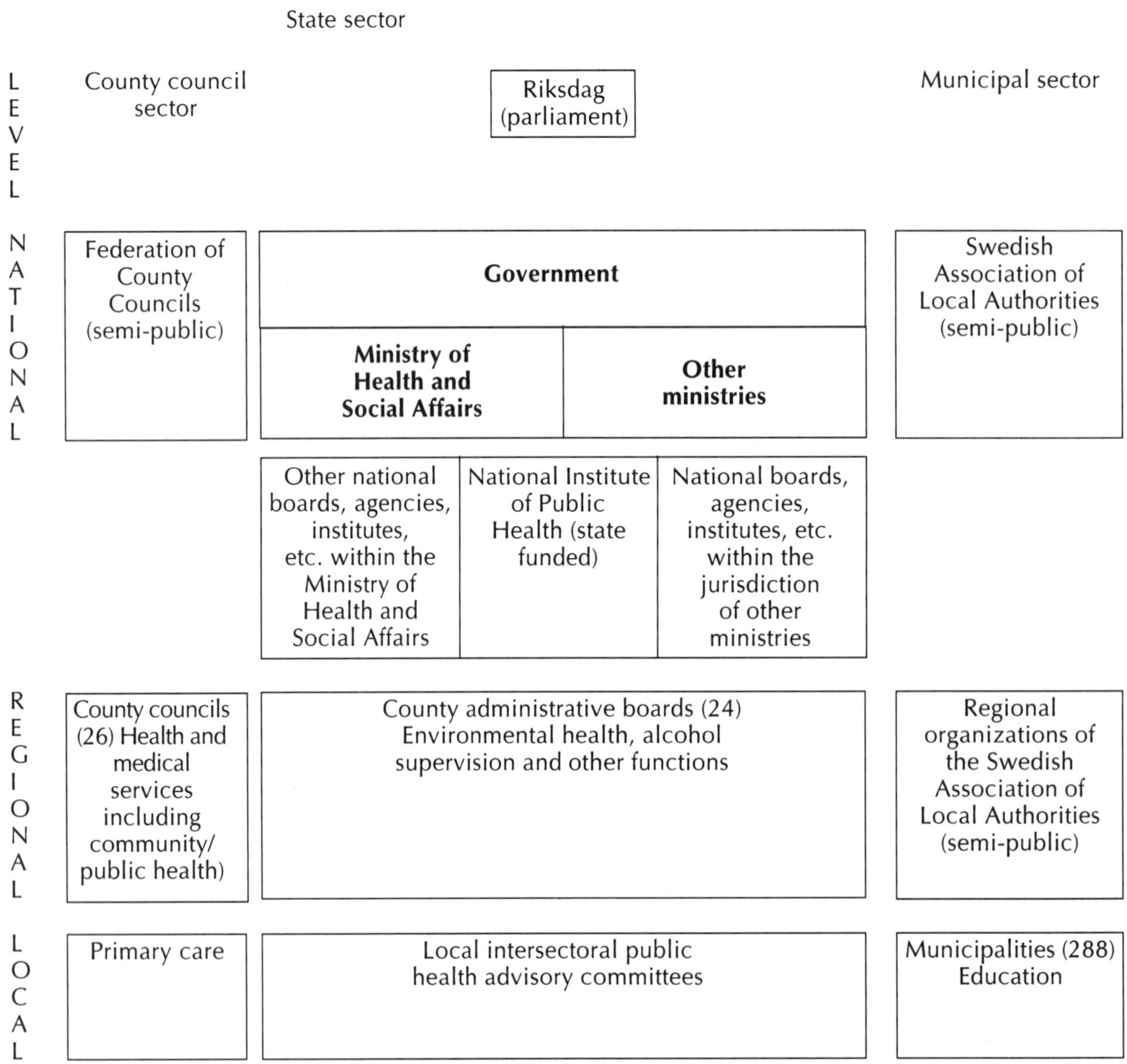

State sector

	County council sector	Riksdag (parliament)			Municipal sector
LEVEL					
NATIONAL	Federation of County Councils (semi-public)	**Government**			Swedish Association of Local Authorities (semi-public)
		Ministry of Health and Social Affairs		**Other ministries**	
		Other national boards, agencies, institutes, etc. within the Ministry of Health and Social Affairs	National Institute of Public Health (state funded)	National boards, agencies, institutes, etc. within the jurisdiction of other ministries	
REGIONAL	County councils (26) Health and medical services including community/ public health)	County administrative boards (24) Environmental health, alcohol supervision and other functions			Regional organizations of the Swedish Association of Local Authorities (semi-public)
LOCAL	Primary care	Local intersectoral public health advisory committees			Municipalities (288) Education

religion, political convictions or economic and social circumstances". This is interesting because it refers to health as a human right and because health is linked with universal equality of dignity and opportunity.

Having a right presupposes that that right can be exercised under given conditions. It is open to question, on rational grounds, who is capable of guaranteeing anyone's health. Guaranteeing a person's health is simply not possible in the widest sense, if only because not enough is known about all the interrelationships of health. The words of the Universal Declaration about everyone being entitled to the highest possible standard of health must therefore be interpreted in a relative sense. That is, society must guarantee the best possible preconditions for the individual to develop good health and must safeguard human health against violations.

Universally equal dignity in opportunities for health reaffirms an accepted ethical principle that is firmly rooted in Sweden's health policy. Few people argue that health differences caused by income, gender, ethnicity or place of residence are fair.

This makes it natural to discuss more equitable health developments in a perspective of justice. Viewed against the background of the Universal Declaration of Human Rights, conditions exemplified by the socioepidemiological data available today provoke the challenging thought that the health of certain groups is, in fact, subjected to greater violation than that of others, which amounts to discrimination. To conclude, much of the debate and focus on equity in health is linked to what is considered as fair in accordance with the ideas of a general welfare system.

Health for all – changing the focus of health policy

The concept of health for all was launched at the World Health Assembly in 1977. At the same time, the WHO definition of health was made more operative with the adoption of a resolution to the effect that "the main social target of governments and WHO in the coming decades should be the attainment by all citizens of the world by the year 2000 of a level of health that will permit them to lead a socially and economically productive life" (resolution WHA 30.43). The health for all ideas were consolidated and further developed through the International Conference on Primary Health Care in Alma-Ata in 1978 *(15)* based on the conviction that, if everyone could be reached by and included in primary health care, this would also effectively influence health developments.

In most of western Europe, including Sweden, however, primary health care has never acquired the meaning intended at Alma-Ata. The difference is clearly revealed by a comparison of the two phenomena of primary health care and primary medical care. In Sweden, the first moves towards primary health care came in the mid-1940s, with the then Director-General of the National Board of Health, Axel Höjer, and an official report on outpatient medical care in Sweden *(16)*. As a result of strong criticism, mainly from the Swedish Medical Association, which was afraid of state control, these ideas were put aside to make room for a strongly hospital-based approach, with the result that health care was given lower priority than medical care. A recent study *(17)*, based on a survey among a sample of more than 2000 members of the

Swedish Medical Association, concluded that lack of time and information and doubts about the impact of individual and group prevention (except on smoking) explain why physicians do not commit themselves to prevention.

The ideas of public health in a modern sense were first brought back into Sweden's health policies in the 1980s. The Lalonde report in Canada *(18)* and the U.S. Surgeon General's *Healthy people* (*19*) were discovered through international exchange and significantly affected professionals working at the national level and some researchers. The concept of prevention was found attractive as such, but it also offered a complementary strategy to reduce the increasing share of gross national product allocated to medical services.

A new perspective on the health of Canadians (18), which was published in 1974 by the Canadian Minister of Health, was probably the first national policy document of its type after the Second World War. The report eventually acquired growing international importance, mainly because it launched the concept of health as being determined by human biology; the organization of health and medical services, including their standard and efficiency; the ambient environment; and lifestyles. These ideas were then further developed in the United States, through *Healthy people (19)*, which drew attention to the question of social conditions and health and the concept of management by objectives. Both these reports, however, strongly advocated diverting efforts to improve public health from medical care to measures to promote health and prevent disease.

The Lalonde report was an important source of inspiration both for the Swedish Commission on Health and Medical Services, set up to review the Health and Medical Services Act, and the HS 90 Commission, which was to lay the foundations for the development of health and medical services in Sweden in the 1990s. A statutory reform gave special responsibility for the health of the population to county councils, and preventive work was enshrined in the Health and Medical Services Act *(20)*, which came into force in 1983. The report of the HS 90 Commission *(4)* addressed socially conditioned health differences. Although medical care in Sweden was generally equally available to all, lack of good care could not account for the health differences that were emerging. The Commission, therefore – albeit for somewhat different reasons – came to endorse the conclusions reached both in Canada and the United States, that public health can mainly be improved by promoting health and preventing disease. The HS 90 report became a cornerstone of what later evolved into a strategy for equity in health in Sweden.

Inequities in health

As a consequence of World Health Assembly resolution WHA 30.43 on health for all, the WHO Regional Office for Europe began to work on a health strategy. This was inspired by Lalonde's health field concept and the *Healthy people* strategy of management by objectives, combined with the primary health care strategy formulated in the Declaration of Alma-Ata.

An overall first European target on equity in health was evolved: differences in health status between Member States and between groups within countries were to be reduced by 25% by the year 2000 by improving the health status of disadvantaged countries and groups. The logic of formulating an overarching target that is very difficult to quantify can be debated, but the target was formulated. This target acquired symbolic importance and is the most distinctly political of the 38 targets.

Sweden endorsed the targets for health for all but, except for the sub-target on alcohol policy of reducing consumption by 25%, the targets never became a direct subject of parliamentary policy-making *(21)*. In fact, the health for all objectives received comparatively little attention in Sweden at the national level. Their impact was much greater at county level, through various regional health programmes and plans such as the policy for Östergötland County. The Federation of County Councils also played a dynamic part at various stages through programming work and other initiatives.

The HS 90 Commission highlighted differences in health status between different groups in Sweden and concluded that further studies were needed, based on better data. These materialized when the Government commissioned the National Board of Health and Welfare to compile a national report on public health *(5)*. That report, presented to Parliament in 1988, confirmed and underscored the HS 90 Commission's conclusions that health differences in Sweden were increasing. It was already observed at the beginning of the 1980s *(7)* that Sweden had substantial data for in-depth analysis of health differences *(22)*, and some of these data were presented in a series of reports *(23,24)* on patterns of illness and causes of death.

Prior to the national reports on public health, a study had been made of health differences between different population groups in Great Britain. The findings on how low income correlated with poor health were first presented in 1980 in *Inequalities in health* (the Black report) *(25)*. The findings presented, however, were not acknowledged by the Government of the time and the report was published very discreetly.

In Sweden, inequality in health status has been regarded as a challenge for health policy. Both Social Democratic and non-socialist governments have highlighted the importance of reducing health differences. The parliamentary debate on the national public health report in spring 1988 resulted in the Government appointing a Public Health Group with the dual mandate of being an expert body but also acting through various initiatives. Half the members of the Public Health Group were directors-general of relevant national agencies and half were professors in various public health disciplines. All were men.

Health promotion and disease prevention
The Public Health Group came to represent a breakthrough in Sweden for health promotion and disease prevention at the national level. Its strategy project responded to the signals emitted by the first national public health report in 1987.

Frames of reference for health promotion evolved internationally, especially in industrialized countries. The ideas came principally from Canada *(26)*, and eventually resulted in the Ottawa Charter for Health Promotion *(27)*, which describes and elaborates a frame of reference for health promotion. This involves a further shift in the definition of health, which can then be regarded not as an end in itself but as a resource in everyday life. Interest focuses on the factors that determine health and on how to make them more equally available. The Ottawa Charter was translated into Swedish and was broadly introduced from 1987 onwards.

The model from the Ottawa Charter was developed further through the Adelaide Recommendations *(28)* on health-oriented social policy. In this way, the approach was broadened from health policy to social policy in general and its importance for health development. For example, in this context tobacco is regarded not merely as a problem related to smokers but as a matter of tobacco growing in developing countries and as a question of how the alternative use of such land could help to improve the food supply. The concept of a healthy public policy cannot easily be translated into Swedish. Even if it can be understood literally, it still has to be explained as a dimension of policies in such sectors as the labour market, education and agriculture.

The third step in the development of international health promotion was the Third International Conference on Health Promotion, in Sundsvall, Sweden in 1991 *(29–36)*. This was guided by the move from theory to practice and the further development of the concept of supportive environments, with a shift of emphasis from lifestyle to creating, through various measures in the social, political, economic and physical environments, the greatest possible equality in the preconditions of human health.

Over the years, public health planners and practitioners in Sweden have become very interested in the concept of a supportive environment. This alternative to victim blaming is much appreciated and also opens for intersectoral collaboration in which the social dimension of human environments can be made very visible. Nevertheless, it took 3–5 years before health promotion, healthy public policy and supportive environments were accepted, used and understood in Sweden.

The political process of building the new public health
In Sweden, the Government's Public Health Group was instructed to compile supportive documentation for a national strategy for public health. The main argument was the growing health differences in the population revealed by the 1987 national public health report. Inequality between socioeconomic and ethnic groups has been confirmed in later public health reports *(6–8)*. At the same time, the other Nordic countries can be said to have made much more headway than Sweden in this respect *(37)*. The Public Health Group's strategy project was operated intersectorally, in close contact with a large number of national authorities, the Federation of County Councils and the Swedish Association of Local Authorities.

In spring 1991, during the final phase of the Public Health Group's strategy work, the National Board of Health and Welfare presented the second national public health report *(6)*, further underlining the growth of health gaps in the population. The Government therefore introduced a special public health bill *(38)*. Drafting work on this bill and the national strategy for health *(39)* proceeded in parallel during the final phase. The Public Health Group's proposals, except as regards a national master's programme in public health and setting up a public health fund, directly influenced the public health bill.

The main organized proposal was the revival of a national public health institute. Unlike other institutes of its kind, the new National Institute of Public Health was to use an operational approach and act in support of local and regional public health work instead of focusing on basically epidemiological research.

Reducing health inequalities – the overall aim

The overall aim of the national public health strategy was formulated as that of reducing socially induced differences in health. The standing instructions for the National Institute of Public Health reflect this by saying that the Institute's task is:

> ... to prevent diseases and other forms of ill health and to promote good health for all. The Institute's activities are aimed at creating universally equivalent preconditions for good health. Special importance should be attached to the conditions promoting health among the groups exposed to the greatest health hazards.

The political proposal to establish a National Institute of Public Health had been raised by the Liberal Party during the 1980s with no success. The Social Democrats proposed establishing such an institute in 1991. After the change in government in autumn 1991, however, the four-party bourgeois coalition carried the proposal through Parliament and also formulated the standing instructions for the Institute.

The principle of everyone having equitable prospects of achieving good health is also strongly rooted among professionals in the public health sector. In Sweden's first public health declaration adopted in connection with a national public health conference in Sundsvall in 1991, parallel to the third International Conference on Health Promotion, the delegates affirmed that (29):

> The aim of public health work is to participate in a sustainable social development, where the living environment offers all human beings the possibility of achieving good health.

The government green paper on investing in health and giving priority to health (40) reaffirmed the national health strategy but also made clear that greater attention was to be to focused on women's health, allergies and the role of the municipalities in public health promotion.

A population strategy

Strategies for health equality rest largely on the theory that the greatest effect on public health can be achieved if policy measures include the entire population. This theory is sometimes known as the epidemiological paradox (41). The most important recommendation is that of working with a population focus as opposed to targeting more-or-less clearly delimited and defined high-risk groups. This is sometimes expressed by saying that it is more effective to support many people in changing their living habits moderately than to support a few people in changing them completely. This includes different means, from structural policies to health education, aimed at influencing individual behaviour. The difficulty in reducing health differences, even with a population-based approach, lies in delivering the input so that it will produce effects among the groups whose needs are greatest.

Another fundamental concept of egalitarian public health work is that everyone must derive health benefits from the measures taken but that the biggest advantages must be gained by the people whose health is poorest. In this way widespread acceptance is created for egalitarian public health work, because everyone derives personal gain from it: no-one's health suffers as a result of somebody else's health improving.

The intersectoral approach continues to have support in Sweden. This is shown, for example, by cooperation, partnership and stimulus being principles of the activities of the National Institute of Public Health and, accordingly, this approach is one of the main instruments of public health promotion. Since it is firmly believed that health differences in Sweden cannot be ascribed to unequal availability of health and medical care, measures to promote health and prevent disease become the choice for a strategy of reducing health differences.

Developing an equity-based policy in practice

The concept of equality in health appears to be firmly rooted among policy-makers, and many people are practically involved in public health work. Several county council documents also contain generally worded goal definitions concerning greater equality in health. Nevertheless, specific, politically based action programmes and strategies for achieving these goals are lacking *(42)*. One difficulty here, presumably, is that many structural preconditions for health are determined at the national level. This, however, can hardly be the whole reason, because environmental measures, educational planning, housing and urban planning have been extensively decentralized to the municipalities.

A study *(13)* among the 288 municipalities in Sweden with a response rate of 86% shows that commitment to public health is growing. Among the responding municipalities, more than 60% had established intersectoral advisory public health committees and a health planner was employed in two thirds of the municipalities. Nevertheless, only 20% had a health planner, a health committee and a comprehensive health plan. At the national level, an intersectoral mechanism has been created by a group of 20 directors-general and executive directors representing national agencies, county councils and municipalities. About 150 municipalities and counties are engaged in various networks similar to the WHO Healthy Cities model in implementing public health action at the local level.

Measures for reducing health differences can proceed in two main ways. They can focus on working directly with and/or for the groups that are more exposed to health hazards than others or have less chance of developing good health. The other option is influencing various structural conditions such that people with the biggest health needs will reap the main benefit. Practice appears to show that there are strikingly few instances of either kind of measure. The Public Health Project of the Swedish Confederation of Trade Unions targeted blue-collar workers from 1987 until 1992 and still remains a unique venture of an integrated kind *(43)*. Youth projects in deprived areas, work with self-help groups and health information specifically targeting young people through the magazine *Glöd* are other examples.

Methods of working with and for different groups need to be developed, and development projects can make important contributions. A health-oriented social policy requires further analysis, of which changes in structural conditions can offer the greatest health benefits.

The position of public health work in Sweden has become both clearer and stronger as a result of Sweden joining the European Union in 1995 and Article 129 of the Maastricht Treaty. Nevertheless, the Treaty does not advocate working to reduce health differences in the European Union. Section 1 of Article 129 lays down that "The Community shall contribute towards ensuring a high level of human health protection ...".

The Ministry of Health and Social Affairs took the opportunity to lay down a strategy for Sweden's action on public health within the European Union (44). Sweden's priorities include combating unemployment and developing strategies to reduce health inequalities within the European Union, so that countries and population groups can achieve the best level of public health represented among the 15 Member States. Three issue-based priorities are also mentioned:

- decreasing tobacco consumption, through such measures as banning advertising and levelling out subsidies for tobacco farming;
- reducing harm from alcohol consumption, initially by creating alcohol-free environments and situations (such as the workplace, driving, pregnancy, childhood and adolescence); and
- reducing drug addiction, based on a restrictive drug policy.

In 1995, the Government decided to set up a parliamentary committee to develop proposals for national health targets. Such targets should guide efforts by society as a whole to promote people's health, prevent ill health and diseases, diminish health hazards and prevent early and avoidable dysfunction, morbidity and mortality. An overall aim is to decrease inequality in health. The National Public Health Committee is expected to propose strategies for how the national health targets can be achieved and procedures for monitoring and evaluation, but also proposals on how to integrate the targets in various decision-making processes. The Committee will also focus on balancing the investment required in relation to the benefits of implementing the targets. The Committee started its undertakings in early 1997 and will publish its results by 2000. The approach of the Committee is two-fold: to stimulate debate by publishing thought-provoking reports on such themes as the importance or not of genetic inheritance and/or environmental factors and the relevance of Sweden's alcohol policy; and to work closely with partners from relevant sectors with the aim of achieving an integrated process of consolidating comments and proposals on draft reports.

In conclusion, Sweden has programmes and plans expressing political will, functions and mechanisms as well as strong national political initiatives that promote public health. Much progress has been made, as reported in Sweden's contribution to the third evaluation of the progress towards health for all in the European Region (45). Nevertheless, the equity target will not be achieved by the year 2000, although the Government is strongly emphasizing this target.

References

1. *Hälsa för alla vårt mål – om sjuksköterskors, barnmorskors och laboratorieassistenters roll i folkhälsoarbetet* [Health for all is our objective – on the role of nurses, midwives and laboratory technicians in public health work]. Stockholm, Swedish Association of Health Professionals, 1995.
2. *Läkare i folkhälsoarbetet – Ett preventionspolitiskt program från Sveriges läkarförbund* [Physicians in public health work – a programme on disease prevention policy from the Swedish Medical Association]. Stockholm, Swedish Medical Association, 1996.
3. *Samhällsmedicin och folkhälsoarbete i landstingen 1995* [Public health work in the county councils in 1995]. Stockholm, National Board of Health and Welfare, 1996 (SoS-rapport 1996:6).
4. *Hälso- och sjukvård inför 90-talet (HS 90). Huvudrapport* [The Swedish health services in the 1990s. Main report]. Stockholm, National Board of Health and Welfare, 1984 (SOU 1984:39) (summary in English: *The Swedish health services in the 1990's.* Stockholm, National Board of Health and Welfare, 1985).
5. *Folkhälsorapport 1987* [The 1987 public health report]. Stockholm, National Board of Health and Welfare, 1987 (Socialstyrelsen redovisar 1987:15).
6. *Folkhälsorapport 1991* [The 1991 public health report]. Stockholm, National Board of Health and Welfare, 1987 (SoS-rapport 1991:11).
7. *Folkhälsorapport 1994* [The 1994 public health report]. Stockholm, National Board of Health and Welfare, 1987 (SoS-rapport 1994:9).
8. *Folkhälsorapport 1997* [The 1997 public health report]. Stockholm, National Board of Health and Welfare, 1987 (SoS-rapport 1997:18).
9. *Om vissa ersättningar till sjukvårdshuvudmännen, mm* [On certain funds granted to the main providers of health care, etc.] Stockholm, Government Printer, 1984 (Regeringens proposition 1983/84:190).
10. *Att förebygga ohälsa* [Preventing ill health]. Stockholm, National Board of Health and Welfare, 1986 (Socialstyrelsen redovisar 1986:7).
11. *Health for all targets. The health policy for Europe.* Copenhagen, WHO Regional Office for Europe, 1993 (European Health for All Series, No. 4).
12. *Targets for health for all.* Copenhagen, WHO Regional Office for Europe, 1985 (European Health for All Series, No. 1).
13. DANIELSSON, M. & MARKLUND, U. *Kartläggning av kommunernas folkhälsoarbete* [Survey of the public health work of Sweden's municipalities]. Stockholm, National Institute of Public Health, 1996 (Folkhälsoinstitutet 1996:88).
14. *Folkhälsa och Agenda 21 – Exempel från 8 kommuner* [Public health and Agenda 21 – examples from eight municipalities in Sweden]. Stockholm, National Board of Health and Welfare, 1996 (SoS-rapport 1996:5).
15. *Alma-Ata 1978: primary health care. Report of the International Conference on Primary Health Care, Alma Ata, USSR, 6–12 September 1978.* Geneva, World Health Organization, 1978.
16. *Den öppna läkarvården i riket* [Outpatient medical care in Sweden]. Stockholm, National Board of Medicine, 1948 (SOU 1948:14, 21.

17. HIMMELMAN, L. & WEINEHALL, L. Preventivt läkararbete viktigt men vanskligt. Brist på tid och kunskap hinder [Preventive medical work is important but difficult. Shortage of time is the main obstacle]. *Läkartidningen*, **93**(8): 694–699 (1996).

18. LALONDE, M. *A new perspective on the health of Canadians*. Ottawa, Department of National Health and Welfare, 1974.

19. *Healthy people – the Surgeon General's report on health promotion and disease prevention*. Washington, D.C., USGPO, 1979.

20. SWEDISH COMMISSION ON HEALTH AND MEDICAL SERVICES. *Mål och medel för hälso- och sjukvården – Förslag till Hälso- och sjukvårdslag* [Objectives and means for health care in Sweden – proposal for a Health and Medical Services Act]. Malmö, Liber/Allmänna Förlaget, 1979 (SOU 1979:78).

21. *Utvecklingslinjer for hälso- och sjukvården mm* [Guidelines for the development of health care etc.]. Stockholm, Government Printer, 1985 (Regeringens proposition 1984/85:181).

22. ERIKSSON, C.G. ET AL. Health problems in a Swedish county – what can we learn from official sources? *Social science and medicine*, **15C**: 143–151 (1981).

23. *Hur mår du Sverige? Ohälsa och vårdutnyttjande i Sverige – undersökningar om levnadsförhållanden (ULF) som underlag för planering* [Do you feel well Sweden? Ill health and care utilization in Sweden – level of living surveys as the basis for planning]. Stockholm, Swedish Institute for Health Services Development, 1982 (Spri-rapport 82).

24. *Dödsorsak? Dödsorsaksstatistik som underlag för planering* [Causes of death? Statistics on causes of death as the basis for planning]. Stockholm, Swedish Institute for Health Services Development, 1983 (Spri-rapport 122).

25. TOWNSEND, P. & DAVIDSON, N., ED. *The Black report. Inequalities in health*. London, Penguin Books, 1992.

26. PEDERSEN, A. ET AL. *Health promotion in Canada – provincial, national and international perspectives*. Toronto, W.B. Saunders, 1984.

27. Ottawa Charter for Health Promotion (1986). *Health promotion international*, **1**(4): iii–v (1986) and *Canadian journal of public health*, **77**(6): 425–430 (1986).

28. The Adelaide Recommendations: Healthy Public Policy, Adelaide 1988. *Health promotion international*, **3**(2): 183–196 (1988).

29. PETTERSSON, B. ET AL. *Playing for time. Creating supportive environments for health. Report from the 3rd International Conference on Health Promotion, Sundsvall, Sweden, June 9–15, 1991*. Sundsvall, People's Health Västernorrland, 1992.

30. BISTRUP, M.L. *Housing and community environments – how they support health. Briefing book for the Sundsvall Conference on Supportive Environments 1991*. Copenhagen, National Board of Health, 1991.

31. *Conditions for life. Towards a sustainable development in Västernorrland. Briefing book to the Sundsvall Conference on Supportive Environments 1991*. Sundsvall, Västernorrland County Council, 1991.

32. DHILLON, H.S. & PHILIP, L. *Health promotion in developing countries. Briefing book to the Sundsvall Conference on Supportive Environments 1991*. Geneva, World Health Organization, 1991 (document WHO/HED/91.1).

33. *Food and agriculture. Briefing book to the Sundsvall Conference on Supportive Environments 1991.* Oslo, Norwegian Directorate of Health, 1991.

34. HAGLUND, B.J.A. ET AL. *Work for health? Briefing book to the Sundsvall Conference on Supportive Environments 1991.* Stockholm, National Board of Health and Welfare, 1991.

35. KUMPUSALO, E. *Social support and care. A briefing book on the subject social support, care and health.* Helsinki, National Agency for Welfare and Health, 1991.

36. WILSON, D.N. ET AL. *Creating educational environments supportive of health. Briefing book to the Sundsvall Conference on Supportive Environments 1991.* Ottawa, Minister of Supply and Services, 1991.

37. PUBLIC HEALTH GROUP. *Folkhälsans villkor* [The prerequisites of public health]. Stockholm, Allmänna Förlaget, 1991 (Folkhäsogruppens skrift nr 9).

38. *Om vissa folkhälsofrågor* [On certain public health issues]. Stockholm, Government Printer, 1991 (Regeringens proposition 1990/91:175).

39. PUBLIC HEALTH GROUP. *Hela folkets hälsa. En nationell strategi* [Health for all. A national strategy]. Stockholm, Allmänna Förlaget, 1991 (Folkhälsogruppens skrift nr 8) (summary in English: *A national strategy for health.* Stockholm, Allmänna Förlaget, 1991 (Folkhälsogruppens skrift nr 13)).

40. *Investera i hälsa – Prioritera för hälsa* [Invest in health – make health a priority]. Stockholm, Government Printer, 1994 (Regeringens skrivelse 1993/94:247).

41. ROSE, G. *Strategies for preventive medicine.* Oxford, Oxford University Press, 1992.

42. *Landstingens folkhälsoansvar* [The public health responsibilities of county councils]. Stockholm, National Board of Health and Welfare, 1994 (SoS-rapport 1994:6).

43. LUNDBERG, B. ET AL. *Rätten till hälsa* [The right to health]. Stockholm, Swedish Confederation of Trade Unions, 1993.

44. MINISTRY OF HEALTH AND SOCIAL AFFAIRS. *Strategi för Sveriges EG-arbete i frågor som gäller folkhälsa och hälso och sjukvård* [Strategy for Sweden's European Union work related to public health and health care]. Stockholm, Fritzes, 1997 (Ds 1997:4).

45. *Third evaluation of the progress towards health for all in the European Region of WHO 1996–1997, Sweden.* Stockholm, Ministry of Health and Social Affairs, 1997.

Comparative analysis of development of health policy in Östergötland County, Sweden

Lena Rydin Hansson

Introduction

Health care administration in Östergötland County

In Sweden, health care is entrusted to regional authorities, the county councils. The Östergötland County Council serves Sweden's fifth largest county, with slightly more than 400 000 inhabitants. The county encompasses 13 municipalities. Ten of these are fairly small, mostly rural and sparsely inhabited. Most of the population lives in urban districts within the three larger municipalities.

The county councils comprise members elected in general elections every 4 years (until 1994 every 3 years). Most county council revenues (60% in Östergötland) come from county council taxation and general state subsidies (12% in Östergötland). Less than 10% of revenue is user fees, although the possibility of increasing these fees is sometimes discussed. Increasing fees might reduce equity and accessibility for poor people. This is in special focus now, since fees for medicine were increased on 1 January 1997. Free medicine for people with chronic diseases such as asthma and epilepsy has been eliminated.

County councils have extensive freedom to operate within the legal framework of Sweden's Health Act from 1983 *(1)*. The Health Act stipulates that health promotion, disease prevention and medical services are county council obligations and that equity and health for all principles should guide the administration and distribution of services.

County councils are also major sources of employment, although a few county council duties have been transferred to municipalities over the last few years (such as care for elderly people). In Östergötland health care workers comprise about 7% of the total work force. Most (83%) of these health care workers are women. The health care sector employs 13% of all female employees in Östergötland.

Most of the 13 000 people employed by the County Council in 1996 were health professionals working at the 4 major hospitals, 36 primary health care units or 36 dental care units.

Development of a policy for health for all

In 1987 the County Council began to realize that it lacked a clear and comprehensive policy and strategy for attaining health for all. Developing the health policy of the Östergötland County Council would harmonize and align regional policies for health for all with national and international policies formulated and approved by the WHO Regional Office for Europe and the national Government.

After many years of committed but relatively ad hoc health promotion activities, the County Council started to develop a target-related health policy in 1987 to achieve regional consistency in health for all policy. For a long time, the County Council had devoted resources to developing preventive and health promotion activities. Collaboration with the Linköping University Faculty of Health Sciences was well established. The County Council politicians, administrators and health professionals were by then already well acquainted with and convinced by the WHO concept of health for all *(2–4)*.

The national report on public health published in 1987 *(5)* described inequities in health between different groups of the population and how part of the population was more at risk because of lifestyle and environmental socioeconomic conditions. In addition, health care supply in relation to need differed in different groups.

The County Council epidemiologist described how the national figures were also relevant to the conditions in Östergötland. This was a crucial condition and background to the decision to initiate a health policy programme.

The 1987 County Council decision stated that a health policy programme should be drafted, which later comprised two programmes. The programme was to explain and formulate the health policy of the County Council. Objectives and targets were to be set and the strategy and direction of health policy implementation was to be described.

Simultaneously, a public health report was developed. Ideally, a public health report should come first and the policy programme should be based on that report. Nevertheless, since the report was not available and the County Council considered it most important to draft its policy programme, the Council decided that both documents should be developed simultaneously. The realities of the policy-making world do not always harmonize with the perfect manual, and one has to learn to deal with that.

The County Council decided to base its health for all programme on the WHO principles of community involvement, public participation and intersectoral collaboration, the principal aim being to improve the health and equity in health of the inhabitants of Östergötland.

The County Council also decided that the health for all policy and targets should be in harmony with the organizational structure and culture of the County Council. This way the policy and targets could be more easily and naturally integrated into the existing internal and collaborative activities of the organization.

The Health Act *(1)* stipulates that health promotion and disease prevention are a concern of the health care sector. But the law does not prescribe how the health care sector is to collaborate with other actors in society, nor does it give the health care sector any right to impose its will over other organizations and authorities that have the power to influence public health. This makes integrating and networking in every stage of the health for all process one way to succeed, and perhaps the only way.

The County Council has built its health for all policy and programme on that conviction. Only by collaborating and networking can one integrate all the skills and experiences necessary to implement a successful health for all policy that really improves the public health in Östergötland.

Political framework and policy environment

For decades, Östergötland County Council had a solid Social Democratic majority. Developing tools for equity in health and serving the population with health care equally accessible to all was a deliberate policy many years before the specific WHO-influenced health policy was developed in the latter part of the 1980s. Nevertheless, tremendous effort was put into involving all political parties in formulating health policy. This was important to ensure that the policy would not change should there be a change in the political majority.

The policy environment when the two basic documents on health policy were formulated and settled in 1988 and 1990 *(6,7)* was the solid Social Democratic majority. In 1992, a coalition of Conservatives and Liberals won the majority in the County Council election and together formed the political majority from 1992 to 1994.

The process by which the health policy was formulated included thorough discussion and negotiation with all political parties represented in the County Council Political Board. All health policy decisions were by consensus. This provided stable support and the health policy has proven to be politically solid and untouched by changes in political majority (now back to the Social Democratic Party since 1995). Political consensus is crucial to developing and setting a stable and long-term health policy.

The Östergötland health policy emphasizes health promotion and disease prevention. This was considered important in an organization that has mainly focused on medical treatment. The long history and tradition of the Swedish county councils is to care and cure. The new emphasis on promoting health and preventing disease requires specific political consideration in a policy environment so strongly focusing on diagnosis, treatment, secondary prevention, rehabilitation and palliative measures.

Criteria used in defining policy and for setting goals, objectives and targets

The main reason for developing the Östergötland health policy was to achieve better health for the county inhabitants. The conviction was that this could be best accomplished following some basic criteria for policy development, and the policy was therefore built on the principles of community involvement, public participation, intersectoral collaboration and a focus on equity in health for all. The following criteria were formulated and are included in the first health policy programme *(6)*.

- To integrate activities in the existing health care system, all County Council health professionals, administrators and politicians should support and participate in policy implementation.
- Health professionals must accept that their role as expert must be replaced by a more advisory and supportive role in health promotion and disease prevention activities, and must embrace a wider view of health in which other actors have a valid contribution to make.
- Policy implementation presupposes intersectoral collaboration, thus promoting community-oriented health activities.
- Four basic ethical rules should guide policy implementation and health activities:
  - not to harm;
  - to respect the integrity of the individual;
  - to use the most effective method possible in health promotion and disease prevention; and
  - to distribute resources equitably.
- Health cannot be measured in monetary terms. The results should be measured in terms of health gain and improved quality of life.
- Promoting health and preventing disease is as important and as high a political priority as medical care and cure.

Equity

Scope of the policy
During 1988, the health problems of the County were defined, goals were formulated and the overall health policy was decided *(6)*. All political parties represented in the County Council Political Board approved the programme and its content. The goals were the following.

Goal 1. Östergötland County Council – a healthy county council.
Goal 2. Health promotion and disease prevention that is equally accessible to all the people.
Goal 3. Health promotion and disease prevention of high quality.
Goal 4. Health activities that satisfy the needs of the population.
Goal 5. Community participation in health activities.

Twenty-six measurable and outcome-related targets were formulated and adopted in 1990 *(7)*. These targets focus on healthy lifestyles, accident prevention and musculoskeletal disorders. The target groups defined were children and youth, pregnant women, young parents and elderly people (Appendix 1).

The strategy for implementation *(7)* emphasizes the community level with intersectoral activities and networking as the foundation on which a healthy county can be built. This is to be supported by countywide activities including mass media strategies, information material, education and training, and research and development projects.

In 1995, the health policy and targets were revised and rewritten *(8)*. The strategy now focuses even more on equity. Measures and activities are now clearly focusing on vulnerable groups. The targets and target groups from 1990 have been sharpened and defined more clearly. The health policy now also defines the arenas in which the County Council can act to promote health for all (Appendix 2).

Special programmes for vulnerable groups

In February 1996, a report on children, youth and health *(9)* was published and in October 1996, a report on workers, unemployment and health *(10)*. The next health report, on women and health, is being written. These health reports describe and analyse the health and environmental conditions of the targeted groups and provide recommendations for future activities. They will form an important basis for the decisions by the County Council Political Board and the contract committees on resource allocation and activities.

Protocols for health have been under development since 1995. The protocol agenda focused on mental health and cardiovascular diseases in the first phase and is continuing with cancers and musculoskeletal disorders in the second phase. Vulnerable groups are being identified and activities to promote health, prevent, treat and cure disease, rehabilitate and palliate will be described. These health gain activities and their economic implications are to be presented.

These protocols were established because the County Council wanted to have a thorough description of major diseases, their incidence, various methods for their prevention and treatment, the cost and the expected outcomes. The protocols for health include relevant parts of the health policy targets and present means and tools to achieve these targets, such as smoking cessation activities and the desired results among risk groups for cardiovascular diseases.

The County Council health policy goals, objectives and targets thus comprise one of the starting points for the protocols and will successively be integrated into the protocols for health as they develop.

Communication with the general public and specific interest groups is taken seriously as part of the process of developing the protocols for health. User groups have been established in which politicians and patients and their relatives meet and exchange experience and opinions on how a specific disease can and should be prevented or treated and how best to involve patients and their relatives in the process. Communication with the general public is mainly developed in specific population surveys in which the County Council asks the population for their opinions, experiences and priorities.

Intersectoral action for equity in health

Many local intersectoral health promotion projects aim at promoting equity in health between different groups. For instance, the County Council has allocated money to the health facilitators project *(11)*. The health facilitators are located in geographical areas in which socioeconomic, health and health insurance statistics show that the population is especially vulnerable to poor health. Health facilitators are County Council employees based at primary health care units. Most of them are district nurses by profession. Ideally they should also have a masters degree in public health. This is not the case today, but since a

Master of Public Health programme has been established in Linköping, all health facilitators are now offered that education. In a few years, all health facilitators in Östergötland should have a masters degree in public health.

The health facilitators project is restricted by three political decisions.

1. The public health service in the area should initiate the formation of a local health group with representatives from the public services and the nongovernmental organizations of the area. This group can map, analyse, decide and perform activities to improve health in the area.

2. The mapping and analysis of health and health conditions made by the local health group should be presented in a local public health report and form the basis for health activities in the area.

3. The activities should successively be more and more integrated into people's lives and the activities of nongovernmental organizations in each local area, to ensure that the activities continue based on the internal resources of the area itself. This will increase public participation, improve self-confidence, and teach people to demand their rights and to feel able to take responsibility for themselves and their families, friends and neighbours, all of which are a good basis for improving health and equity in health.

Health facilitators are meant to be the key people in supporting this intersectoral action for health and equity in health in the local area. Skills and training are important ingredients of the professionalism appropriate to health facilitating.

The Faculty of Health Sciences at Linköping University offers good opportunities for education and training in this direction. The Faculty was created as a joint organization by Linköping University and Östergötland County Council. The focus is a stronger emphasis on preventive medicine and primary care, and on problem-oriented team training and integration. Health promotion and disease prevention have been given a more prominent role, as has special training to identify and analyse disease patterns in the community for early preventive measures.

The County Council Centre for Public Health Research, the Faculty of Health Sciences, the Faculty of Political Science and the Faculty of Theme Research collaborated to found a Master of Public Health degree programme within the county at Linköping in 1994. The programme is based on the principles of health for all and with the Östergötland health policy programme as the basis for practice and training. This degree programme will strongly support the County Council efforts to achieve health for all in Östergötland.

Equal access to healthy lifestyles, environment and health care

Vulnerable groups can be defined and described based on statistics and the results of population surveys. In Östergötland, a County Council population survey has been conducted every two years since 1989.

Together with other official statistics, the results from the population surveys form a good basis for epidemiological description and analysis. The official figures reveal:

- how many people live in socioeconomically disadvantaged conditions
- how many people smoke and drink
- how many people live in substandard housing
- which diagnoses form the pattern of morbidity
- who utilizes how much health care
- the mortality panorama
- who is struck by early and avoidable death.

Promoting health by supporting healthy lifestyles and healthy environments and by making health care equally accessible means transforming these statistics into real-life activities that reach the right groups and individuals at the right time with the right messages and support.

Implementing the health policy so that activities really reach the people in most need is the most difficult and crucial part of health promotion. But since this is the only way to actually improve equity, much effort must be put into finding useful tools to make equity policy a reality. International, national and local longitudinal health studies and reports show too little progress in this direction. The results of the Östergötland County Council health policy are no exception.

Equity in health is not achieved by equally distributing health promotion activities to every person. Even a local community has great differences between groups of the population, and accessibility to services must be organized to account for this.

Equity in health is achieved by special efforts to reach those most in need, and to support them when they are permanently or temporarily unable to help themselves. People in disadvantaged economic, social, cultural and emotional conditions must receive support and knowledge from professionals, to enable and encourage them to choose healthy lifestyles and supportive environments for themselves and their children.

People with little education and low socioeconomic status often benefit less from health-promotive and preventive information than do people with more education and higher socioeconomic status.

The County Council believes that equity is best achieved in the local community, in small-area settings where people can meet on a more personal basis. Here individuals and groups can get involved and even the small-scale results of joint efforts can be clear and evident. This is why resources have been put into the health facilitators project *(11)*. Support for health and for equity in health should be integrated into the ordinary everyday life of the community.

In the local community the primary health care units can promote health together with social care units, schools, business and commerce and nongovernmental organizations (interest groups). The role of society should be supportive: helping individuals to develop a healthy lifestyle and to live in a healthy environment with health care easily accessible to everyone.

The County Council subsidizes study circles on various health issues and for different groups (such as elderly people, young single mothers and unemployed youth) where people can learn, gain experience and meet others in the same situation. An example is healthy cooking for young parents or elderly people. The financial support of these study circles from the County Council makes them accessible to everyone regardless of their private finances. Lack of money is often combined with cultural, social and intellectual poverty as well – a good basis for poor health.

Supporting equity through research and development

In-depth analysis of statistics and self-reported health status and lifestyle from the County Council population survey (12) is a basis for the protocols for health (described previously). In-depth studies of the latest survey from 1995 examine the correlations between unsatisfied need for health care, excessive utilization of health care, drugs, self-assessed health and other parameters. Longitudinal comparisons are made with previous surveys (1989, 1991 and 1993) to study the changes over time for different groups. This information can be used to formulate equity policy, and resources can be allocated to specific efforts for specified population or patient groups.

The Primary Health Care Research and Development Unit in Linköping is developing a method to use all County Council general practitioners in collecting and analysing population health data by interviewing a randomized sample of the population in depth. This will give information on differences in health and health conditions between different groups of the population and add to the knowledge of the County Council population surveys.

The County Council Centre for Public Health Research, established in 1995, pursues research and development projects that focus on the underlying factors that can explain why some individuals or groups are more vulnerable to ill health than others. They especially focus on the gender perspective and also look for early biochemical markers and environmental factors in the fetal period and early childhood that might explain health differences in the adult population.

Participation

During 1988, the health problems of Östergötland were defined, goals were formulated and the overall health policy was decided (6). This process was very much led by experts, since the programme was drafted by a working group of seven senior health professionals employed by the County Council or the Faculty of Health Sciences of Linköping University, in close cooperation with the leading politicians of the County Council. All political parties represented in the County Council Political Board approved the programme and its contents by consensus.

During 1989, the 26 specific measurable targets were defined, strategies for action were outlined and a target-related and specific health policy was adopted (7). The process by which this was accomplished was quite different from the one mentioned above. It took the form of a project involving about 50 experts and lay people from governmental and nongovernmental organizations throughout the county and with whom the County Council wanted to establish collaborative participation in the future health for all intervention.

This part of the policy formulation process was also regarded as the first step of the implementation process. From society's point of view, the most important thing is to achieve results, and the first prerequisite to achieving results is that organizations and people know, accept and implement the policy.

When the policy and targets were being formulated, Östergötland County Council arranged hearings and seminars to give professionals from health care, the social sector, education and other sectors, as well as nongovernmental organizations and the general public, the opportunity to discuss and influence the development and content of the programme.

When the County Council Political Board unanimously approved *Better health for all in Östergötland (7)*, they knew that numerous health for all agents were already associated with the policy and targets and ready to make intervention and activities for health the business of regional and local communities. This was a result of the comprehensive collaboration process the County Council had initiated when developing the target programme.

Participation by the politicians

The deliberate and regular discussions and meetings with the County Council politicians during the policy formulation process aimed at bringing the political and professional communities into agreement. The politicians were confronted with the policy and target formulation process, both as parliamentarians and as members of different political parties.

The regular dialogue between County Council politicians and health professionals has continued throughout the implementation and activity process. The County Council health policy can only survive and influence progress towards health for all in Östergötland if the politicians stay closely engaged and bound to the policy they have adopted.

The senior health professionals must nourish the political agenda with feedback, evaluation of progress towards achieving health targets and reports on the health policy process.

Participation by the general public

When health policy or a programme in any health area is being developed and formulated, the group of people for whom the policy is defined should participate. Confronting professionals with the general public often vitalizes the discussion and brings new angles and impulses to the activities planned.

The County Council experience is that young children can be involved in processes of this kind. Children, who may have difficulty in making their voices heard in professional discussions and planning, can draw or write down their experiences and feelings *(13)*. Thus, their contributions can be integrated into the policy and planning.

In Östergötland, communication started even during the health policy planning process. For instance, elderly and retired people were invited to public discussions advertised in the local newspapers on the content of health policy and the means and methods of implementation.

An important question is how to involve the silent minority of the population in policy discussions and activities. Reaching them is vital when equity is on the agenda. One way could be population surveys *(12)* in which a representative sample of the population is asked for their experiences and opinions. More people may dare to express their feelings, experiences and opinions anonymously than in open discussions. The average response rate in Östergötland is 70%.

Acting locally is a successful practice to communicate with the general public. Many primary health care units in Östergötland have formed local health groups within their catchment areas. This is one of the strategies decided in the health policy programmes *(6–8)*. Local health groups, in which professionals from different sectors of the local community meet with lay people from the same area, provide a good basis for equitable health work.

The Linköping University Hospital, the three general hospitals and all primary health care units in the County from time to time conduct open-house activities with public lectures and presentations of preventive programmes and medical care. These popular arrangements have two functions. They inform and teach the general public on self-care, lifestyle and early symptoms, and the health professionals have an informative and valuable opportunity to meet and discuss with the healthy general public as a complement to the clinical experience of meeting people who are usually already sick.

These arrangements also provide opportunities for the clinicians to get a community perspective. Medical knowledge should be integrated into community health activities, and communication between professionals and the general public should be promoted.

The perspective of patients and the general population is guiding the County Council political process more and more. The specific orientation towards purchaser and provider, with politicians more and more focusing on the perspective of patients and the general population, will require greater focus on public participation and orientation towards users in health policy development. This is a general reorientation within official services in Östergötland and in Sweden as a whole.

This perspective focuses on the responsibility of the population to express their opinions and to participate in the political debate, but it also focuses on the responsibility of the politicians and professionals to let public opinion carry weight in the planning and developing process. Health policy and activities must be based on professional and political decisions, but communication with the general public could improve these decisions.

Intersectoral action

Review of existing intersectoral policy
Intersectoral groups on specific intervention areas were established during the 1980s. For example, the County Council participates in groups on alcohol and drugs (with social care authorities, the police, social insurance authorities, nongovernmental organizations and others) and accident prevention (with road agencies, nongovernmental organizations, trade unions and others). The composition of each group depends on the topic. The policy formulated for these specific intersectoral groups was integrated into the County Council health policy programmes *(6,7)*.

The broad intersectoral framework in which the County Council health policy was developed, with participation from professional and voluntary organizations, disseminated knowledge of existing health-related policies in other sectors. Representatives of other organizations integrated policies, knowledge and experiences from the County Council policy panorama into the policy-defining project.

Intersectoral collaboration was not a totally new concept invented in the development of health policy, but the collaboration became more intense and structured at that time. This was a result of the policy development process.

Fitness activities were developed and started in the early 1980s in collaboration between the County Council, municipalities and sports organizations. Contracts were written between these actors that define and regulate responsibility, financing, goals and target groups for the county-wide fitness movement. When the County Council health policy programmes were formulated and adopted *(6,7)* the existing policy was integrated.

Intervention measures adopted
The strategy of Östergötland County Council on health policy strategy since the very first policy document from 1988 is based on a mixture of research and development, clinical and intersectoral practice, informing and educating employees, and informing and educating the general public.

All these strategic components emphasize intersectoral collaboration as a means for successful and effective intervention for health for all.

Examples of intersectoral activities
By tradition, research and development builds on the close collaboration with the Faculty of Health Sciences of Linköping University, other University departments and the County Council. Many of the

intervention projects related to health policy are supervised, supported and evaluated by these collaborating units, especially the Department of Community Medicine, the Primary Health Care Research and Development Unit and the County Council Centre for Public Health Research.

A County Council fund (2 million kronor per year) supports local projects that develop new methods to reach the right groups and to change attitudes, behaviour and the pattern of disease. Such a project could, for instance, aim at reducing risk among men in their forties with multiple risk factors for heart attacks.

Intersectoral projects involving County Council units together with external organizations are given the highest priority, although projects accomplished by one unit may be funded if substantial benefits are expected.

The County Council also funds large research projects of national and international interest, such as one on accidents and injury prevention (resulting in Motala: a WHO Safe Community, a project coordinated by WHO headquarters) *(14)*. This research project involves Linköping University (the Department of Community Medicine), the County Council (Motala Hospital), a municipality (the Municipality of Motala) and other organizations.

Another intersectoral research project of major impact funded by the County Council is a project on osteoporosis prevention, with population strategies for general prevention (such as physical exercise promoted by nongovernmental organizations), lifestyle consultations at primary health care centres and research on osteoporosis markers in blood and urine (at Linköping University), which allows for early screening to detect high-risk populations *(15,16)*.

An example of clinical practice with intersectoral overtones is the accident registration that all Östergötland County Council acute wards are contracted to perform regularly. They are also contracted to feed risk information back to the municipalities as the basis for measures on safer housing, roads and institutions.

Information is disseminated to the general public through local television, newspapers and information leaflets. Health articles on various topics and information on health-related activities are published in local newspapers and produced through collaboration among health professionals, patient associations, other voluntary organizations and journalists. Information on tobacco use is produced, and support for smoking cessation is being offered in collaboration with the pharmacies.

One example of intersectoral education activities is the Health Adventure at the Linköping Science Centre, at which computerized or hands-on stations and interactive pedagogics are used to teach schoolchildren about health and how they can promote or retard health through everyday choices even at a young age. Specially trained teachers work in the Health Adventure to teach the children how to use the material at hand, and also to understand and discuss how they can integrate their new knowledge into their own lifestyles.

All pupils from 7 to 16 years of age in Östergötland come to the Health Adventure for lectures and experiments. Study kits are lent and can be used for follow-up in the classroom after a visit to the Health Adventure. The Health Adventure has 180 000 visitors each year (Östergötland has about 400 000 inhabitants). The Linköping Science Centre is funded and operated by the University of Linköping, the Municipality of Linköping and the County Council.

Formal intersectoral councils and teams

The County Council has made an effort to establish local health groups in every municipality in Östergötland. The biggest cities, Linköping and Norrköping, are divided into smaller primary health care areas. Each one should have a local health group. The strategy from 1990 *(7)* stipulated that each primary health care unit would take responsibility for initiating a local health group in its catchment area (municipality or urban area).

A local health group is a collaborating body consisting of representatives from different local governmental and nongovernmental organizations. A core of organizations is usually permanently represented, with others co-opted depending on the current activities. The local health group formulates a local action programme within the policy framework of the County Council health policy programmes *(6–8)*.

Local health groups were unevenly developed in different parts of the county because County Council senior administrators and politicians did not apply direct pressure. The local health group strategy was to be executed by senior general practitioners who headed primary health care units, a group of professionals with very diverse views on intersectoral health promotion and health for all activities. Since 1994 the annual contracts of the primary health care units within the purchaser–provider system have more directly mandated the establishment of local health groups as a basis for budgeting, activities and evaluation.

As of January 1997, more then half of Östergötland was covered by local health groups dealing with a wide spectrum of intersectoral issues decided on a local basis within the framework of the County Council health policy programmes *(6–8)*. During the last few years health for all has more and more become an evident interest and ambition for municipalities and social insurance offices, which also support the establishment of local health groups.

At the regional level, intersectoral groups on specific topics have been established as a mechanism to promote intersectoral health activities (described previously). During 1995, the County Council initiated discussions with other regional government organizations and municipalities to constitute a County Health Council in the next few years, in which the wider spectrum of health for all issues can be discussed, adopted and supported.

Existing intersectoral groups on specific topics could then become committees to the County Health Council. The County Health Council is expected to lead to all major organizations in initiating, formulating and accepting mutual health for all policies in Östergötland. The effects of the County Health

Council on various sectors, especially its influence on various policy sectors and their impact on population health, should be evaluated and reported.

Other alliances and partnerships
Alliances are being built continually as a natural effect when local health activities are started. Needs and project ideas are driving forces to seeking alliances. Intersectoral partnership ennobles and enriches health activities.

For example, the foremost strategy for healthy lifestyles is to work with young families and with children and youth. The school is a very important arena under municipal authority. Children and youth are the most important target groups for the County Council health policy targets on tobacco, alcohol and other drugs, healthy eating and exercise.

The school is probably the most important arena for reaching these groups. Thus alliances have been and are being built between health professionals from the County Council Centre for Public Health Research and elsewhere, school authorities and social service authorities to promote tobacco-free schools, accident-free schools and healthy schools.

In a housing area in Linköping, the local health group, the health facilitator, the County Council Centre for Public Health Research and the municipal social services received government funding in 1995 to develop a method to build alliances in school and around the school in the housing areas and to integrate supportive activities to promote healthy living and healthy lifestyles among young people.

Health status orientation

Health status includes quantitative outcomes such as morbidity and mortality and the more qualitative aspects of health such as quality of life and wellbeing. The County Council has conducted population surveys *(12)* to collect qualitative data on self-reported health. For a period of years the population survey was performed every two years. The future focus will be on analysing and presenting information from data already collected instead of collecting new data. The interval between future general population surveys will probably be four or five years.

The newly established County Council Centre for Public Health Research includes the County Council Epidemiological Unit, which has been involved in public health reporting since the early 1980s. Morbidity and mortality are analysed and reported regularly.

Geographical patterns and differences between socioeconomic groups, age groups and females and males are reported. A new technique to study the geographical dispersion of information, including studies of covariation between environmental and lifestyle factors and morbidity and mortality is being developed *(17)*. A geographical information system might prove to be the best method for determining health status, with monitoring, analysing and reporting on health as a basis for planning, purchasing and evaluation.

A geographical information system offers a technique to map information, thus making covariation very visible to the observer. Geographical information systems can be used in environmental epidemiology to show the association between environmental exposure and health outcome.

The County Council decided that all health status presentations and public health reporting should support the development and revision of the health protocols (described previously), focusing on population groups, morbidity and mortality patterns, lifestyle and health factors and other factors such as socioeconomic variation that are important in describing, weighting and analysing various aspects of the different disease groups that are the focus of the protocols.

The second health policy document *(7)* outlined how health policy and target implementation could be monitored. When the targets were formulated, it was explicitly demanded that they be measurable and that possible methods of evaluation be presented in the document.

Every project, small or large, that is funded by the County Council and planned and accomplished based on the County Council health policy and targets is analysed, evaluated and reported. The results are integrated into the political and professional knowledge base so that these new experiences and results can be integrated and allowed to adjust policy successively. In 1994 a report was written that described the process of health policy progress and the implementation of policy *(18)*. This, together with the measurable target-related project outcomes, formed a basis for the 1995 revision of the County Council health policy programme *(8)*.

The revision resulted in some of the targets being eliminated. Some other targets were more clearly defined, and new targets were put into the programme. Instead of only defining target areas and target groups in the revised programme, arenas were also defined. Not only the content of the programme but also its structure was revised. The correspondence between the Östergötland programme and the WHO European strategy for health for all was made more visible in the revised version.

Policy formulation and target-setting, implementation, monitoring and evaluation of process and outcomes, feedback of results and the review and revision of policy are linked together in a continuous process to develop future policy based on experiences and the results achieved (Table 2.5 and Fig. 2.7).

International influence and collaboration

The Östergötland experience is an example of regional health policy development inspired by and based on the WHO model. Throughout the process of County Council health policy development, the WHO regional targets for health for all have been a very important model in guiding development. The principles of equity, community involvement, intersectoral collaboration and public participation permeate the County Council health policy programmes *(6–8)* and activities.

The Faculty of Health Sciences of Linköping University is a WHO collaborating centre. Specific research and development projects on health promotion, policy implementation and international networking are proceeding within this framework.

Östergötland County Council is a member of the WHO Regions for Health Network, which means a very specific and close interaction between WHO and the County Council in health policy development. The County Council is a founding member of the Network and finds this close relation with the WHO Regional Office for Europe and other European regions for health extremely inspiring and supportive to the continuous development of the County Council health policy and activities. The Regions for Health Network was founded in 1992 with the aim of facilitating the exchange of experience and knowledge as well as collaboration between European regions to develop the WHO European health for all policy.

Conclusion

WHO has offered countries and regions a good source of inspiration and served as a model for developing a health policy *(2, 3)*. WHO strategies for health for all and their pioneering target-setting has influenced the Östergötland County Council throughout the policy development process, from the first initiative of formulating strategies and goals through to evaluating and revising the targets.

Developing a health policy with all its components is not easy. It cannot be done by implementing experiences, knowledge and recommendations from available models without the model being adapted and redesigned to fit local conditions and need. The very process of developing regional health policy is an important tool through which local politicians, organizations and people become engaged and true participants.

A regional health policy must build on existing prerequisites, be integrated into everyday political life and permeate professional actions. Formulating a health policy requires time, so that the strategies, objectives

Table 2.5. The process of health policy development
of Östergötland County Council

1988	Health policy, strategies and goals
1990	Objectives and targets for health for all in Östergötland
1994	Report on health policy progress
1995	Review and revision of health policy targets; target groups and arenas defined or redefined

Fig. 2.7. The Östergötland policy development cycle

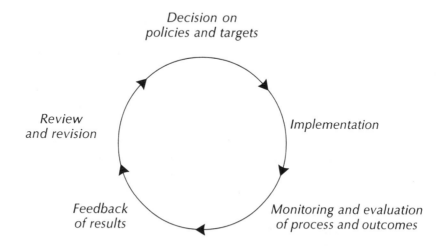

Decision on
policies and targets

Review
and revision

Implementation

Feedback
of results

Monitoring and evaluation
of process and outcomes

and targets adopted are well prepared and supported by both politicians and professionals as well as by the professional and voluntary organizations with whom collaboration is desired.

When the health policy programme is formulated, its strategy, objectives and targets should be completed with guiding principles for monitoring and evaluation. Even the most well prepared health policy must be open to revision when circumstances show that the course should be adjusted.

Even if it is concluded that a regional health policy should be comprehensive and specific to serve as a tool for guiding and supporting health for all activities, the policy must not be too detailed. Local health authorities and their allies must have freedom of action within the policy framework to stimulate enthusiasm, energy and creativity. Here the top-down and the bottom-up perspectives must be tied together to complete the link between the centre and periphery. A health policy with substantial influence on equity in health, health status and the environment can only be implemented by autonomous, cross-sectoral activities and collaboration between local professional and voluntary organizations.

References

1. *Hälso- och sjukvårdslagen HSL 1982:763* [The Health Act]. Stockholm, Ministry of Health, 1982.
2. *Formulating strategies for health for all by the year 2000.* Geneva, World Health Organization, 1979 ("Health for All" Series, No. 2).
3. *Health for all targets. The health policy for Europe.* Copenhagen, WHO Regional Office for Europe, 1993.

4. Ottawa Charter for Health Promotion. *Health promotion*, 1(4): iii–v (1986) and *Canadian journal of public health*, 77(6): 425–430 (1986).

5. *Folkhälsorapport 1987* [Public health report, 1987]. Stockholm, National Board of Health and Welfare, 1987 (Socialstyrelsen redovisar 1987:15).

6. *Hälsopolitiskt program 1988* [Health policy programme, 1988]. Linköping, Östergötland County Council, 1988 (English summary available).

7. *Bättre hälsa för alla Östgötar. Effektmålsprogram för landstingets hälsoarbete 1990–2000* [Better health for all in Östergötland. Measurable outcome target programme for County Council health work 1990–2000]. Linköping, Östergötland County Council, 1990 (English summary available).

8. *Bättre hälsa för alla Östgötar – reviderat målprogram för landstingets folkhälsoarbete 1995– 2000* [Better health for all in Östergötland – a revised target programme for County Council health work, 1995–2000]. Linköping, Östergötland County Council, 1995.

9. *Barns och ungdomars hälsa 1995* [Health of children and young people, 1995]. Linköping, Östergötland County Council, 1995.

10. *Arbetsvillkor, yrke och ohälsa i Östergötland – en antologi* [Working conditions, occupation and ill health in Östergötland – an anthology]. Linköping, Östergötland County Council, 1996.

11. HANSSON, R.L. Investment for health in Östergötland – with the help of "health facilitators". *In: Investing for health*. Report of a WHO Meeting, Bolzano, Italy, 13–14 October 1995. Copenhagen WHO Regional Office for Europe, 1996, pp. 53–54 (RHN Conference Series No. 3, document EUR/ICP/HSC 424).

12. *Landstingsenkäten 1991, 1993 och 1995 i CMT rapportserie* [Reports on County Council population surveys in 1991, 1993 and 1995]. Linköping, Linköping University, 1992, 1994, 1996.

13. *Vi mår bra av vänner 1993* [Friends make us feel good]. Linköping, Östergötland County Council, 1993.

14. LINDQVIST, K. *Towards community-based injury prevention. The Motala model*. Linköping, Linköping University, 1993, (Linköping University Medical Dissertations, No. 404).

15. WALLER, J. ET AL. Logic and logistics of community intervention against osteoporosis. An evidence basis. *Journal of medical systems*, 21: 33–48 (1997).

16. MAGNUSSON, P. ET AL. Determination of bone alkoline phosphatase isoforms in serum by a new high-performance liquid chromatography assay in patients with metabolic bone disease. *Acta orthopædica scandinavica*, 66 (Suppl. 266): 202– 204 (1995).

17. *Geografiska InformationsSystem – något för landstinget?* [A geographical information system – something of interest to the County Council?]. Linköping, Östergötland County Council, 1994.

18. *Bättre hälsa för alla Östgötar. Landstingets folkhälsoprogram 1990–2000. En avstämning av de första årens verksamhet 1995* [Report on health policy progress and the implementation of policy]. Linköping, Östergötland County Council, 1995.

Appendix 1. Targets for health for all in Östergötland County, Sweden[a]

Measurable outcome target area 1: reducing lifestyle-related health risks

Targets 1–4
- The proportion of 12- to 16-year-olds using tobacco should be minimized; the reduction should be at least 20% by 1995.
- Alcohol consumption should be reduced among ninth-grade pupils; a marked reduction should have occurred by 1995.

Target 5
- Women should refrain from using tobacco and alcohol during pregnancy.

Target 6
- From 1992 onwards, no-one other than inpatients will be permitted to smoke in County Council premises.

Targets 7–8
- The proportion of the population who exercise regularly should rise by 10% by 1995.
- Everyone 65 years of age or over should be offered a health check every five years as an introduction to a healthy lifestyle. This should be available countywide by 1995.

Target 9
- By the year 2000, fat consumption should be reduced and fibre consumption increased to bring 90% of all the residents of Östergötland within the limits recommended by the National Food Administration.

Target 10
- By 1996 the proportion of the county's inhabitants with an appropriate calcium intake should have increased by 15%.

Targets 11–12
- By 1997 at the latest, study circles should be available to pensioners throughout the county, combining instruction, preparing food and spending time together.
- By 1996 at the latest, dental care for elderly people should be of such a standard that no 80-year-old will be unable to eat nutritious and good food because of poor dental status.

---

[a] Adapted from *Bättre hälse för alle Östgötar. Effektmålsprogram för landstingets hälsoarbete 1990–2000* [Better health for all in Östergötland. Measurable outcome target programme for County Council health work, 1990–2000]. Linköping, Östergötland County Council, 1990.

Measurable outcome target area 2: reducing the accident rate

Target 13
- To reduce by 25% the number of accidents resulting in injury or death by the year 2000.

Target 14
- To reduce the number of accidents among children by 25% by 1996.

Target 15
- To reduce the number of physical exercise and sports accidents by 25% by 1996.

Target 16
- To reduce accidents among elderly people by 20% by 1996.

Measurable outcome target area 3: reducing musculoskeletal disorders

Targets 17–18
- To stop the rise in the proportion of people with hip fractures by 1996.
- To reduce by 10% the proportion of people with hip fractures over a 10-year period beginning in 1996.

Targets 19–20
- To reduce the number of persons reporting sick with neck, shoulder or lower back symptoms by 15% by the year 2000.
- By 1993 to halt the rise in, and by 1995 to reduce by 10%, the number of persons reporting sick with neck, shoulder or lower back symptoms.

Targets 21–22
- To restore more rapidly the functional ability of patients with neck, shoulder or lower back symptoms and to reduce the number of working days lost through illness by 25% by the year 2000.
- By 1993 to halt the rise in the number of days people are absent from work due to neck, shoulder or lower back symptoms.

Targets 23–24
- To reduce by 15% exclusion from working life in the form of early retirement due to functional impairment in the neck, shoulder or lower back by the year 2000.
- To halt the rise in the number of those retiring early due to functional impairment in the neck, shoulder or lower back by 1995.

Measurable outcome target area 4: improving health care for elderly people

Target 25
- By the year 2000 at the latest, all pensioners-to-be should have the opportunity of participating in programmes preparing them for retirement.

Target 26
- Development in care for elderly people during the 1990s should aim at preventing unnecessary passivity and functional impairment during periods of treatment

Appendix 2. Revised targets, target groups and areas for health for all in Östergötland[a]

During 1995, the County Council health programme from 1990 was thoroughly examined and its content and targets reviewed from an organizational and environmental point of view. Experience and knowledge from five years of policy implementation and health for all activities were structured and analysed and taken into consideration in the revision.

The revised programme emphasizes that the political priority is disadvantaged groups – a high-risk strategy to support equity in health and health conditions. This strategy should be combined with broad health activities for the county population in general – a population strategy. The population strategy emphasizes children and youth as the most important target group. A supportive environment must be created as a basis for health for all. A supportive environment is of specific importance to high-risk individuals.

In October 1995, the County Council Political Board adopted the revised health for all programme for County Council health work in Östergötland. The overall content and strategies from 1990 were maintained. The whole County Council organization is still obliged to participate in the implementation and activities. Contracts with primary health care units, hospitals and dental care units include health promotion and disease prevention activities. Intersectoral action, alliance building, public participation and equity in health are County Council health policies firmly integrated in the revised health for all programme.

The following broadly outlines the main targets and directions of the revised health for all programme with reference to the corresponding WHO European targets for health for all.

Targets have been formulated within the following areas

Lifestyles conducive to health with special focus on:
- reducing the use of tobacco (European target 17)
- reducing the use of alcohol and other drugs (European target 17)
- improving healthy eating patterns (European target 16)
- promoting appropriate and healthy physical activity (European target 16).

Reducing unintentional and self-inflicted injuries and death by:
- reducing accidents (European target 11)
- reducing suicides and attempted suicides (European target 12).

---

[a] Adapted from *Bättre hälse för alle Östgötar – reviderat målsprogram för landstingets folkhälsoarbete 1995–2000* [Better health for all in Östergötland – a revised target programme for County Council health work, 1995–2000]. Linköping, Östergötland County Council, 1995.

Preventing widespread and/or chronic diseases such as:
- cardiovascular diseases (European target 9)
- allergies (European target 4)
- diabetes (European target 4)
- cancer (European target 10)
- osteoporosis (European targets 11, 16 and 17).

Target groups

Target groups for County Council health policy work are individuals and population groups that particularly need support to achieve and retain health. This strategy aims at achieving equity in health and health conditions for the population.

Health of children and youth (European target 7) with special focus on:
- children who might be at particular risk, such as those from families who abuse drugs, those who have a low educational level, those who have one or two parents unemployed or who have a single parent with a low educational level, and those of first-generation refugees or immigrants
- unemployed youth with a low educational level.

Women (European target 8) with special focus on:
- women with strenuous and monotonous manual work
- first-generation refugees or immigrants
- single mothers with poor social support
- women with the burden of multiple roles that lead to psychosocial stress.

Elderly people (European target 6) with special focus on:
- elderly people who need substantial medical care
- elderly people with poor social support
- elderly relatives of people with senile dementia and other chronic diseases.

Healthy environment, focusing on the arenas in which the County Council can act

Healthy schools (European target 14) can be achieved by:
- building alliances with the municipalities to support health activities within schools; the initial stage focuses on alcohol, tobacco and other drugs but aims at future broad health promotion activities
- developing supportive environments to strengthen health education such as the Health Adventure, a science centre in Östergötland.

Healthy workplaces (European target 25) with a special focus on:
- healthy County Council workplaces
- collaborating with municipalities and companies to support healthy workplaces in which a healthy lifestyle and a healthy psychosocial environment can be promoted.

Health-promoting County Council organization (European targets 26–29 and 31) with a special focus on:
- health-promoting health care that emphasizes health gains for patients and employees when outcomes and quality are evaluated.

Intersectoral action and partnership (European target 37) with a special focus on:
- building community-oriented alliances for collaboration with voluntary organizations and the general public
- a County Health Council focusing on supporting activities.

Healthy City Gothenburg: the work of the Public Health Advisory Committee in evaluating the European regional targets as they relate to Gothenburg

Per Haglind & Willy Nilsson

Introduction

WHO has always clearly stressed that preventive health programmes are desirable and beneficial and constitute an important part of social planning. Sweden was one of the 26 countries that participated in creating WHO. From the very start, WHO chose a broad definition of health.

In 1984, the Member States in the European Region of WHO adopted a European strategy for health for all including 38 targets *(1,2)*. This means that all these countries accept the idea of working towards changing health policies and ensuring that health considerations influence every area of social planning.

The health for all strategy is visionary in many respects. Health for all does not mean intrinsically that, in the year 2000 or later, people will always be healthy and will not require health services. The strategy is based on the belief that people can influence and improve their own health, can understand the value of health, can help to prevent ill health and illness, and should have equitable access to health and medical care when they need it.

International and national public health reports, such as city public health reports in Gothenburg *(3–6)*, provide broad-based, basic factual documentation, but the descriptions themselves do not always provide guidance on how these data should be used in public health programmes. The first stage is therefore to translate the public health data via an action plan on health policy into practical strategies and priorities for public health programmes.

At the local, national and international (WHO) levels, public health data and factual information must form the basis of developing health policy action programmes and practical strategies. Health targets and plans of action for implementation, follow-up and evaluation must therefore be based on correct and specific data. This creates both understanding and respect for public health programmes.

Developments in Gothenburg

The developments in Gothenburg have been based on the framework of the European and national policy discussions. This is important, since translating an ideological document into an operating system with indicators and time schedules is demanding, is sometimes unmanageable and calls for continuity.

National reports

In Sweden, the prerequisites for national health policy include a report on Swedish health services in the 1980s (HS 80) *(7)*, followed by HS 90 *(8)*, both examples of target realization. Work on HS 2000 is in progress. The national Public Health Group, which acted as an advisory body for the Health and Medical Service Planning Committee, is one example of national intersectoral collaboration that has gradually been established. Developments were slow in the 1980s but have been more effective in the 1990s, partly as a result of the activities of the Institute of Public Health and, at the local level in Gothenburg, the Department of Public Health.

The National Board of Health and Welfare's programme on the Swedish health services in the 1990s (HS 90) *(8)* and the Public Health Group's reports and, first and foremost, its policy document on Sweden's national strategy for health for all *(9)* comprise important basic documentation for future public health programmes, completely in line with the European health for all strategy. The National Board of Health and Welfare's public health reports *(10–13)*, especially the latest one from 1997 *(13)*, and the National Board of Health and Welfare's social report from the same year stress the importance of target-oriented health policy programmes with the opportunity for follow-up and evaluation using different measurement and gauging methods.

Delegating to the local level

During the late 1970s, the Gothenburg City Council commissioned the Health Care Promotion Committee to define and document the ill health situation in Gothenburg. The Committee submitted its final report in 1980 *(14)*.

Problem areas of strategic significance for the continued development of health services were analysed for the first time, with the focus on the period 1990–2000. Other local reports highlighted the situation in Gothenburg most impressively and thus formed the basis of later local public health programmes.

As a result of the 1980 report, the Gothenburg Health Council was set up in 1981 to draft public health reports. The Council included committees from the Social Welfare Board, the Health Care Board, the School Board and the Environment and Health Protection Agency.

The Gothenburg Public Health Advisory Committee is a broadly based group of experts from the University of Gothenburg, the Nordic School of Public Health, the Health Service in Gothenburg, Statistics Sweden and the City of Gothenburg. The Committee has produced four public health reports on behalf of the City of Gothenburg Health Council. These reports describe the public health situation in Gothenburg and put forward proposals for improving the health of the people of Gothenburg.

Public health report No. 1 from 1987 *(3)* presented information on population structure, ill health, the utilization of institutional care, and mortality from various diseases and groups of diseases.

Public health report No. 2 from 1989 *(4)* focused on health promotion programmes, health education and an assessment of the health situation in Gothenburg. Special sections dealt with ill health among middle-aged men and the health of women, children, adolescents and elderly people. The relationship between social problems and ill health was spotlighted. In addition, variations in health status in different areas of Gothenburg were reported, and clear-cut proposals for possible action were made based on summaries and conclusions.

Public health report No. 3 from 1991 *(5)* presented a detailed report on the health of children, adolescents and families in Gothenburg. All the public health reports emphasized the substantial variation in health in Gothenburg, and the special significance of health education was stressed.

Public health report No. 4 from 1996 *(6)* applied the 38 regional targets for health for all to Gothenburg.

Other international and national developments were also influencing the process of developing health policy.

In 1988, Gothenburg became a member of the WHO Healthy Cities project and is therefore part of a worldwide network of cities working towards implementing health for all by the year 2000. The project aims to place health high on the agenda of decision-makers at every level and in every sector of society, build powerful platforms and alliances for health in cities, spotlight health in the social debate, and create broadly based popular involvement and participation in health work.

In 1990, the city district council reform was introduced. It represented a great organizational change in working with health in Gothenburg. In connection with this reform, the city district councils assumed responsibility for social services, elementary education, health care activities and local cultural and recreational programmes.

The city district council reform was designed to promote greater local democracy and offered an opportunity for streamlining through integration and local solutions and a holistic approach to local services. The quality and content of the city district council activities is vitally important in public health programmes.

In 1994, the City Council decided to set up a Public Health Delegation comprising city councillors and a Department of Public Health. The Department of Public Health works to improve public health in

Gothenburg, provides a base for supporting strategic decisions related to health policies, and extends collaboration on public health and strengthens intersectoral activities.

The Department of Public Health is a joint knowledge centre and interaction body for the city. Its principal task is to initiate, support and maintain the development and growth of knowledge to promote good health and prevent illness within city and other activities in Gothenburg.

Formulating a policy for health at the city level

Adapting international and national targets to the city level

The 38 European targets for health for all define health broadly. WHO has pointed out that commitment is needed in every sector of society if the fundamental objective of equal health for everyone is to be realized. WHO has also stressed that this calls for political determination and stamina, changes in the distribution of resources, more intersectorality and the creation of networks for health.

The health for all targets are designed to be implemented at the national level, but it is also interesting to apply them at the local level This was done in Gothenburg and is reported on in the fourth public health report for Gothenburg *(6)*.

The evaluation process

The latest public health report *(6)* was produced on the initiative of the Public Health Advisory Committee and has been revised several times based on suggestions from individuals or groups on the Committee. People who are not members of the Committee have also participated. The Committee has linked to each target between one and four proposals for priority action.

The report assessed the current situation in the form of comments on the targets. Every set of comments on the targets comprises the updated target, and different possible interpretations of the target are described.

The Public Health Advisory Committee suggests indicators, including some indicators provided by WHO. The developments relating to the target since the starting point in 1980 are described wherever data are available. Developments are then forecast for the year 2000 with existing data as the starting point.

Using this forecast, the report assesses whether the target can be achieved for all groups, in part or for certain groups, or whether it is not expected to be achieved in any group. Indicators, developments and forecasts are then analysed. Action to assist in achieving the targets is proposed and the action for each target is then placed in order of priority.

The target group for public health report No. 4 comprises politicians, civil servants and decision-makers in the commercial sector, voluntary organizations and the city's agencies and companies.

The fourth public health report is presented in two parts: a summary containing the proposals of the Public Health Advisory Committee for priority action and the full text, including interpretation, development, analysis and more detailed suggestions for action.

The health for all targets for Europe and for Sweden were used as a benchmark to assess the situation in Gothenburg. This enabled consideration of areas in which progress has been less than satisfactory and additional efforts were needed.

According to the assessment of the Public Health Advisory Committee, Gothenburg has been more successful in achieving these targets than Sweden and the European Region.

Results

Sixteen health for all targets will be achieved by the year 2000, according to the Public Health Advisory Committee, provided that – and this is important – the level of resources applied remains the same as it was until the mid-1990s. Six of these 16 targets fall within the area of healthy environment.

The assessment that 16 targets will be realized is based on the situation in Gothenburg, which is located in an affluent and well structured society with a level of awareness and knowledge that allows continual attention to be paid to health and the environment. There is still, however, a great deal of scope for improving the health of the people of Gothenburg.

The Public Health Advisory Committee believes that 20 targets can be achieved in part: to some degree and/or within certain groups. The Committee states that future public health programmes in Gothenburg should focus primarily on achieving six targets:

- WHO target 7: health of children and young people
- WHO target 8: health of women
- WHO target 14: settings for health promotion
- WHO target 16: healthy living
- WHO target 17: tobacco, alcohol and psychoactive drugs
- WHO target 24: human ecology and settlements.

The Public Health Advisory Committee concludes that two targets will not be achieved:

- WHO target 1: equity in health
- WHO target 2: health and quality of life.

These two targets play a fundamental part in social planning and public health programmes. At the same time, they are the most difficult to realize and are perhaps even utopian.

The Public Health Advisory Committee proposed priority action to achieve these targets. For target 1 on equity in health, the Committee proposed:

- giving priority to meaningful work and meaningful employment and stimulating the creation of effective social networks and support structures, including identifying and reducing the health consequences of the fact that certain groups of young people and immigrants do not have access to the labour market;
- focusing on trends in segregation by combining the percentages of non-Swedish citizens; unemployed people; people participating in employment programmes; single-parent households; people with disability pensions; and refugees in relation to the composition of the population in different areas to produce a social index; and
- following up and presenting these indices systematically with the aim of reducing negative segregation, and developing and using in parallel measurements of effect, which indicate the quality of life and wellbeing.

For target 2 on health and quality of life, the Committee recommended:

- organizing local public health programmes to realize the vision and requirements of the city district council reform on local responsibility for the population in combination with local democracy;
- increasing the interaction between working life, schools, social services, recreation, social care and primary care with the aim of creating increased involvement, participation and commitment on the part of the inhabitants; and
- training staff and volunteers in a new way of thinking, better methods and more clearly defined targets in health education and local public health programmes, with the focus on health and quality of life, health and protection factors and supportive environments (Table 2.6).

The Public Health Advisory Committee's public health reports constitute broad-based, interesting documentation that describes the public health situation in Gothenburg. In this context, Gothenburg has made great progress compared with some county councils in Sweden. There is one important difference, however: most county councils have drawn up public health and environmental policy programmes that are politically established and accepted by the county council's executive bodies based on their public health reports. So far, Gothenburg's public health reports have not formed the basis of well planned, politically approved health policy programmes.

Nevertheless, the political management bodies and the Public Health Delegation have a joint task: to develop a comprehensive, integrated policy programme to create the conditions for developing supportive environments for sustainable development. The Department of Public Health and other city departments have the important task of jointly drawing up the basic documentation for a health policy programme and constantly promoting its implementation at the local level. To this end, the

Table 2.6. Assessment by the Public Health Advisory Committee
of Gothenburg's progress in achieving the 38 targets for health for all

WHO target	Description	This target will:		
		not be achieved	be achieved in part[a]	be achieved[b]
1–13	**Achieving better health**			
1	Equity in health	*		
2	Health and quality of life	*		
3	Better opportunities for people with disabilities		*	
4	Reducing chronic disease		*	
5	Reducing communicable disease			*
6	Healthy aging			*
7	Health of children and young people		*	
8	Health of women		*	
9	Reducing cardiovascular disease		*	
10	Controlling cancer		*	
11	Accidents		*	
12	Reducing mental disorders and suicide		*	
13–17	**Lifestyles conducive to health**			
13	Healthy public policy			*
14	Settings for health promotion		*	
15	Health competence			*
16	Healthy living		*	
17	Tobacco, alcohol and psychoactive drugs		*	
18–25	**Healthy environment**			
18	Policy on environment and health			*
19	Environmental health management			*
20	Water quality			*
21	Air quality			*
22	Food quality and safety			*
23	Waste management and soil pollution			*

Table 2.6 (contd)

WHO target	Description	This target will:		
		not be achieved	be achieved in part[a]	be achieved[b]
24	Human ecology and settlements		*	
25	Health of people at work		*	
26–31	**Appropriate care**			
26	Health service policy			*
27	Health service resources and management			*
28	Primary health care		*	
29	Hospital care			*
30	Community services to meet special needs		*	
31	Quality of care and appropriate technology		*	
32–38	**Health for all development strategies**			
32	Health research and development		*	
33	Health for all policy development			*
34	Managing health for all development			*
35	Health information support			*
36	Developing human resources for health		*	
37	Partners for health		*	
38	Health and ethics		*	

[a] To some degree and/or in certain groups.

[b] Provided that the same resources as are available now continue to be available.

Department of Public Health has now allocated special resources to producing a joint public health programme for the City of Gothenburg as part of a broad-based, intersectoral process. This work also supports the development of local health councils.

References

1. *Health for all targets. The health policy for Europe.* Copenhagen, WHO Regional Office for Europe, 1993 (European Health for All Series, No. 4).

2. *Targets for health for all*. Copenhagen, WHO Regional Office for Europe, 1985 (European Health for All Series, No. 1).

3. *Folkhälsorapport 1. Hälsoutvecklingen i Göteborg 1970–1985* [Public health report 1. Health trends in Gothenburg, 1970–1985]. Gothenburg, Public Health Advisory Council on behalf of the City of Gothenburg Health Council, 1987.

4. *Folkhälsorapport 2* [Public health report 2]. Gothenburg, Public Health Advisory Council on behalf of the City of Gothenburg Health Council, 1989.

5. *Folkhälsorapport 3. Barns, ungdomars och familjers hälsa* [Public health report 3. The health of children, young people and families]. Gothenburg, Public Health Advisory Council on behalf of the City of Gothenburg Health Council, 1991.

6. *Folkhälsorapport 4. WHO's 38 hälsopolitiska mål för Europa tillämpade på Göteborg* [Public health report 4. WHO's 38 European targets for health for all applied to the City of Gothenburg]. Gothenburg, Public Health Advisory Council, 1996.

7. *Hälso- och sjukvård inför 80-talet* [The Swedish health services in the 1980s]. Stockholm, National Board of Health and Welfare, 1973.

8. *Hälso- och sjukvård inför 90-talet (HS 90). Huvudrapport* [The Swedish health services in the 1990s. Main report]. Stockholm, National Board of Health and Welfare, 1984 (SOU 1984:39) (summary in English: *The Swedish health services in the 1990's*. Stockholm, National Board of Health and Welfare, 1985).

9. PUBLIC HEALTH GROUP. *Hela folkets hälsa. En nationell strategi* [Health for all. A national strategy]. Stockholm, Allmänna Förlaget, 1991 (Folkhälsogruppens skrift nr 8) (English summary in: *A national strategy for health*. Stockholm, Allmänna Förlaget, 1991 (Folkhälsogruppens skrift nr 13)).

10. *Folkhälsorapport 1987* [The 1987 public health report]. Stockholm, National Board of Health and Welfare, 1987 (Socialstyrelsen redovisar 1987:15).

11. *Folkhälsorapport 1991* [The 1991 public health report]. Stockholm, National Board of Health and Welfare, 1991 (SoS-rapport 1991:11).

12. *Folkhälsorapport 1994* [The 1994 public health report]. Stockholm, National Board of Health and Welfare, 1994 (SoS-rapport 1994:9).

13. *Folkhälsorapport 1997* [The 1997 public health report]. Stockholm, National Board of Health and Welfare, 1997 (SoS-rapport 1997:18).

14. *Friskvårdsberedningens rapport* [Report of the Health Care Promotion Committee]. Gothenburg, City of Gothenburg, 1981.

The development of national health policy in Turkey

Gül Ergör & Zafer Öztek

Introduction

Since 1984, when the first European health for all policy and targets were adopted, many of the Member States and the Region as a whole have gained valuable experience in developing and implementing national health policies. Turkey joined these countries relatively late. Several weak attempts were made in the early 1980s, but serious initiative was first taken in the late 1980s, and the first draft of a document on Turkish national health policy was issued in 1990 *(1)*.

The historical development of Turkey and the particularities of its political environment and administrative structure may help in understanding Turkey's progress towards achieving health for all.

Historical development

Despite being considered a conservative country, Turkey has undergone many social, administrative and economic reforms since the Turkish Republic was founded in 1923. Turkey has changed from totalitarianism to democracy, from Islamic rules to secularism, from the Arabic to the Latin alphabet and from an agricultural to an industrial economy. The Turkish nation is not the same as it was 70 or even 20 years ago, and Turkey will also be changing substantially in the near future.

Before 1950, national health policy gave priority to preventive health services. Curative services were not seen as the direct responsibility of the Ministry of Health, and the municipalities were authorized to provide hospital services. The Ministry of Health, however, did establish five public (model) hospitals to encourage municipalities and the private sector and to demonstrate how a hospital should be managed.

The other major priority of health policy prior to 1950 was that health services were predominantly mobilized towards controlling hyperendemic diseases such as malaria, tuberculosis, trachoma, syphilis and leprosy through vertical programmes similar to those popular in many countries before the Second World War.

The year 1950 was an important milestone in Turkish development: the starting point of a western-type democracy. Similar to other public services, national health policies and strategies changed fundamentally at that time. The Ministry of Health began to take responsibility for curative services. Almost all municipal hospitals were nationalized and attached to the Ministry of Health. New government hospitals were built, initiating a shift of health personnel previously employed in preventive and promotion services in rural areas to employment in urban hospitals. Higher salaries and permission to engage in private practice helped to attract personnel to urban areas, with the result that many left the network of preventive services and joined hospitals. By the end of the 1950s, the inappropriate distribution of human resources was a major problem in Turkey's health services.

After the Army overthrew the Government in 1960, an intersectoral body entitled the State Planning Organization was set up. Under its coordination, each sector, including health, was reorganized to meet planned social and economic targets. As early as 1961, the Government established health objectives emphasizing the integration of public health services (referred to as socialization) and increased coverage in rural areas. Services formerly provided by separate agencies were unified under the same health care delivery system. Health centres were to provide basic medical care, integrated maternal and child health care and family planning services, prevention and treatment of contagious diseases, environmental health care and school health services, all of which were organized to reach even the most peripheral localities.

Turkey's health sector is extremely complex. Many public, semi-public and private institutions finance and deliver health services. The public sector, for instance, is not limited to the Ministry of Health. Medical schools, through their university hospitals, provide substantial health services. The Social Insurance Organization not only operates its own hospitals but also purchases services for its members from public and private facilities. The Army has a large network of facilities and covers the health needs of its active members and retirees and their dependents. Other ministries (such as the Ministry of Education), public organizations (the national post and telecommunications organization and the state railways) and state economic enterprises operate their own hospitals.

Turkey has a very active private hospital sector, and many hospitals are funded by nongovernmental organizations. Most health services are supplied under three largely autonomous systems: the Ministry of Health, medical schools and the social security system.

Turkey's health care system has improved substantially in the last three or four decades. Nonetheless, the overall level of public health, the fertility level and access to health services still differ between eastern and western Turkey and rural and urban areas of the country. Large segments of the population still have a surprisingly high rate of infant mortality (the overall rate was 53 per 1000 live births in 1993), malnutrition and unsanitary environmental conditions, and Turkey's overall health status is unacceptably lower than other middle-income and neighbouring countries.

Administration
The Turkish Republic is a parliamentary system. The President and the Cabinet exercise executive power. Turkey's national administration is centralized, with all crucial decision-making powers given to Ankara-based ministries. The country is now divided into 80 provinces. A governor is appointed by the

Government as the highest-level administrative and political officer in each province and represents the state as a whole, the Government and each ministry. The governor is therefore responsible for directing and coordinating the work of ministries, including the Ministry of Health, in the province. Each provincial agency, such as the directorate of health, has contact with the relevant ministries through the provincial governor. All budget requests must be submitted to the governor first.

A second organ is the provincial council, whose members are elected from the districts proportional to their population for a term of 5 years. This council constitutes the provincial local administration and is also chaired by the governor. Its decisions can be put into effect only with approval of the governor.

Provinces are further divided into districts, which are subdivisions of the province and not incorporated bodies. The sub-governor, head of the district, acts on behalf of the provincial governor and is directly responsible to him or her. The districts have no budgets, but have a council similar to that of the provinces.

Districts are divided into villages. These are settlements with fewer than 2000 inhabitants, on average 500. The villagers elect the head of the village and the council of elders, which is the executive organ of the village, for a period of five years. The village teacher and the imam are *ex officio* members of the council of elders. The village head, like the provincial governor, has the dual role of head of the village and the executive agent of the central government.

Municipalities are incorporated administrative units, whose status is defined by their population, that serve communities with populations of more than 2000 inhabitants. Today, Turkey has approximately 2000 municipalities. The municipalities have legal authority and are responsible for providing various services, including preventive measures for the environment and food inspection. They can also provide curative medical services at the primary and secondary levels if they so decide. The mayor is elected for five years and exercises executive power on behalf of the municipal council and the municipality as a whole. Nevertheless, the provincial governor has the right to supervise the mayor, and the Ministry of the Interior can terminate a mayor's term of office if necessary. Such cases have been rare in the past.

Political environment
The Grand National Assembly has final authority to decide matters at the national level. In the past it controlled administrative agencies directly, but a substantial part of this power has been given to the Government, which has been the executive organ in the last decade.

The Grand National Assembly has a system of standing committees, one being the Committee on Health and Social Affairs. The political parties are proportionally represented in the committees.

All proposals are referred to related committees before being discussed by the Assembly. Most lobbying activities and interaction between parties take place in the committees. The committees may invite civil servants and experts for consultation. Their meetings are open to journalists provided that no confidential matter is on the agenda.

In the past, health was not a priority for any political party. The first priority has tended to be to economic development. Although some parties may have announced health policies and proposed clear solutions, as these solutions generally depend on economic and other social developments, they are often postponed and obscured by other issues that are given higher priority.

The Supreme Health Council, chaired by the Minister of Health, formally advises the Minister on health policies. It has permanent members who are also senior administrators of the Ministry of Health and members selected by the Minister for a two-year period. The Council meets at least once a year to discuss national health policies and problems. Since it is only an advisory body, however, its meetings have become more of a formality recently. As in every democratic country, nongovernmental organizations influence policy-making. However, the interaction between nongovernmental organizations, the Government and the Grand National Assembly is not formally defined in most cases.

The nongovernmental organizations, including professional associations (such as the Turkish Medical Association), trade unions, related societies and charity organizations, declare their views and use the mass media and bilateral meetings to try to reach their counterparts. Nevertheless their voice is not as loud as that of the organizations in many other western countries.

Policy environment
Turkey has had six five-year development plans starting from the early 1960s. These plans were made centrally and represented the views held by the Government at the time they were made. One of the major difficulties with the plans was that none of the past governments stayed in power during the planning and implementation phases. Subsequent governments amended the plans, which weakened their reliability. Moreover, the policies outlined in the plans were occasionally contrary to what actually happened. For example, although one government announced the objective of reducing the number of very small hospitals, the number of such hospitals actually increased during its period of governance. This reflects the fact that most policy intentions have been inadequately specified: the objectives have not been translated into precise, short-term policy measures. None of the plans (except, to some extent, the sixth plan) defined measurable targets. This might be because health services and their quality are not assessed. Above all, however, the major weakness of the planning procedure in Turkey has been the failure to develop health plans on a regional basis. Provincial health directors and regional and local institutions are not involved sufficiently in the planning process. This creates problems in adapting the plans to regional and provincial circumstances.

Developing health for all policy
Governments in Turkey have been considering revising the health care system since socialized health services were introduced in the early 1960s. The WHO-supported project for strengthening primary

health care in Turkey, which started in 1979 soon after the Alma-Ata Declaration, provided hope for those who favoured change, but the project went no further than theoretical work.

There were some efforts to strengthen primary care and especially the health centres, but there were no attempts to implement fundamental changes in the system until the late 1980s. Recent attempts in Turkey started as independent projects by three separate groups. These projects arrived at a common conclusion: health care reform is needed.

Collaboration between the Ministry of Health and the World Bank

At an international meeting, the Turkish participants were informed that the World Bank was interested in supporting health development activities in individual countries. Meanwhile, Turkey's Treasury Undersecretariat had already signed a credit agreement with the World Bank and asked several ministries whether they would like to take part. After returning to Turkey, the group of civil servants made an agreement between the Ministry of Health and the Undersecretariat that enabled a World Bank mission to assess health status in Turkey. The assessment was carried out in 1987 and led to a further agreement for developing primary health care in Turkey. Thus, the first World Bank project was drafted in 1988 and an agreement was signed one year later. A total of 32 World Bank projects on education, agriculture, municipalities, health and other areas are being carried out in Turkey.

Some 80% of the World Bank loan was devoted to developing health infrastructure in eight provinces and the rest to institutional development such as reorganizing the Ministry of Health, developing managerial capacity and conducting operational research. The project was first started in 1991. Interim reports until then stated that achieving many of the project aims required changing the health care system.

Master plan study of the health sector

The State Planning Organization is officially responsible for planning all public sector developments. In 1988, the Organization decided to conduct a master plan study of the health care sector to explore the problems of the sector and alternative solutions. The study was carried out by a consortium of firms from Turkey and elsewhere and was completed in 1990. The report outlined comprehensively the current situation of the sector and indicated the urgent need for changes in health care services. It produced four strategy options for developing the health care sector: improving the status quo; a free market strategy; a national health service strategy; and an intermediate option. The State Planning Organization chose the last option. Financial resources and technical support were needed to carry out further work and planning. The Ministry of Health had control of both the World Bank loan and the technical staff.

Collaboration between the Ministry of Health and WHO

In the 1980s some European countries adapted the regional targets for health for all to their own situations. The WHO Regional Office for Europe supported such developments and made efforts to motivate other countries to define their own targets. Turkey joined these activities in 1989 and drafted its health for all targets in 1990 with the technical support of WHO experts, producing a document called

National health policy of Turkey (2). Many of the targets seemed impossible to achieve, however, unless the health care system was changed.

Thus, these three separate studies, which were very much related to each other, coincidentally but fortunately drew common conclusions. In 1991, the Ministry of Health therefore decided to integrate them in a package of projects and redefined the tasks of the World Bank Health Project Coordination Unit in the Ministry. Now, the Unit is responsible mainly for three tasks: carrying out the World Bank projects, reform activities and activities to produce a document on national health policy.

A committee within the Ministry of Health was established to adapt the regional targets for health for all to the conditions in Turkey, and then ten subcommittees were developed. The subcommittees identified experts and scientists who would be invited to the discussions. Experts from Turkey and elsewhere contributed to the studies. Thus, more than 400 experts and representatives of other sectors and institutions were identified and invited to a two-day meeting to discuss the draft document in committees. Each committee prepared a report on its subject, and individuals and institutions also submitted their opinions. A consolidated report was developed evaluating the committee reports, various options, the policies of other European countries and the advice of WHO. After the opinions of various institutions about the first draft document were received, a revised document was prepared.

At this stage the Government changed. The new Minister of Health wanted a new policy document as a product of a continuous and long-term consensus-building process. Thus, the First National Health Congress was convened in March 1992 and attended by more than 500 people from the health care sector and other sectors. All other ministries, medical and dental associations, health-related nongovernmental organizations, political parties, the mass media, insurance organizations, the State Planning Organization, universities, private enterprises and pharmaceutical companies were represented at the Congress. Many came from areas outside the capital. In particular, the health directors of some provinces in which a World Bank project was in progress were invited. The participants discussed the national health policy draft document and the draft health sector reforms in working groups and plenary sessions for five days.

The reports of the working groups were published soon after the Congress and distributed to all participants and the mass media *(3)*. Thus, the health policy options and proposed reforms were opened to public discussion. Within six months of the Congress, articles appeared in newspapers and several panel discussions were broadcast on television. Many participants and institutions sent their objections and alternative solutions to the Ministry of Health. All these comments were published and distributed to all interested parties. Most of the discussions focused on the reform and proposed health care system changes, including the general health insurance system. The strongest objection to the health reform came from the Turkish Medical Association *(4)*, which published its approach as a separate report. The Turkish Medical Association was mainly objecting to the financing system on which the general health insurance system was to be based. This system proposed that extra premiums should be collected for health insurance. During this discussion period, groups from institutions and the Ministry of Health had several small meetings to explain their views in detail.

A select group of experts redrafted the document on national health policy *(1)* taking all these discussions and Congress reports into consideration. It was a distinctly Turkish approach to health for all, and not only defined the health for all targets but also explained the activities needed to achieve the targets comprehensively.

This document was then sent to the WHO Regional Office for Europe for evaluation. The Regional Office had some comments on the format and some targets, principles and strategies. Taking these comments into consideration, the *National health policy of Turkey* was finalized and published in April 1993 *(2)*.

The aim of the national health policy is to attain a healthy population with healthy individuals. The policy takes into consideration that healthy individuals and a healthy population cannot only be attained by services provided by the health care sector but that intersectoral policies are required.

The document has five chapters dealing with support for health development, environmental health, lifestyles, health services delivery and targets for a healthy Turkey. The ten targets in the fifth chapter are directly related to health, such as reducing mortality and morbidity rates. The previous chapters include the prerequisites and infrastructure for the final targets, and they are defined and written in the format of targets. Thus, the policy document includes 30 targets.

In contrast to the procedure in some other countries in the European Region, this document was presented to all members of the Grand National Assembly but was not to be discussed. If it had been, the discussions would have led to legislation that would then have prohibited the necessary modifications of the policy afterwards.

Equity

Equity in health is defined as:

- equal access to available care for equal need
- equal utilization for equal need
- equal quality of care for all.

This definition suggests a stepwise approach to equity. Each step has to be attained before the next can be achieved. If there is no health facility to which people can gain access, neither equal utilization nor equal quality of care could be an issue *(5)*.

Although substantial progress has been made in the past two or three decades in providing health care services throughout Turkey, access still needs to be made more equitable, especially in rural areas. The other components of the definition are also important in the areas of the country in which the access problem has almost been solved. Equal utilization is especially a concern in the outskirts of the metropolitan areas. The health care services are available at all levels in the metropolitan areas. Nevertheless, people who live in slum areas are of the lowest socioeconomic status, and most have no social security or health insurance and therefore cannot use the health care services that exist. This is mostly true for the secondary health services because the primary health services such as immunization and family planning are free of charge. Some disadvantaged people who have recently moved from rural areas and who do not know how to access the services may have difficulty accessing even the primary health services in the metropolitan areas.

Quality of care in terms of equity will probably be discussed at a later stage, but meanwhile, quality itself is being discussed. These discussions are oriented towards the most developed services, especially hospital care, which will broaden the current equality gap between urban and rural areas and between west and east. In conclusion, the national health policy recognizes equity as a main principle underlying attempts to achieve health for all. The document even emphasizes equity as a target (target 30) *(2)*.

The national health policy discussed equity at large, in financing issues, the development of health care facilities and human resources for health. Nevertheless, the policy document does not emphasize equity throughout. Further, even when equity is recognized as an essential principle, no explicit action is described than can lead to equity. The main instrument intended to achieve equity is the general health insurance system. Based on this policy, a law on a general health insurance system was drafted and proposed to the Grand National Assembly in 1995. The national health policy document had advocated that the law on a general health insurance system be enacted in 1993. This delay shows that there are some obstacles to the process. The policy requires commitment by the Government and activists to carry out activities to gain public and political support. Above all, political will to make changes is necessary. Unfortunately, the minister for health has been replaced four times, as have other high-level officials, since the policy document was prepared, which has greatly hampered the process.

A "green card" system was introduced as part of the proposed general health insurance system to attempt to reduce inequity. The poorest and uninsured individuals were to be given a card entitling them to free health care services. This model is far from satisfactory. Because of budgetary restrictions, the cardholders get free services only if they are hospitalized: outpatient services are not free of charge. Further, the procedure for issuing these cards is not uniformly equitable. The applicants' income must be under a certain level, which is very difficult to assess. Some of the poor people who really deserve the green card are not aware that they are entitled to it, and therefore do not even apply or cannot get over the bureaucratic hurdles to obtain the card.

The specific health targets in the policy document are intended to reduce inequity in a broad sense. Most of the targets are aimed at vulnerable groups: infants, children, women and elderly people. Health indicators show major differences between the regions and between the urban and rural settlements of

Turkey. The infant mortality rate is 44 per 1000 live births in the urban areas and 65 per 1000 in the rural areas. Almost all the health indicators are worse in eastern Turkey than in the rest of the country. Therefore, even if equity is not mentioned explicitly, it definitely needs to be attained to improve the health of the most vulnerable groups.

The document mentions specific programmes aimed to reduce the results of inequity, but the strategies for resolving them are not clear. Everything is related to financing, which is planned to be solved with a general health insurance system. To develop a model for the general health insurance system, research and data collection was designed. The results would show the extent of the uninsured population, and the premiums could then be calculated. The Ministry of Health therefore carried out a utilization survey and a cost analysis. The results and findings of these studies were taken into consideration in preparing the draft law on the general health insurance system.

A number of interest groups, such as the Turkish Medical Association and several experts from the universities, objected to the proposed law. Most of the objections arose from the principles of financing. The proposed system requires separate insurance financing instead of tax financing. Many of the opposing parties strongly advocate that the health system should be financed by tax revenues. These objections created a controversy around the new health policy and delayed the legislative process. The Grand National Assembly gave higher priority to other issues, and the general health insurance system was given low priority. The objections to the financing system are based on the fact that collecting health insurance premiums is difficult. Some 40% of the population are unemployed, do not receive payment for their work or are self-employed. This makes it difficult for the insurance system to determine the level of income of such individuals and hence to assess their premium and collect it. The concern is that the only groups paying the correct premiums will be government and private-sector employees. They will in effect be subsidizing all the others. In addition, about 10% of the population cannot pay any premium, which will be subsidized by the Government and thus constitute a burden on the budget.

Public participation

Turkey's national health policy recognized the concept of public participation long before the health for all principles were recognized internationally. At the national level, public participation was established through the National Health Services Committee in 1961. The Committee had members from all health-related sectors, as well as distinguished experts. It met regularly to review health problems and challenges to recommend solutions to the Ministry of Health. At the peripheral levels, each health centre had to establish a health committee formed by community leaders such as teachers, religious leaders and the village headman. This committee had to meet once every three months under the leadership of the health centre physician to discuss local health problems and to decide how to solve them. Nevertheless, neither the central nor the peripheral committees functioned effectively, probably for several reasons. The underlying factor is the traditional hierarchical and vertical managerial system, not only for health care services but for all the public sector. Thus, the central and provincial managers could not succeed in achieving public participation, which was relatively new; another crucial reason was the fact that the public is used to being obedient and passive, which resulted in unwillingness to participate.

When the need for a new health policy was recognized in the late 1980s, participation from a variety of groups became essential. Several interested parties, such as the professional associations, insurance organizations, universities and the mass media, defined the need. The Ministry of Health sparked action for change. One of the first efforts was to prepare a national health policy. Collaboration and participation in forming the policy was on a very large scale. The Ministry of Health created a committee that established ten subcommittees to identify experts and scientists. Thus more than 400 experts and representatives of health-related sectors were invited to a two-day meeting to discuss the draft document on national health policy (6). The document was reviewed several times by the participants and then sent to the WHO Regional Office for Europe, which responded in detail with proposed changes, suggestions and comments. This response was translated into Turkish, published as a booklet and disseminated (4). The comments of the Regional Office on the policy document were taken well and revisions made accordingly.

The participants in developing national health policy include all ministries, medical and dental associations, nongovernmental organizations working in health, political parties, the mass media, private and public insurance agencies, the State Planning Organization, universities, private enterprises and pharmaceutical companies. Most of these groups were represented at the national level, but the provincial governments and the health directorates were also involved locally. The participation in formulating policy was extensive, but the same collaborative effort was not organized or maintained for implementation, monitoring and evaluation activities and for converting the policy into legislation. Further, all responsibility for policy development was given to the Health Project Coordination Unit, which was initially established in the Ministry of Health for coordinating the health projects supported by the World Bank. Additional participation in the policy development process at the implementation and monitoring stages required proper channels between the Unit and the other directorates involved in delivering health care services.

Participation in policy formation has traditionally been limited to experts. The general public and other non-expert interest groups do not usually participate and there are no channels to involve the public. The opinions of experts outside Turkey, however, are valued and taken into consideration. In contrast to the usual practice, great effort has been made to involve as many experts and interest groups from as wide a variety of backgrounds as possible in formulating this policy, which resulted in a unique example of participation.

The proceedings of the policy formulation were disseminated to the public through the mass media. Articles in newspapers presented a global attitude but did not include in-depth criticism. If there had been well organized client and other interest groups, public opinion would have been reflected more explicitly. Thus, the opinion of the public (external parties) was not properly taken into account. The policy was discussed more by the health care providers (internal parties). The health providers and provincial officers had the chance to express their views and affect the policy formulators.

Intersectoral policy

Many sectors outside the health care sector are also interested in health for all. They are also willing to collaborate in activities planned to reach these goals. According to the Constitution, the Ministry of Health is responsible for health care services, but other ministries and institutions are involved in community health. The Ministry of Health is legally responsible for setting standards and coordinating activities. Therefore, the Ministry develops the main policies for health. The Ministry of Health defines the role of the other sectors, and they are asked to collaborate.

In 1983, an attempt was made to involve other sectors in making national policy by forming a council consisting of the ministers responsible for health, food and agriculture, social security, education and finance. This council would make decisions on setting priorities and strategies for health care services. The Minister for Health found this proposal unacceptable because it was thought to minimize and delegate the ministerial power to the other ministries. At that time Turkey was under military rule. In that political environment the legislative process was fast, and it would have been easy to legitimize this council if it had served as an advisory board rather than a decision-making body. This can be regarded as a missed opportunity.

Nevertheless, a recent trend is to include other sectors in the process of developing policy. In addition, other sectors also develop their policies related to health with the collaboration of the health care sector.

There have been several examples of intersectoral policy development in health care; one is the national activity plan for women's health and family planning (7). This was initiated by the General Directorate of Family Planning and Maternal and Child Health and supported by WHO, the United Nations Fund for Population Activities and the US Agency for International Development. They organized a meeting with five working groups focusing on infrastructure and logistics, health personnel, service provision, public education and information. The participants were health service providers from the hospitals, central level officials of the Ministry of Health, universities, the State Planning Organization, UNICEF, the Ministry of Education, foreign and local nongovernmental organizations and members of mass media organizations. Each group presented a report related to objectives and strategies. This comprehensive policy helped to start a strategic planning process. This intersectoral collaboration created new alliances, especially between the Ministry of Health and the nongovernmental organizations, and strengthened the old partnerships. This procedure for policy formulation is encouraging, but the results have not yet been seen.

Another example of intersectoral policy formulation for healthy lifestyles was related to smoking. In the late 1980s the Ministry of Health decided to take initiatives to reduce smoking, which was triggered by a WHO initiative on smoking. To brainstorm and develop various solutions, the Ministry organized a workshop and invited representatives of all related groups to express their views. As a result of this meeting, a permanent intersectoral committee was formed to take action. This intersectoral approach was successful in creating public awareness, but failed to be as effective after a few years. The main reason was that the programme manager, who truly believed in the programme and collaboration, left the programme. This is a common weakness of many programmes. The success and maintenance of policies and programmes depend on the leaders who believe in the issue and take the initiative. One might imagine opposition to an anti-smoking campaign because Turkey cultivates tobacco. Nevertheless, at the time, the Government owned all the cigarette companies and therefore had a monopoly; now private multinational companies have entered this market. Therefore, since the initiative came from the Ministry of Health (the Government), the tobacco industry could not oppose it, at least openly.

The Turkish Medical Association later considered this issue. They called a meeting and invited representatives from the ministries responsible for health, labour and education, nongovernmental organizations, universities and the mass media. This group called themselves the National Smoking and Health Committee and are still active in policy development. The members of the committee that represent the ministries are not as eager to participate as are the members representing nongovernmental and professional organizations. This is partly because the ministerial representatives are appointed to the committee by their superiors, in contrast to the voluntary participation of the others, and because the ministerial representatives do not have the right to take decisions for their ministries.

One of the most powerful coordinating bodies in Turkey for forming intersectoral policy is the State Planning Organization. The Organization's main task is to prepare the five-year development plans with an intersectoral approach. Health is one of the components of the plan. For each component, an expert committee meets that is coordinated by the State Planning Organization. The members of the committee are selected based on their expertise and on the principle of representing a diverse group of institutions and sectors. Each committee discusses the issue extensively from the perspective of every sector and prepares a report. The State Planning Organization consolidates the reports of the committees and prepares a five-year development plan to be submitted to the Grand National Assembly. The role of the State Planning Organization continues after the plan is approved, all through the implementation stage. At this stage, the Organization is responsible for and has the power to form links between the sectors to prevent duplication and establish the necessary cooperation. Any investment has to be approved by the Organization so that it is in accordance with the plan.

Turkey is under its seventh five-year development plan until the year 2000. Unconventionally, the seventh plan states in detail the principle and direction of reorganization of health care services. These statements reflect the previous efforts for health reform as described earlier.

Intersectoral collaboration is not an easy process. Nevertheless, each experience provides valuable lessons. Skills in defining the role of the health care sector in negotiations and in striving for common objectives have certainly been improved. The process has to be examined systematically to define the mechanisms for achieving intersectoral action.

Orientation towards health status

Monitoring and evaluation are the most important steps in policy development. In Turkey, the task is usually considered to be completed after a policy is formulated. There is great enthusiasm and participation in defining the policy and setting targets and strategies, which dies off gradually in implementation and monitoring. The policy document mentions that monitoring was planned. Some of the targets were quantified. These quantified targets were set for the reduction of infant, child and maternal mortality, mortality due to cancer and cardiovascular diseases and morbidity caused by communicable diseases and accidents. The indicators for these targets were the only ones to be monitored, because data collection and monitoring is very difficult.

Data are not collected uniformly and completely all over Turkey. Nationwide surveys are carried out every five years on fertility, family planning, infant mortality and some illnesses such as diarrhoea and acute respiratory infections. In addition, several surveys are carried out on specific topics. Unfortunately, data are not available on health-related lifestyles and behaviour, except some small- scale surveys on these topics. The large-scale surveys are very costly and usually conducted with the support of nongovernmental organizations and international agencies. These organizations are mainly interested in family planning and fertility in Turkey. The topics related to lifestyle and behaviour are regarded as secondary issues.

Thus, extensive monitoring is not possible and no specific group or division is held responsible for these activities. The related divisions of the Ministry of Health will conduct routine data collection and evaluation, but they are not expected to perform evaluation in conjunction with the national health policy.

The Ministry of Health is attempting to improve the managerial capacity of the provincial directors. Courses on epidemiology are conducted with the collaboration of Hacettepe University and the Ministry of Health to expand the capacity of health personnel in evaluation and monitoring. The Ministry of Health is allocating significant resources and efforts for these training activities. The trainers attended the Epidemiology Intelligence Service course at the Centers for Disease Control and Prevention and Emory University in the United States prior to organizing a similar course in Turkey. Eighty health officers have been trained in this course.

Another activity to develop the capacity of other health personnel is orientation courses. The aim of these courses is that the local health officials can orient the new staff in a province. The permanent local health officials were therefore trained in Ankara, to form a core group of trainers at the provincial level. When they returned to their provinces, they started to conduct their training programmes with central support. Although the effects of these two courses cannot yet be measured, it is believed that they provide an infrastructure for better management, including monitoring and evaluation.

As mentioned earlier, a major part of the health policy depends on health reform, without which most of the strategies cannot be implemented and targets realized. The first section of the policy related to support for health development depends totally on health reform. Since the Grand National Assembly did not approve the legislation and regulations, the reform could not be achieved. Although there has been some action towards achieving some of the targets concerning infrastructure, progress in these targets is not being monitored. One of the major barriers is that reform is perceived as a whole and there is not much will to achieve targets in part; everything seems to be pending until reform is complete.

One of the major general handicaps of policy-making is the fact that when the administration changes, the successor does not follow up on the previous progress. A similar situation was faced in the development of national health policy. A group of experts invited by the Ministry developed this policy but when the minister and the high-level officials changed, the new minister and his group did not feel obligated to monitor the health policy.

Since the policy could not be regarded as fully implemented, it did not appear to need to be revised. However, some parts of the policy have already been implemented in the current health services and are being evaluated.

Summary and conclusions

A written policy is an essential starting point for any administration. Objectives and targets should then be established and strategies to achieve these objectives should be developed. This general approach is also recognized in Turkey, but the policy formulation process is not linked to implementation. The administration does not feel obliged to work according to a plan. Another reason for not adhering to the policy could be that some of the policy principles and targets are too ideal and unrealistic. The targets and objectives are consciously set at an unachievable level to motivate the health workers, but this discourages the health administrators.

Services are not evaluated routinely, and the data collected are not processed into usable information and are therefore not used in decision-making. Decisions are usually based on the previous experience of the individuals involved in the policy formulation process or on political will.

The high turnover of administrators at the national and provincial levels of the Ministry of Health is another major barrier to adopting and implementing the health policy. If the core of administrators is not stable, a stable policy cannot be established.

One of the obstacles to progress was the poor communication between the newly developed Project Coordination Unit and the well established general directorates of the Ministry of Health. Each directorate is autonomous: all deal with different issues. The Unit functions overlapped in many ways with those of the general directorates. This created an awkward situation for them, and sometimes they felt left out from decisions that affected them profoundly. The Unit reports to the undersecretary of state and the minister; therefore, the link with the general directorates was intended to be established through these offices, but sometimes this linkage failed, which resulted in duplication of decisions and activities. Instead of working together towards a common goal, which would strengthen their efforts, they usually work separately.

The future is not easy to predict. Change is still needed, but the political environment and level of stability cannot be foreseen. The new Government is pursuing reform activities. The Grand National Assembly has not yet discussed the proposed legislation. New discussions will start at the Assembly, and the policy could be reformulated as a result. This may take some time, which will delay the process. One can hope that the achievements attained so far will be considered and built upon.

References

1. *Health for all by the year 2000. Turkish national health policy*. Ankara, Ministry of Health, 1990.
2. *National health policy of Turkey*. Ankara, Ministry of Health, 1993.
3. *Çalisma Gruplan Raporu Saglik Kongresi 23–27 Mart 1992* [Report of the Working Groups, First Health Congress, 23–27 March 1992]. Ankara, Ministry of Health, 1992.
4. *"Ulusal Saglik Politikasi" Taslak Dökümani Üzerine Görüsler* [Comments on the draft document *National health policy*]. Ankara, Ministry of Health, 1992.
5. *Glossary of terms used in the "Health for All" Series No. 1–8*. Geneva, World Health Organization, 1984 (Health for All Series, No. 9).
6. *Çalisma Gruplan Raporu Ikinci Saglik Kongresi 12–16 Nisan 1993* [Report of the Working Groups, Second Health Congress, 12–16 April 1993]. Ankara, Ministry of Health, 1994.
7. *Ana Sagligi ve Aile Planlamasi Ulusal Aktivite Plani Hazirlik Toplantisi Raporu, 26–27 Mayis 1994* [Report of the Preparatory Meeting for the National Activity Plan for Maternal Health and Family Planning, 26–27 May 1994]. Ankara, Ministry of Health, 1994.

England: a healthier nation

Diana McInnes & Ruth Barnes

This case study was originally written in 1996, when the Department of Health was about to commission a review of *The health of the nation (1)*, the health strategy for England. The timing was good, as the paper not only provided a case study for this publication but also an account of health policy to date as background information for the review. It was, fortuitously, a way of taking stock, describing the history of *The health of the nation* and giving examples of how it had been implemented up to that time.

Since then the Government of the United Kingdom has changed, and the values on which health policy is based have changed fundamentally. A much wider health perspective is now being taken; the Government is really committed to improving health status in the longer term by tackling inequality and the root causes of ill health.

As a result, a line has been drawn under *The health of the nation*. Although it has been important in raising awareness of health and many valuable programmes and projects have been developed under its banner, the policy is now being recast to broaden its perspective and scope even further. The Government published its proposals for a new health strategy in a consultative green paper *Our healthier nation (2)* in February 1998. It has a number of new themes as its focus, reflecting the Government's commitment to address the challenges of social cohesion and its effects on health. This is an exciting and challenging time of change. With health policy development progressing apace, we can never hope to give an entirely up-to-date or comprehensive account of progress in England. The case study therefore provides a descriptive historical account of *The health of the nation* from its inception to the time when the new policy initiative was launched in July 1997. The original text has, however, been revisited and revised in places with the aim of showing how the achievements of *The health of the nation* can be built upon and integrated into the new policy.

Introduction

History: main stages and political environment
Interest in and awareness of health among the general public in England has increased in the 1980s and 1990s. This was reflected at the Department of Health by a shift towards assessment of health needs and health care services oriented towards health outcome, which can be traced back to such publications as *Promoting better health (1987) (3)* and the 1988 Acheson report on public health in England *(4)*.

Promoting better health set out the programme of the Government at that time for improving primary health care. It focused on general practitioners, proposing significant changes in primary health care with regard to health promotion and disease prevention, and recognized the need for more extensive and better integrated work between and across disciplines. Fees were introduced for screening, immunization and vaccination targets were set, and additional resources were made available for the development of multidisciplinary primary health care teams. This initiative clearly marked the beginning of a shift towards a National Health Service (NHS) led by primary health care. This trend of reorientation will be continued by the new Government, as indicated in its white paper *The new NHS (5)*.

The Acheson report *(4)* set out the findings of a committee of inquiry into the future development of the public health function. The committee was set up in 1986 in response to two major outbreaks of communicable disease but, as a departmental committee, it could interpret its remit more widely to address not only the control of communicable diseases but also issues related to health authority responsibilities *(4)*:

- to review regularly the health of their populations and to define objectives and targets to deal with problems accordingly in the light of national and local guidelines;
- to relate their decisions about resource use to their impact on the health status of the population;
- to monitor and evaluate progress towards their stated objectives; and
- to work with other agencies and organizations to promote health.

These responsibilities were set out in a health circular *(6)* requiring health authorities to take action on the main recommendations of the report. The circular was also sent to local authorities.

There is evidence, especially in the form of annual reports on the health of local populations, that the Acheson report had a wide-reaching effect and that it greatly shaped the development of the public health function during the 1990s.

A further shift towards the assessment of health needs took place with *Working for patients (7)*, a white paper published in January 1989 and enshrined in the NHS and Community Care Act 1990 *(8)*. This brought health and health service issues to the forefront of the political and public arena.

Working for patients argued that, because demand is rising and advances in medical technology enable an ever widening range of treatment, public expectations of the health service have not been matched by an increase in resources. It was argued that tackling this problem required reviewing and reforming how health care was structured and managed. The specific recognition that health authorities are responsible for health in a defined geographical community was a key measure of the reforms, especially in relation to public health, although health care services became the dominant feature of health authority activity.

The NHS in the United Kingdom is based on the principle of universal access, regardless of income, to care financed mainly by general taxation. *Working for patients (7)* reiterated these principles but recognized that there were was wide variation in the quantity, quality and cost of health services across the country. It aimed to raise the performance of all hospitals and general practices to that of the best. The means of achieving this were controversial – the creation of an internal market and general practitioner fundholding. Its stated objectives were *(7)*:

- to give patients, wherever they live in the United Kingdom, better health care and greater choice of the services available; and
- greater satisfaction and rewards for those working in the NHS who successfully respond to local needs and preferences.

The ways in which these objectives were pursued via the NHS and Community Care Act 1990 were controversial. The introduction of an internal market did create some evidence that it led to a strong competitive culture in the NHS and that, in turn, led to greater inequality in access to health care. Nevertheless, although the Government at that time was mostly interested in health care rather than in health, discussions began within the Department of Health that were to mark the start of the development of a formal health (as opposed to a health service) policy. A "green paper", a consultative document on a strategy for health for England *(9)*, was published in 1991 followed by *The health of the nation* white paper in 1992 *(1)*. Health policies have also been developed in Wales, Scotland and Northern Ireland.

Criteria used in defining policy and in setting goals, objectives and targets
England's health policy acknowledged the health for all approach of WHO *(10)*, albeit only in passing, which is reflected by the overall goal of *The health of the nation (1)*:

> to secure continuing improvement in the general health of the population of England by:
>
> adding years to life: an increase in life expectancy and reduction in premature death; and
> adding life to years: increasing years lived free from ill-health, reducing or minimising the adverse effects of illness and disability, promoting healthy lifestyles, physical and social environments and, overall, improving quality of life.

The consultative document *(9)* proposed three criteria for selecting key areas within this overall goal:

- the area should be a major cause of premature death or avoidable ill health;
- effective interventions should be possible, offering significant scope for improvement in health; and
- it should be possible to set objectives and targets, and monitor progress towards them.

The criteria were restated in *The health of the nation (1)*.

Emphasis of the health policy
The consultative document *(9)* identified 16 possible areas in which objectives and targets could be set. They were selected from the many ideas put on the table, and more were proposed during the consultation

period. Each area was carefully considered; trends in England and abroad, the potential scope for improvement through prevention, treatment and rehabilitation, and the possibility of setting realistic objectives and targets by which progress towards them could be monitored were examined.

Although there was scope for improvement in many fields, it was considered impractical to have a large number of target areas. It was decided initially to focus efforts on five key areas, which represented the beginning of a rolling programme for priority action. The key areas were:

- coronary heart disease and stroke
- cancers
- mental illness
- HIV infection, AIDS and sexual health
- accidents.

Political considerations were also important when the criteria were applied, and some weight was given to the views of groups wielding power and influence in the policy-making process. As a result, close scrutiny of the key areas, and especially of the objective and target areas within them, reveals that not all the target areas meet the three criteria for selection, although all can be considered important within the overall spirit of the policy.

The framework for implementation programmes within each key area especially emphasized *(9)*:

- public policies: by policy-makers at all levels, not only across government but also in other public bodies and industry, considering the health dimension when developing policies;
- healthy surroundings: by the active promotion of physical environments conducive to health – in the home, in schools, at work, on the roads, at leisure and in public places;
- healthy lifestyles: by increasing knowledge and understanding about how the way people live affects their health, and enabling families and individuals to act upon this; and
- high-quality health services: by identifying and meeting the health needs of local populations and securing the most appropriate balance between health promotion, disease prevention, treatment, care and rehabilitation.

The wider policy environment

When the first discussions about the possible shape and content of a national health policy were held, indicators of health service activity such as hospital waiting lists and ambulance response times were emphasized. This closely matched the *Working for patients (7)* approach and ideas relating to health service delivery and individual patient care. It was followed up through the *Patient's Charter (11)* and the Patient's Charter targets, for which *The health of the nation* had set the scene. In terms of health policy, however, the focus of thinking subsequently shifted towards wider health issues, and health policy was put firmly on the agenda alongside health care reform.

The health of the nation (1) was published in July 1992; it had a broad appeal and received a positive response within the Government as a whole as well as gaining cross-party support, at least for the principles and concepts underlying it. In addition, professional organizations such as the British Medical Association provided a high level of support.

The WHO Regional Office for Europe also welcomed the policy document and has used it in its policy development work with other European Member States.

Equity

Health policy largely emphasized the individual, and it was not widely acknowledged in government that socioeconomic factors affect the health of individuals or communities. The new Government has a quite different approach, being firmly committed to a more socially equitable and cohesive society, and working towards this goal is a major theme running throughout all its policies. It has established a Social Exclusion Unit for the purpose of addressing inequity in all areas, including health. This approach has been welcomed in most quarters, not least in health and health services, where it legitimizes a health for all approach with existing initiatives and allows new ones to be developed.

This section on equity does not attempt to look into the future but rather describes the base, laid by *The health of the nation*, on which England can now build.

Scope of the policy

The health of the nation recognized that, in framing action within the key areas, the needs of specific groups of the population had to be considered, and the challenges addressed within each key area needed to be disaggregated to ensure that the policy was relevant to all sectors of the population.

The health of the nation referred specifically to infants and children, elderly people, women, people from black and other ethnic minority groups, people from specific socioeconomic groups, people with physical or sensory disabilities or learning disabilities and others.

For example, the differential morbidity and mortality rates between ethnic minority groups and the white population and between individual ethnic minority groups in many of the key areas were recognized. A report on ethnicity and health *(12)* was published in 1994 as part of the series of documentation related to *The health of the nation*.

The Black report *(13)* and *The health divide (14)*, published in 1980 and 1988 respectively, documented in detail the inequalities in health status between different population groups and especially those between people in different socioeconomic categories.

The previous Government considerably underplayed this evidence, and especially that related to the socioeconomic determinants of health, but *The health of the nation* did acknowledge that inequalities in health status persisted as of the early 1990s in England, as they did in all other industrialized countries. The rates of illness and death are generally higher in social classes III(M), IV and V, and this pattern holds for all the key areas except for breast cancer (for which the rates are higher among women from social classes I and II), malignant melanoma and possibly HIV infection, for which hard evidence is less readily available.

Recognition and concepts of equity

Although inequality in health status was acknowledged initially, it was referred to subtly. The concept of equity was not defined explicitly and thus equity was not given high priority at the national level. The Government was reluctant to concede the inequitable nature of some types of variation in health status and to recognize the need to tackle such variation by implementing wide-ranging, intersectoral health and social policies.

As a result, *The health of the nation* was strongly criticized in some quarters for merely paying lip service to equity, and the term used – inequity and inequality were referred to as "variations" – reflects this. Nevertheless, given the ideological climate, the fact that *The health of the nation* mentioned inequality at all was an achievement for health campaigners.

The Chief Medical Officer produces an annual report on the state of the public health as part of a series that began in 1858. Each year the report documents changes in the health status of the population, tries to interpret and explain the changes and identifies areas for improvement. Specific issues are usually highlighted for special mention. In 1994, one of the four key issues identified for broader discussion during the coming years was equity and equality *(15)*.

In addition, Priorities and Planning Guidance issued to the NHS in 1994–1995 (EL(93)54, Section A, 29 June 1993) was explicit that inequity in health needed to be addressed. It asked health authorities to "address variations in health status between regions and between social groups", and the 1995–1996 Guidance (EL(94)55 Paragraph 5, 22 July 1995) stated that "services should not only improve the health of the population as a whole, but should aim to reduce variations by targeting resources where needs are greatest". The Priorities and Planning Guidance in subsequent years (1996–1997 and 1997–1998) underlined this policy, with equity continuing to be of central importance to the NHS and *The health of the nation* being seen as a major vehicle for policy implementation.

Locally, within the NHS and elsewhere, existing initiatives were designed to tackle inequity in health, but there was little practical central guidance on effective intervention to address inequity, and the initiatives tended to be piecemeal and at the margins of mainstream health service activity. Given the great deal of evidence about the differences in health status, the paucity of information on evaluated interventions, and the Department of Health's central role in achieving the overall goals of *The health of the nation*, the

Chief Medical Officer established a working group in 1994 to investigate what the Department of Health and the NHS could do to address inequity in health status. The working group published its findings in October 1995 as *Variations in health (16)*. The publication was publicized via a parliamentary question and a press release was issued; 3500 copies were printed and circulated freely and widely. A second print run had to be ordered within a week, reflecting the level of interest in the issue among the NHS and the public. The publication was free of charge and went to a third print run in February 1996.

Objectives and targets: identification of vulnerable groups

In the last two decades, extensive research has been published showing continuing – and sometimes increasing – differences in mortality and morbidity rates between socioeconomic groups, men and women, regions of the United Kingdom and ethnic groups. *Variations in health (16)* started to compile information from numerous studies that identify vulnerable groups and the underlying reasons for their vulnerability.

A subsequent research initiative has sought to commission further work emphasizing understanding and tackling the wider socioeconomic determinants of health.

Programmes for vulnerable groups

Health status is unequal between different groups within all the key areas of *The health of the nation*. The experience of the most healthy group within each area indicates what can be achieved. An important way of achieving the targets set by *The health of the nation* was by bringing the health experience of those in the least healthy groups closer to that of the most healthy groups. Indeed, without specific attention to vulnerable groups, inequality in health would prove a potentially serious barrier to achieving the targets.

National initiatives

At the national level, action was taken across a number of areas and is likely to be continued and strengthened when *Our healthier nation (2)* comes into play.

For some years the formula for allocating funds to health authorities has taken account of the characteristics of the resident population by weighting by needs indices, which include socioeconomic factors. General practitioners prepared to work in deprived areas also receive additional payments. This is potentially an excellent instrument for improving health, especially as additional payments could be made for activities directly related to health policy priorities.

General measures such as public health intervention and health promotion and disease prevention programmes directed at the whole population influence the most vulnerable groups. Although inequity in health status and differences between population groups persist, the health of all groups has been influenced by taking a population-based approach to health promotion and by promoting healthy public policies. Nevertheless, the benefits of this approach are differential and tend to increase inequality rather than reduce it.

The establishment of the Chief Medical Officer's Working Group on Variations and the publication of its report *(16)*, together with the launch of a £2.4 million research initiative in 1996, are key to the further understanding of variations in health status and how they can be dealt with effectively.

Before *The health of the nation* was published, such initiatives as campaigns to stop rickets and to promote health among Asian mothers and babies targeted specific population groups. Since *The health of the nation* was launched, a much wider range of activities has been encouraged, including:

- central funding for 35 projects to deliver primary care services to homeless people, refugees and travellers and to help them integrate into mainstream health services;
- an anti-smoking campaign targeting social groups III(M), IV and V;
- funding of services for young people experimenting with drugs or at particular risk of drug misuse; and
- the Ethnic Health Unit, which was established to help the NHS improve access to services for ethnic minorities and to provide services sensitive to their needs.

Local initiatives: making local health policy successful

At the local level, initiatives and implementation programmes involve alliances between a range of groups such as housing associations, voluntary organizations, social services and other local authority departments, schools and employers.

The NHS takes action in a number of areas, independently and in partnership with other organizations. In particular, health authorities may be concerned with assessing health needs to identify the groups at greatest risk, monitoring and improving access to services, and targeted health promotion.

For example, an initiative in south-east England is establishing two health think tanks to identify the reasons for poor health in three electoral wards. The members of the think tanks are people who have special knowledge of the area. Interviews have been held with local people, and an extensive public consultation exercise was held to draw up proposals for intervention.

A London health authority assessed the health needs of black and ethnic minority people and refugees in its area. Its report *(16)* is based on a review of the literature as well as local studies and consists of four sections: a demographic profile, health and lifestyle survey, health care provision and recommendations for action.

The Liverpool health authority and local authority have launched a joint five-year city-wide health strategy that places poverty, unemployment and housing at the centre of their policy objectives.

Intersectoral action

A wide range of organizations are responsible for moving towards the goal, objectives and targets set out in *The health of the nation*. Nevertheless, the unique management relationship between the Department of Health and NHS Executive and the NHS has been used to drive *The health of the nation* forward at the local level through the NHS, which has been given responsibility for mobilizing local action through health alliances and exploring the common ground on health issues with other organizations and groups.

Variations in health (16) cites some instances of intersectoral action to address inequity in health. For example, the Coventry City Council and local health authorities have been working together to improve the level of health in a local housing estate with high rates of unemployment, single-parent families, crime and accidents and a lower average life expectancy than in other areas of the city.

The Exeter and North Devon Health Commission has produced an action for health plan in partnership with about 60 other agencies. Each section of the plan identifies a project, the project's objectives and which partner is responsible for taking action, by major setting and each key area from *The health of the nation*. This approach distils a broad interagency strategy into discrete projects with clarity about who is responsible for taking action. It also provides a framework for annual monitoring and implementation.

Research and training
Variations in health (16) supports equity policy and goes some way towards fleshing out the Policy and Planning Guidance to the NHS. In addition, it advises on the research needed to underpin the policy. At the end of 1994, the Variations Sub-Group of the Chief Medical Officer's Health of the Nation Working Group presented a preliminary report to the Director of Research and Development of the Department of Health, indicating that several types of research would be needed:

- evaluation of NHS-based interventions aiming to reduce health variations;
- research studies to inform the development of policy and practice to target action on population groups at higher risk of poor health; and
- longer-term theory-based work on the causes of inequalities in health.

These recommendations have been adopted, and the Department of Health has made significant funding (£2.4 million) available for research into health variations. It is also working with other groups such as the Medical Research Council to promote work in this area.

Some work has already been done in compiling information on the effectiveness of intervention to reduce inequalities in health status. The NHS Centre for Reviews and Dissemination at York carried out a literature review commissioned by the Variations Sub-Group *(16)*. The aim of the review was to identify types of intervention for which there is evidence of effectiveness in reducing variation in health status between different population groups. The types of intervention examined were broadly related to public health, including those that promote equitable access to services that could be provided by the NHS, whether alone or in collaboration with other agencies. The types of intervention covered sought to reduce inequities in the key areas from *The health of the nation*, general health, and other relevant areas affecting general health such as child health and development, health in pregnancy and nutrition *(16)*.

The findings demonstrate how limited is the evidence of the effectiveness of interventions in reducing inequities and how few tried and tested types of practical public health intervention exist for the NHS to use (or at least how few have been reported in journals). This indicates that more research is needed and that future studies need to be evaluated fully. The research initiative funding mentioned previously aims to address these needs.

Public participation

Central, regional and local groups

The formulation of *The health of the nation* was characterized by extensive consultation. Although the consultative document *(9)* was drafted within the Department of Health, it drew on a wide range of expertise. There was a formal consultation period of three months between the time the consultative document was published and the time the white paper *(1)* began to be drafted. A similar process will occur with *Our healthier nation*: a green paper to be published in January or February 1998 followed by three months of consultation before the white paper is prepared. For *The health of the nation*, a particular aim of the consultation was to involve a very wide range of organizations, including not only the NHS but also local authorities, voluntary organizations and others that had not normally been regarded as being of interest in health policy. More than 2000 written responses to the consultative document were submitted – a large number for a green paper – and many commented in some detail. In addition, many organizations published their own responses to the consultative document, and a series of related articles appeared in such publications as the *British medical journal* and the *Health services journal*.

The Chief Medical Officer and his staff compiled the responses, and 30 issues for possible selection as key areas were identified. Expert papers on all 30 issues were commissioned.

In addition to this written consultation, a series of regional conferences was held in which the Minister for Health, the Chief Medical Officer and the NHS Chief Executive participated. The idea was not only to disseminate the concept and idea of a national health policy using a cascade method, but also to invite comment from health authorities, local authorities and others on the content of the policy and on how it might be implemented.

More than 80% of the responses were positive. They confirmed that the concept being proposed was on the right track – developing a health policy at that stage was appropriate, and the timing was right. As a result of the consultation exercise, some of the targets set were probably more challenging than they would otherwise have been, although some, disappointingly, represented little more than an extrapolation of existing trends.

After the consultative document *(9)* was published, three national-level working groups were established:

• the Chief Medical Officer's Health of the Nation Working Group on health priorities;

- the NHS Chief Executive's Health of the Nation Working Group on Implementation in the NHS; and
- a Wider Health Working Group chaired by a health minister.

With the publication of the white paper *(1)*, a Cabinet Sub-Committee on Health Strategy was also established.

The Cabinet Sub-Committee and the Wider Health Working Group are discussed in more detail in the section on intersectoral policy (see page 223).

The Chief Medical Officer's Working Group comprised eminent professionals and academics from a range of health-related disciplines, together with representatives from the Ministry of Agriculture, Fisheries and Food, the Department of the Environment and the Department of Health. Its terms of reference were to advise on *(17)*:

- the monitoring and review of progress towards the achievement of targets in the five key areas;
- the more general epidemiological and public health issues concerned with the development of the health strategy, including identification and assessment of the effectiveness and cost–effectiveness of interventions; and
- the identification of new key areas.

Activity can be monitored in accordance with these terms of reference, but assessing the tangible effects of the Working Group is difficult. Nevertheless, anecdotal evidence suggests that the Working Group was worthwhile and was commonly referred to as a useful tool.

The Chief Executive's Health of the Nation Working Group on Implementation in the NHS was responsible for considering how the NHS should implement a health strategy in England, including how the NHS should be accountable for and deliver its contribution to the strategy *(17)*.

The NHS Management Executive (now the NHS Executive) also commissioned five focus groups, one for each of the key areas, to produce handbooks *(18–22)* on possible local approaches to the key areas. The aim of the handbooks was primarily to assist health service managers and directors in purchasing authorities and, for mental illness, local authority social services departments in developing local strategies for reducing mortality and morbidity. The handbooks also aimed to disseminate information about local initiatives and other relevant information. They were intended as practical guides to be used selectively and adapted to local circumstances.

Who has used the handbooks and how was not monitored, but anecdotal evidence suggests that they have been helpful reference and idea-promoting documents for health authorities and others involved in implementing health policy.

The recommendations of the focus groups were also compiled in *First steps for the NHS (23)*, which set out the range of possible actions for each level of the NHS.

Consultation continued on strategic implementation issues and on the future development of the policy. In July 1997 the newly appointed Minister for Public Health – the first ever such appointment in the United Kingdom – set out the new Government's proposals for health policy development. Although a line was to be drawn under *The health of the nation*, its achievements were acknowledged and the new policy will build on the best aspects of the old policy where appropriate.

Balance of central, regional and local responsibility and accountability

All government ministries were accountable for meeting the targets set out in *The health of the nation*, although the Department of Health, and especially the health promotion division, took the lead. Similarly, implementing programmes intended to ensure progress towards achieving the targets depended on shared responsibility for action with a range of sectors.

There has been only limited progress in practice at the national level in establishing a common agenda with a focus on health, partly because of competing priorities and the financial disincentives built into the organizational structure of national and local government. *Our healthier nation* and other initiatives by the new Government, notably the establishment of an interdepartmental Social Exclusion Unit, will address this issue.

Despite this, and the fact that the NHS agenda in recent years has been dominated by health services, on paper at least, *The health of the nation* remained at the top of the NHS management agenda as a central plank of policy for the NHS and formed a main context for NHS planning. The health strategy was reflected in service delivery contracts and in local initiatives. Meeting the targets was part of the baseline activity required of all health authorities, and was set out in the Priorities and Planning Guidance issued to the NHS each year. Equally, promoting health and preventing ill health were explicitly highlighted in some of the six medium-term priorities selected for particular management attention in 1996–1997. For example, in relation to the development of local health strategies, a move was made to promote more cost-effective purchasing and influence the shape of medical education and higher specialist training.

Local targets were agreed between the regional offices of the NHS and health authorities, and were reflected in corporate contracts. They were built into performance management arrangements with the use of fast-moving Health of the Nation indicators featured in the quarterly monitoring report to the NHS Executive. The NHS Executive worked closely with NHS colleagues to develop a performance management framework. This identified key questions on developing, implementing and monitoring local strategies to deliver objectives related to *The health of the nation*. Regional offices used these in their performance management discussion with health authorities. This was and still is seen as a crucial component in integrating health into the performance management agenda. Until now, it has had to compete against other initiatives such as the Patient's Charter and Waiting Times, which are easier to measure. It is hoped that the new *Our healthier nation* initiative, coupled with the white paper *A new NHS*, will start to redress this balance. In some regions measures have already been put in place to establish health as a high priority on the public policy agenda.

Health authorities had a key role to play in delivering Health of the Nation targets by emphasizing prevention and promotion more, both through the priorities they chose and through the contracts they negotiated with providers. The annual report of the director of public health of each health authority is an important component of such assessment and usually features local progress towards Health of the Nation targets.

NHS Trusts and everyone who works in them were well placed to deliver the health service components of the Health of the Nation strategy by involving all groups in the community they served – patients and their carers, visitors and staff – in the active participation and delivery of health care. Opportunities for this existed through the initiatives Health at Work in the NHS and Health Promoting Hospitals.

This shared responsibility for health as well as health care will continue to be important in the future.

Interest groups
Despite these clearly defined responsibilities and lines of accountability, neither the Government nor the NHS works in isolation towards the goals, objectives and targets of health policy. For *The health of the nation*, there was ongoing consultation with relevant interest groups, and local implementation programmes were established to tackle specific aspects of the policy in which employers, schools, voluntary organizations and others take the lead.

In addition, the key area focus groups were crucial in generating shared ownership of the policy within the NHS and among the health professions.

Communication with the public
When *The health of the nation* was published in 1992 it received wide-ranging media coverage and continued to do so, for example, in television programmes related to health. This was initially facilitated by press releases, conferences and advertisements in the national press. A short version of the white paper was produced for the general public and was available in a range of minority languages – Bengali, Chinese, Greek, Gujarati, Hindi, Polish, Punjabi, Turkish, Urdu and Vietnamese as well as in English. The uptake of these short versions is not known.

A year later, in 1993, in order to maintain momentum and keep the profile of *The health of the nation* high, the Chief Medical Officer issued "a challenge to every person in the country to take one small step to improve their own health". The challenge was printed on a leaflet with a list of suggestions for how people might change their health-related behaviour and was made available through general practice surgeries, health centres, libraries and other public places. Health authorities, local authorities and other organizations adapted the challenge to local needs as a focus for health promotion initiatives. Almost all government departments accepted the challenge widely and circulated it among their staff. About 2 million leaflets were printed, and the challenge also appeared in Manchester United Football Club's programme at one of its most important matches.

A range of further initiatives have since disseminated information about the health policy and raised awareness of health issues. Examples include the publication of a series of booklets on mental health, the establishment of the Young Quit programme to combat smoking among young people, and Health Education Authority campaigns to raise public awareness of the importance of physical exercise and of preventing skin cancer.

The Department of Health published a quarterly Health of the Nation calendar that listed some of the larger events planned for each year. The calendar was distributed to health authorities and voluntary organizations so that their staff had a constant reminder of *The health of the nation* on their office walls. Schools also had access to the wall chart following the launch of the Health of the Young Nation initiative in July 1995.

The Department of Health published a bulletin called *Target* every two months for those directly involved in developing and implementing health policy: 30 000 copies were circulated to voluntary organizations, health authorities, NHS trusts, health promotion units and others. It listed forthcoming Health of the Nation events across the country. As an example of the level of locally coordinated activity, the list of regional events for June 1995 showed more than 60 events in 17 health authorities and trusts, ranging from sun awareness weeks aimed at general practitioners, primary health care workers and pharmacists and the launch of a survey of young people's health-related behaviour, to a sponsored walk to promote exercise.

To raise the public profile of the Health of the Nation further, ministers approved action to enable the Department of Health to engage the services of a sponsorship company to secure private sector support for a limited number of Health of the Nation projects. Part of its brief was to adapt the Health of the Nation Meeting the Challenge logo, which could be awarded to companies whose aims and objectives met those of the Health of the Nation. This enabled the Department of Health to benefit significantly from unpaid publicity at events and on leaflets and posters.

International factors

The role of international organizations in developing health policy in England was limited under the previous Government, although the WHO health for all policy informed *The health of the nation*, especially in formulating its overall goals. Also, in setting targets, comparisons were made with other countries within and outside Europe *(24)*.

The new Government has a positive approach to international affairs and to the European Union. Greater international cooperation and collaboration in health policy development is expected in the future, and the United Kingdom is expected to be playing a fuller and more positive part in shaping European public health policies.

After the publication of both the green paper *(9)* and the white paper *(1)*, the Secretary of State for Health and the Chief Medical Officer visited the WHO Regional Office for Europe to discuss *The health of the nation* and received a positive response to it. Subsequently, the Department of Health welcomed visitors from abroad interested in the process of developing health policy and contributed to a number of international conferences and meetings.

Within the United Kingdom there is international cooperation, as the four countries – England, Scotland, Wales and Northern Ireland – work together and all were represented on the Cabinet Sub-Committee on Health Strategy.

The United Kingdom as a whole also has a role to play internationally. Following the signing at Maastricht of the Treaty on European Union, which introduced an article on public health, the United Kingdom advocated a coherent programme of action on all aspects of public health through the European Union and Council of Europe. This led in 1993 to the European Commission producing a Communication on the framework for action in the field of public health *(25)*, which identified eight specific areas (including AIDS, health promotion and drug dependence) in which European Union activity in support of Member States would have maximum impact on public health.

Some local health authorities have developed strong international links. For example, some regions have European coordinators, and the North West Region has worked jointly with the Valencia autonomous region of Spain in developing its Healthy Cities programme in Liverpool. More recently, London has joined Megapoles, a network of European capitals working together to develop health policies appropriate to the special circumstances encountered in capital cities, and is taking the lead in developing policies to tackle inequity in health status.

Intersectoral policy

Mechanisms to put health on the wider public agenda

Intersectoral policy was central to *The health of the nation*, and government commitment to it at the very highest level was demonstrated by the existence of the Cabinet Sub-Committee on Health Strategy. Its members included ministers from most government departments, including the Scottish, Welsh and Northern Ireland Offices. Their remit was broad: to coordinate government policies on issues affecting health.

The Wider Health Working Group, one of the three original working groups, also worked at the national level. Its members represented a wide range of organizations interested in health. These included public and voluntary sector groups such as the Sports Council, the National Council for Voluntary Organisations, Age

Concern, the National Federation of Women's Institutes, Rotary International as well as the mass media. Local government was involved through the Association of County Councils and the education sector through the National Association of Schoolmasters and Women Teachers. The Health and Safety Executive and the Health Education Authority had members on the group, as did many of the health professional organizations such as the Royal College of General Practitioners, the Royal College of Nursing and the Royal Pharmaceutical Society. Public health experts represented the NHS, and representatives from private industry, including an occupational health physician, also took part.

The terms of reference of the Wider Health Working Group, which was chaired by a health minister, were to advise on the wider public dimensions of developing and implementing the health policy.

The Cabinet Sub-Committee and the Wider Health Working Group contributed significantly to giving health policy and *The health of the nation* a firmer footing on the wider public agenda and helped to build national alliances. It is to their credit that many conflicting interests were resolved and that most of the organizations contributing to health policy locally as well as nationally now have good relationships. Although these developments are mostly intangible, they set the scene well for the new *Our healthier nation* strategy under the new Government.

Intersectoral policy was also promoted under *The health of the nation* by making healthy settings a major cross-cutting theme and advocating joint action in such settings as cities, schools, hospitals, workplaces, homes, environments and prisons. Taken together, these settings offer the potential to involve a high proportion of the population of England.

Alliances and partnerships

The formation of the Wider Health Working Group marked the first stage in identifying health-related interests and, in some cases, health-related policies in sectors not traditionally associated with health. In 1993 the Wider Health Working Group contributed to a publication called *Working together for better health (26)* concerned with alliances, recognizing that the greatest advances in health can be achieved most effectively when individuals, groups and organizations work together on common ground with shared objectives. *Working together for better health* gives many examples of alliances in action and also gives some guidance on how alliances and partnerships might be established. It outlines the contributions various organizations or sectors can make and reviews the likely benefits to these organizations of working in partnerships for health.

The Department of Health facilitated alliances for health professionals by publishing a series on targeting practice aimed at nurses, midwives, health visitors and dietitians. These publications set out the contribution health professionals could make to the key areas and overall goals, the implications for training and principles of good practice, with examples of what could be done. The Chartered Institute of Environmental Health Officers produced a similar document for its members with support from the Department of Health.

In many places the idea of intersectoral policies was not new. Some health authorities and local authorities, for example, have had joint planning groups for the care of elderly people for many years, and many health professionals have developed close working partnerships with personnel from other sectors, notably voluntary organizations. What *The health of the nation* did, however, was to recognize formally the value of such alliances and to give them more status and power.

In April 1995 the first Health Alliance Awards ceremony was held to celebrate the achievements of health alliances across the country. The awards were designed to encourage innovative partnerships for promoting good health. In the first year they attracted over 300 entries from more than 2600 organizations. The awards covered each of the five key areas, and there was an open category for alliances spanning more than one key area. In addition, there was a special national category and two prizes for long-standing excellence, which went to No Smoking Day and Healthy Norfolk 2000. All the winners were presented with a cheque for £2000 and a plaque. The other short-listed entries received certificates.

In 1996 an additional theme for the Health Alliance Awards was the health of young people, to tie in with the Health of the Young Nation initiative launched in July 1995.

National-level examples of intersectoral policies and ways of working

Healthy settings offer some examples of intersectoral work at the national level. For example, an initiative on healthy schools is being developed jointly by WHO, the European Union and the Council of Europe. This offers opportunities to reach pupils, parents, staff and everyone associated with schools and education. In England the Health Education Authority is working with its European partners to establish a pilot network of health-promoting schools. The United Kingdom formally joined the European Network of Health Promoting Schools in January 1993, and since then progress has been made in developing and assessing the effectiveness of strategies for shaping pupils' health-related behaviour, with the aim of safeguarding their long-term health *(27)*. A research programme to evaluate the programme, comparing 16 schools in the network with 32 other schools, ran until March 1997.

In May 1992 the former Prison Medical Service was relaunched as the Health Care Service for Prisoners, signalling an increased commitment to health promotion, disease prevention and treatment in a healthy prisons setting. All prisons are now required to develop health promotion programmes, and initiatives are being piloted in five of them *(27)*.

The quality of the environment significantly influences health. Alongside the promotion by *The health of the nation* of healthy environments as a setting, the white paper *This common inheritance (28)*, produced under the previous Government, set out targets for improving air and water quality. It highlighted such challenges as air quality standards, indoor air quality, drinking-water quality and exposure to ultraviolet radiation. All these are relevant to health in general, but ultraviolet radiation is linked specifically to the target of halting the year-by-year increase in the prevalence of skin cancer *(1)*. Building on this, consultation began in early November 1996 on the addition of the environment as a sixth key area. *Our healthier nation* will continue to give the environment high priority in the new policy.

In addition to the healthy settings initiatives, special time-limited Health of the Nation task forces were established at the national level to tackle individual challenges such as health in the workplace, smoking, nutrition (including its relationship to low income and patterns of food consumption), accident prevention and physical activity. All these have now completed their work.

Local examples of intersectoral policies and working

Many local examples of intersectoral policy for health already existed before a national health policy was formulated. The most well known of these are probably the Healthy Cities projects set up in Liverpool and Camden (London) as part of the WHO Healthy Cities project, which began in 1987. In addition, there are unofficial healthy city programmes, such as the one in Sheffield, and a nationwide network of about 75 cities, towns and rural areas throughout the United Kingdom.

The City Challenge scheme sponsored by the Department of the Environment aimed to address the problems of run-down urban areas and involved local partnerships of local authorities and the public, private and voluntary sectors. Health programmes were incorporated into many of the City Challenge schemes. Many were capital programmes, such as building new health centres, and several projects encouraged broad participation in activities that tackled key determinants of health, including the local environment and housing conditions *(1,16)*.

Middlesbrough provides one example of how the City Challenge scheme could coordinate and integrate programmes and stimulate local partnerships to improve environmental conditions. A comprehensive health package was developed to include a health superstore, four healthy houses, ten health councillors from the local community, health education programmes, an epidemiological study and an air quality survey.

The health of the nation provided a national framework into which these programmes fit and boosted local intersectoral action, often coordinated through public health directorates of health commissions or through health policy officers within the local authorities. *Our healthier nation* will take this idea much further by emphasizing the determinants of health and the root causes of ill health.

A further demonstration of the extent to which *The health of the nation* influenced local thinking comes from a previous Lord Mayor of London, a consultant surgeon, who took up health as a theme for his term of office. The aim was to raise the profile of health, focused on *The health of the nation*, in the City of London. In support of this initiative, the Department of Health seconded a member of staff to the Lord Mayor's office. Now, in an ideological atmosphere in which health inequalities and the importance of a wider health agenda are seen as a top priority of the Government, even more effective partnerships are expected to develop to improve the health of local populations.

Support, research and training

Intersectoral policy is initiated locally according to identified need. Financial support may be provided from local or national funds. For example, about £500 000 was earmarked to support health policy development by voluntary organizations.

Training explicitly related to national health policy is piecemeal, although some medical schools, schools of nursing and social science faculties include the national health policy as an optional course on the syllabus. In some regions, however, discussions are beginning that aim to integrate medical and non-medical public health training.

There are also national initiatives to support and foster training based on health (as opposed to ill health). In October 1995, to promote debate about health policy in the medical schools, the Chief Medical Officer launched an essay prize for medical students on Health of the Young Nation. The Department of Health also produced a special Health of the Nation pack for hospital doctors *(29)* and a similar one for general practitioners.

The Health Education Authority, in its professional education programmes, is producing training modules on health policy and health promotion for a wide range of health professionals, and the Standing Conference on Postgraduate Medical and Dental Education has produced reports on the implications of *The health of the nation* for postgraduate medical and dental training.

Orientation towards health status

Monitoring

The health of the nation had 27 targets relating to mortality, morbidity and risk factors. The targets were identified by a variety of processes, such as review of recent and projected trends; examination of international data relating to current levels, recent past trends and existing or proposed targets; consideration of possible effects of current and future interventions; and review of recommendations made by experts. National progress towards the targets was monitored by the Central Health Monitoring Unit of the Department of Health in collaboration with the Statistics Division.

Immediately after *The health of the nation* was launched, the Central Health Monitoring Unit published a document *(30)* setting out key information that would form the basis of monitoring national progress towards the achievement of targets. *Specification of national indicators (31)* was also intended to be of use to those responsible for assessing and monitoring progress at local level. The document presented for each target detailed information on the indicators to be used, definitions, baseline years, monitoring frequency and proposed subsidiary analyses of national trends. The major sources of monitoring data identified were routine statistics, national surveys and other indicators.

Routine statistics include:

- mortality statistics (Office of National Statistics): 11 targets;
- cancer registration statistics (Office of National Statistics): two targets;
- cigarette consumption data (H.M. Customs and Excise);
- gonorrhoea incidence rates (Department of Health); and
- conception rates (Office of National Statistics).

National surveys include:

- a health survey for England (Office of National Statistics, Social and Community Planning Research and Department of Health);
- general household survey (Office of National Statistics);
- a national food survey (Ministry of Agriculture, Fisheries and Food);
- an infant feeding survey (to determine the prevalence of cigarette smoking in pregnancy) (Office of National Statistics); and
- a survey on smoking among children in secondary school (Office of National Statistics).

Other indicators for which regular national monitoring data are not yet available include:

- health and social functioning of mentally ill people;
- suicide rates among severely mentally ill people; and
- sharing of equipment among injecting drug users.

The information sources identified were those required to obtain information for the direct monitoring of the 27 targets identified in *The health of the nation*. A new health survey for England was initiated at around the time the Health of the Nation strategy started. This survey, initially based on a sample of 3000 adults and focused primarily on cardiovascular disease, has developed in recent years in sample size and topic coverage. The availability of interview and examination data means that this survey programme now represents a key source of data for monitoring and developing the health strategy.

Two of the targets in the mental health key area lacked immediate sources of monitoring data. The Health of the Nation strategy provided an important stimulus for intensive development work since 1992 to develop quantifiable and robust data on the health and social functioning of mentally ill people and on the suicide rate among the severely mentally ill. This work is now at a stage at which quantified targets can soon be specified.

In addition to the sources already identified, a wide range of others were used to provide supplementary information on progress towards the achievement of the targets. Examples include:

- the National Psychiatric Morbidity Survey, which examined the prevalence of mental illness, social disabilities associated with mental illness, and service use and precipitating factors associated with mental illness *(32)*;
- the Confidential Enquiry into Homicides and Suicides by Mentally Ill People;
- the survey on diet and nutrition carried out by the Department of Health and the Ministry of Agriculture, Fisheries and Food *(33)*;
- the Health Education Authority health and lifestyles surveys *(34)*;
- the Health Education Authority health and lifestyles surveys of black and ethnic minority communities;
- the Health Education Authority Health Education Monitoring Survey; and
- the Department of Health statistical returns on screening for breast and cervical cancer.

Data relating to progress towards *The health of the nation* targets were presented and disseminated in a number of ways. Monitoring data were clearly an essential component of the two progress reports *(17,27)*. More detailed and more frequent reports were presented to the Chief Medical Officer's Health of the Nation Working Group so that progress could be reviewed and assessed in depth. Reports were also presented to the other Health of the Nation working groups and the Cabinet Sub-Committee on Health Strategy.

Detailed data relating to progress at the health authority level were disseminated by way of the Public Health Common Data Set *(35)*. This work, commissioned annually by the Department of Health, is derived mainly from Office of National Statistics (previously Office of Population Censuses and Surveys) sources, and provides comparative health data for a wide range of health indicators, including data on demography, fertility, mortality and morbidity. The data set is wider than the Health of the Nation indicators, and these now represent a major component and a key source of relevant data for local monitoring of health policy. The entire data set is disseminated on computer disks, but national volumes are also published, providing a summary of the key data and a range of graphic presentations of the data to enable informed comparisons. Local directors of public health use data from the Public Health Common Data Set in producing their annual public health reports, which draw attention to the major health challenges facing local populations. The five key areas often received substantial coverage in these reports; it is expected that *Our healthier nation* will continue to feature in them.

Many additional indicators were used at the local level to monitor performance in the five key areas. A recent survey by the NHS Executive identified about 500 indicators. The NHS Executive subsequently identified a limited subset of these to enable better tracking of implementation in and through the NHS. The indicators identified are generally readily available from current national data collection systems. Many annual reports of public health directors, at the health authority level, use the indicators and are important as part of the monitoring process locally.

Evaluation
The Department of Health provided support for local evaluation of Health of the Nation programmes and their influence on health status in the form of a set of health outcome indicators covering, for example,

maternal and child health and mental health, and through the Central Health Outcomes Unit, which played an important part in providing a framework for mapping the principal factors that can affect health outcomes *(27)*.

There is also a United Kingdom Clearing House on Health Outcomes, jointly funded by the four Departments of Health. The Nuffield Institute for Health at the University of Leeds was commissioned to set up the Clearing House, which collects, collates and disseminates information on assessment of health outcome. The Clearing House complements the work of such organizations as the Health Education Authority and the Centre for Reviews and Dissemination at York University.

In addition, the NHS Executive has produced two publications on assessing the effectiveness and cost–effectiveness of a range of interventions for coronary heart disease and stroke *(36)* and cervical cancer *(37)*. These aim to guide health commissioners in developing local strategies to assess the potential contribution that specific health interventions could make towards meeting Health of the Nation targets. Both publications draw on a wide range of recent research.

In 1996 the Department of Health produced a guide on *Policy appraisal and health (38)* as part of the Health of the Nation series of publications. It provides guidelines on health impact assessment, primarily in economic terms, for all areas of public policy and has received a good reception from health commissioners.

Review and revision
Two publications reported on progress in implementing *The health of the nation*: *One year on (17)*, an overview of progress in the first year, and *Fit for the future (27)*, the second progress report.

Fit for the future reported that the concepts set out in the white paper had become accepted as a central part of health strategy: health is no longer seen as the exclusive property of the health care sector. Instead, health professionals, hospitals, the NHS and the Department of Health have gained powerful and innovative partners and are working with them to develop health policy with the overall aim of improving health.

Fit for the future also reviewed progress towards the targets outlined in *The health of the nation* and concluded that the general trends were encouraging, with movement towards achieving the targets in many key areas. This might have been expected given the existing trends, but one notable success was the target for reducing the incidence of gonorrhoea which, because it indicates trends towards safer sex, acts as a proxy for HIV infection. This had been set for 1995 and was achieved ahead of schedule.

Nevertheless, for two targets movement has been in the wrong direction: the prevalence of smoking among schoolchildren had increased since the baseline year of 1988, and obesity had become more prevalent among men and women since the mid-1980s. The reasons for these trends are unclear, but the lack of committed policies on tobacco advertising and the heavy emphasis on individual responsibility for healthy lifestyles without considering the importance of opportunities, or lack of them, for healthy choices must be implicated to some extent.

The findings of both progress reports were presented at national conferences, and the Department of Health and other ministries provide continuous feedback to the Government. The mass media also retained a strong interest in health policy and frequently reported on issues related to *The health of the nation*.

A formal external review of the policy of *The health of the nation* was announced in early 1996.

Summary and conclusions

Hints and tips

Several difficult challenges have had to be tackled in developing a health policy for England. Although not all the answers have yet been found and the learning process continues, some lessons can be drawn from experience to date.

Consultation

Public consultation and the involvement of a wide range of individuals and groups at all levels and stages is crucial to implementing the policy. Without it, *The health of the nation* would have remained a paper exercise and the local ownership of the policy that has been achieved in some places could not have come about. This principle has been adopted for *Our healthier nation*, which will benefit from extensive consultation.

Communication

Communication of the concepts underlying the policy and of ideas about its strategic implementation is also crucial. A wide variety of mechanisms have been used in England, and this has helped to maintain momentum and to keep health policy high on the agenda. Anecdotal evidence suggests that the Health of the Nation calendar and the *Target* publication have been especially popular. *Target* in particular has been and continues to be an effective medium for disseminating ideas and examples of successful implementation strategies. In addition, publication of *The health of the nation* material on the Internet widened its potential audience considerably.

Timing

The publication of *The health of the nation* was especially timely, not only in terms of gaining support and commitment from the leadership of the Department of Health and other government departments, but also across the political spectrum. In addition, the then-recent NHS reforms gave new opportunities for health policy to be incorporated into health service practice. *Our healthier nation* is also being launched in tandem with a white paper on health services, and the links between them are being stated explicitly.

Commitment

As indicated above, commitment from the top is essential to the success of the strategy; this applies not only to the Department of Health but to all government departments, local authorities, voluntary organizations and others with a role in developing health policy. Such commitment, especially at the local level, has been achieved in part through the fervent efforts of enthusiastic individuals and in part through extensive consultation.

Content and focus of the policy

The scope of *The health of the nation* is very wide, but focusing on a limited number of priorities or key areas with challenging but achievable targets has been vital in ensuring progress. In addition, to avoid concentrating exclusively on a small number of challenges, overlying themes such as healthy settings and health alliances allow flexibility and encourage innovation in implementation programmes.

Incorporation of existing programmes

When the Health of the Nation initiative began, other activities were already taking place locally and within other government departments that could be described as health policy development: for example, at the national level, the Department of Transport's accident targets and, at a local level, the Healthy Cities programmes. One issue that had to be addressed was how to harness these programmes and to bring them under the Health of the Nation banner when there was already strong ownership in other sectors. This was done through communication, consultation and the promotion of intersectoral working. In many cases the pre-existing programmes continued as before but with stronger intersectoral links and with a wider health perspective.

Continuity

Maintaining continuity in the overall direction of the health policy despite changes in personalities, politically and across the board, has been a challenge and a problem. This has been particularly true at the Department of Health where, as staff tend to move between directorates, corporate knowledge of the process of developing health policy needs to be maintained. The importance of continuity is at least well understood now by ministers, who have ensured that the new health strategy builds on and expands the work done under *The health of the nation*.

Monitoring

Monitoring progress towards the targets was facilitated by the position of the Central Health Monitoring Unit, which is housed within the Department of Health. This was also advantageous in terms of having readily available statistical and analytical resources for setting targets.

Structure of the Department of Health and the NHS

The organizational structure of the Department of Health and the NHS has advantages and disadvantages for health policy development. On the one hand, the line of command from the Minister through the Department of Health to the Regional Offices of the NHS and, through them, to the health authorities means that it was relatively easy to disseminate the policy and to encourage the incorporation of *The health of the nation* into management structures within the NHS. Care had to be taken, however, to ensure that *The health of the nation* was not seen only as a national Department of Health initiative or, locally, as falling only within the remit of public health departments. This potential pitfall was overcome somewhat through the continued consultation and communication that underpin the process of health policy development.

The future

Keeping a longer-term strategy on the agenda and finding new mechanisms for maintaining momentum are probably the biggest challenges for the future of health policy in England. Internal and external reviews of *The health of the nation* are now underway, and these are expected to play an important role in supporting *Our healthier nation*, which is already revitalizing and encouraging interest in and enthusiasm for health and offering new opportunities for publicity and the launching of fresh implementation initiatives.

A second challenge is posed by target areas in which there has been little or no progress, and efforts need to be redoubled. In 1986–1987, for example, 7% of men and 12% of women aged 16–64 years were classified as obese, and the targets to be achieved by 2005 are 6% and 8%, respectively. There is evidence, however, that more people in this age range are becoming obese, as the current rates are 13% for men and 16% for women. This presents a problem to which no solution has yet been identified *(27)*.

Increasing teenage smoking rates (up to 12% among 15-year-olds in 1994, from 10% in 1993) are also disappointing, especially given the continuing reduction in smoking prevalence among adults and in the number of women smoking during pregnancy. The Chief Medical Officer has noted in recent reports on the state of the public health that the general acceptability of smoking is falling, but a more marked reduction in adult smoking may be required before teenagers' attitudes are affected significantly *(27)*. A solution to this problem is especially difficult to identify, as many options, such as legislation and fiscal measures, are politically sensitive.

References

1. *The health of the nation: a strategy for health in England*. London, H.M. Stationery Office, 1992.
2. *Our healthier nation: a contract for health*. London, II.M. Stationery Office, 1998.
3. *Promoting better health: the government's programme for improving primary health care*. London, H.M. Stationery Office, 1987.
4. *Public health in England*. The report of the Committee of Inquiry into the Future Development of the Public Health Function (Acheson report). London, H.M. Stationery Office, 1988.
5. *The new NHS*. London, Department of Health, 1997.
6. *Health services management: health of the population: responsibilities of health authorities*. London, Department of Health, 1988.

7. *Working for patients.* London, H.M. Stationery Office, 1989.

8. *NHS and Community Care Act.* London, H.M. Stationery Office, 1992.

9. *The health of the nation: a consultative document for health in England.* London, H.M. Stationery Office, 1991.

10. *Health for all targets. The health policy for Europe.* Copenhagen, WHO Regional Office for Europe, 1993 (European Health for All Series, No. 4).

11. DEPARTMENT OF HEALTH. *Patient's charter.* London, H.M. Stationery Office, 1991.

12. *Ethnicity and health: a guide for the NHS.* London, Department of Health, 1993.

13. *Inequalities in health: report of a working group* (the Black report). London, Department of Health and Social Security, 1980.

14. Whitehead, M. *The health divide.* London, Penguin Books, 1988.

15. DEPARTMENT OF HEALTH. *On the state of the public health: the annual report of the Chief Medical Officer of the Department of Health for the year 1994.* London, H.M. Stationery Office, 1995.

16. *Variations in health: what can the Department of Health and the NHS do?* London, Department of Health, 1995.

17. *One year on ... a report on the progress of the health of the nation.* London, Department of Health, 1993.

18. *Health of the nation key area handbook: CHD and stroke.* London, Department of Health, 1993.

19. *Health of the nation key area handbook: cancers.* London, Department of Health, 1993.

20. *Health of the nation key area handbook: mental illness.* London, Department of Health, 1993.

21. *Health of the nation key area handbook: HIV/AIDS and sexual health.* London, Department of Health, 1993.

22. *Health of the nation key area handbook: accidents.* London, Department of Health, 1993.

23. *First steps for the NHS.* London, Department of Health, 1992.

24. BARNES, R. *Setting strategic health goals: experience in other countries.* London, Department of Health, 1990.

25. EUROPEAN COMMISSION. *Commission communication on the framework for action in the field of public health.* Luxembourg, Office for Official Publications of the European Communities, 1993 (COM(93) 559 final).

26. *Working together for better health.* London, Department of Health, 1993.

27. *Fit for the future: second progress report on the health of the nation.* London, Department of Health, 1995.

28. DEPARTMENT OF THE ENVIRONMENT. *This common inheritance: Britain's environmental strategy.* London, H.M. Stationery Office, 1990.

29. PAINE, C. ET AL. *What you can do about it: an information pack by hospital doctors for hospital doctors.* London, Department of Health, 1995.

30. *Information to support health of the nation.* London, Department of Health, 1994.

31. *Specification of national indicators.* London, Department of Health, 1992.

32. DEPARTMENT OF HEALTH. *National psychiatric morbidity survey.* London, H.M. Stationery Office, 1996.

33. GREGORY, J. ET AL. *The dietary and nutritional survey of British adults.* London, H.M. Stationery Office, 1990.

34. OFFICE OF POPULATION CENSUSES AND SURVEYS. *Health survey for England.* London, H.M. Stationery Office (annual).

35. *Public health common data set.* Surrey, University of Surrey (annual).

36. *Assessing the options: CHD/stroke. Target effectiveness and cost effectiveness of interventions to reduce CHD and stroke mortality.* London, Department of Health, 1995.

37. *Assessing the options in the cancer key area: cervical screening.* London, Department of Health, 1995.

38. *Policy appraisal and health.* London, Department of Health, 1995.

Health gain investment for the 21st century: developments in health for all in Wales

Morton Warner

Introduction

Wales and its health service

The National Health Service (NHS) in Wales serves a population of 2.8 million people of diverse social backgrounds who are concentrated in the south and north of the Principality. Geographically, Wales represents great diversity within its territory, which is about 370 km from north to south and 240 km from west to east. Industrially, the tradition of coal mining has declined from 80 000 employees a decade ago to less than 1000 now. But the Welsh Development Agency has successfully attracted high-technology inward investment, which now operates alongside the farming, timber and leisure industries.

Through its 65 000 employees, the NHS provides a full range of health care services, including preventive and promotive activities, diagnosis, treatment, care and rehabilitation. Its total budget for the fiscal year 1995/1996 was £2.34 billion (US $3.74 billion).

For most of the period addressed by this case study (1980–1996), health care was managed through nine district health authorities (for hospital and community care) and eight family health service authorities (for general practitioner services – medical, dental and optical). Each authority had its own chief executive and a board made up of professional executive directors and government-appointed non-executive directors. These executives were responsible to the NHS Director for the performance of services in their areas.

From 1 April 1996, only five authorities remained responsible for all aspects of commissioning care. In contrast to previously, the geographical boundaries between health and social care services, which are run by 21 local authorities, are no longer contiguous, making joint planning very difficult.

Managerially, Wales maintains a health service separate from that of England, but the health service in Wales operates within a common policy framework established for the United Kingdom. Thus, the provisions of the National Health Service and Community Care Act 1990 *(1)* apply and, in particular, the purchaser–provider split, contracting and general practitioner fundholding dominate the scene. Some 53% of the population were covered by fundholding by April 1996; and three total purchasing pilot schemes, in which general practitioners control budgets that include provision for emergency as well as elective care, began on the same date. Money for the NHS and other public activities in Wales is voted by the national Parliament and allocated to the Secretary of State for Wales, a member of the Cabinet.

Care is provided by health care personnel working in 158 hospitals, 1800 general practitioners offering primary health care, 800 dentists and a wide range of community-based workers, all supported by a post-secondary health professional education system operating through universities and colleges in Wales.

Health for all in Wales

Three main events signalled the start of the health-for-all-type thinking in Wales. The Heartbeat Wales programme was set up in 1985 in response to very poor morbidity figures and high mortality from cardiovascular disease. In 1987, the Health Promotion Authority for Wales was initiated, which built on and considerably expanded the activities of Heartbeat Wales. In 1988, the Secretary of State for Wales decided to establish the Welsh Health Planning Forum which, chaired by the NHS Director, produced two significant documents in 1989 concerning:

- setting a strategic direction for the NHS, focusing on achieving health gain (reducing unnecessary premature death and improving the quality of life) across the spectrum – from health promotion to rehabilitation and monitoring *(2)*; and
- implementation at the local level, brought about by weaving the strategic thinking into the actual management of the health service *(3)*.

The Welsh Health Planning Forum comprised NHS personnel, civil servants and academics and developed the strategic intent and direction. The Planning Forum was an advisory subgroup of the Executive Committee of the Health Policy Board of the NHS. Its role was to give expert advice on the planning of health services. The Secretary of State for Wales chairs the Policy Board and the Director of the Welsh Office Health Department chairs the Executive Committee.

The political climate in the early and mid-1980s allowed official documents to refer to European and WHO activities, but this was much less the case by 1989 when these overall strategic documents were published. Thus, health for all was certainly central in the minds of those involved in constructing the strategy content and the implementation processes, but little reference to health for all was possible.

The broader context in the United Kingdom

The National Health Service and Community Care Act 1990 *(1)* and the discussion paper, *The health of the nation (4)*, which followed it in 1991, were the most important indications of overall policy shift in the United Kingdom since the NHS was created in 1948. The 1990 Act identifies how health care services are to be changed; and to complement this, *The health of the nation* begins to make more explicit why. Here, then, in public documents for the first time in the United Kingdom, there were overt signs of the influence of the WHO European strategy for health for all and its target-setting approach. Some of this influence had come via the experience in Wales and visits by representatives of the Government of the

United Kingdom to the WHO Regional Office for Europe. At a meeting of the Parliamentary Health Committee in 1990, members of parliament of all parties had asked the Secretary of State for Health why England did not have a strategy equivalent to the Welsh strategy for health for all. Indeed, the Welsh proposals received further endorsement when their more comprehensive approach began to be implemented in 5 of 14 regions in England and in Northern Ireland. Later, a number of regions and countries used the Welsh design in helping to format their own strategies, including Australia, Germany (North Rhine-Westphalia), Ireland, Lithuania, New Zealand, Spain (Catalonia, Valencia and the Basque Country) and Sweden (Östergötland County).

The strategic vision for Wales – equity and health

The key early contribution was the production of *Strategic intent and direction for the NHS in Wales (2)*. This document was published for consultation in November 1989. Following favourable comment by all respondents, the Secretary of State for Wales endorsed the document in July 1990. Specifically, he cited the strategic intent and direction as the management[a] target for the NHS to the end of the century and beyond:

> *Working with others,*
> *the NHS aims*
> *to take the people of Wales into the 21st century*
> *with a level of health*
> *on course*
> *to compare with the best in Europe.*

We must move, he said, "from the present National Illness Service to a fully comprehensive National Health Service". Echoing the document, he stated that, from now on, the NHS in Wales would need to concentrate effort on achieving health gain (adding years to life and quality of life to years), developing a genuinely people-centred service (valuing people as individuals and managing its services to this end) and achieving the best health return from the resources invested in it – in essence getting more and better out of what we have. Commitment from the top became self-evident. The vision, giving priority to health gain, was identified.

Health gain was seen as the key to achieving the strategic intent and direction. But the three themes – health gain, people-centred services and effective use of resources – were recognized as being interdependent and therefore had to be pursued concurrently (Fig. 2.9).

---

[a] Public administration in the United Kingdom, as elsewhere, often has a traditional divide between policy-makers and senior managers. Wales was no exception at this time; and the NHS management was seen as initiating a new policy thrust – which of course it had! The conflict was resolved by referring to the strategic intent and direction as a management target, thus using the best approaches of the satirical television programme *Yes! Prime Minister* to resolving internal conflict.

Fig. 2.9. Strategic intent and direction for the NHS in Wales, 1989

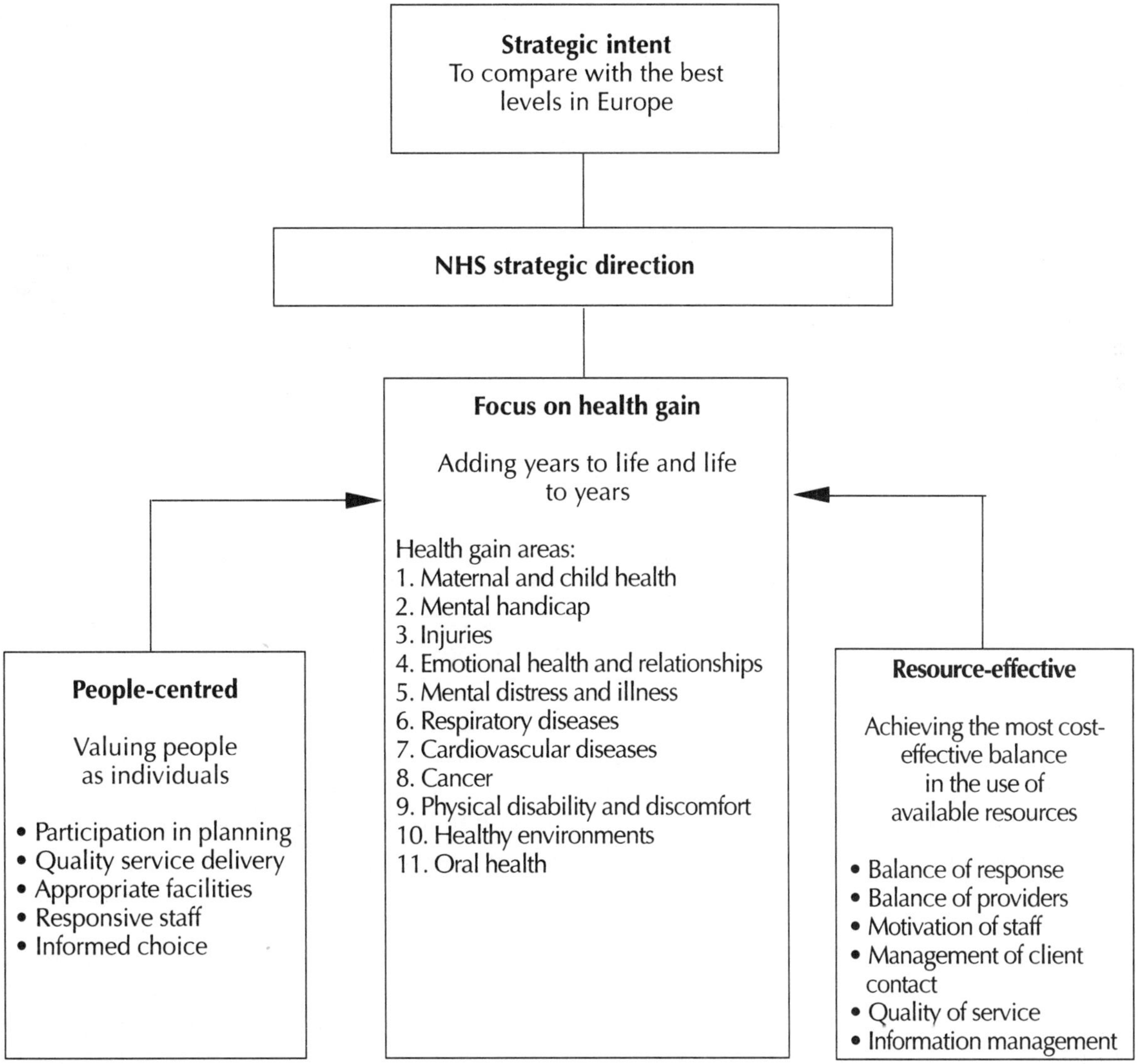

Strategic intent
To compare with the best
levels in Europe

NHS strategic direction

Focus on health gain

Adding years to life and life
to years

Health gain areas:
1. Maternal and child health
2. Mental handicap
3. Injuries
4. Emotional health and relationships
5. Mental distress and illness
6. Respiratory diseases
7. Cardiovascular diseases
8. Cancer
9. Physical disability and discomfort
10. Healthy environments
11. Oral health

People-centred

Valuing people
as individuals

• Participation in planning
• Quality service delivery
• Appropriate facilities
• Responsive staff
• Informed choice

Resource-effective

Achieving the most cost-
effective balance
in the use of
available resources

• Balance of response
• Balance of providers
• Motivation of staff
• Management of client
  contact
• Quality of service
• Information management

Note: Some titles were changed in the subsequently produced protocols for investment in health gain. Area 1 became maternal and early child health, other child and adolescent health being contained in Area 4. Area 2 became mental handicap (learning disabilities) to recognize the changing nomenclature and political climate. Area 4 became healthy living; as required by the Ministry of Health, the Government did not want to be seen to be interfering in individual freedom in relationships. Area 5 became mental health, to align with current nomenclature. Area 9 was disaggregated into physical and sensory disability, and pain, discomfort and palliative care, (*a*) to satisfy the disability lobby that the special nature of their problem was being accounted for and (*b*) to ensure inclusion of general aches and pains as well as pain control. Area 11 was later included as an important area that had been excluded for no good reason.

The NHS, like other health care systems globally, is not free from resource constraints. Priorities always need to be set. An emphasis on health gain helps clinicians and managers make good, cost-effective choices and releases resources to increase the pace at which gains can be secured. A focus on user involvement sharpens the management process and is an additional spur to effectiveness. A people-centred approach underpins health gain by encouraging a partnership between the individual and the NHS. As always, trade-offs often need to be made between policy directions, and this vital decision-making process remains at the heart of good strategic management. Nevertheless, there is a down side. Although it is possible, and perhaps desirable, to undertake planning (the protocol development process outlined in the next section) while applying the requirement not to increase spending (otherwise clinicians and managers would say "we can do anything if we get more money"), maintaining this stance when attempting a transition to the new way of operating was inhibiting.

The Welsh Health Planning Forum agreed that, although the Government of the United Kingdom had not yet decided to formally adopt the numerical targets contained in the WHO strategy for health for all, the starting point for Wales should be the principles of health for all: equity, access, quality of care, targeting (a form of positive discrimination) and community involvement. The Forum wove these solidly into the fabric of NHS planning in Wales.

The Forum identified 10 (later 11) key areas of health gain (Fig. 2.9). Although the list is extensive, the Forum did not suggest that all aspects of each area should or could be tackled at once. Objectives and priorities were to be set at the local level, guided by the actual or potential incidence and prevalence of illness and the corresponding requirements for promotive, preventive, treatment or rehabilitative services.

Throughout this time and beyond, the Health Promotion Authority for Wales continued to lead in developmental work and research. Its focus, however, was not confined to actions that the NHS might undertake; rather, it looked intersectorally. This gave rise to a perception of "separateness" from the NHS, of which the Authority was a special health authority, and to an apparent reduction in support for the NHS.

Achieving the most effective mix and use of providers within and outside the NHS was seen as being of key importance. Individuals, their families and voluntary and community associations were recognized for the role they play alongside the public and private organizations concerned with health and social services.

Several other notions formed the bedrock of the strategic intent and direction. Fundamentally, it outlined a new approach for the United Kingdom at that time: putting health need first and health services second. And even when services were being considered, the question of facilities was to be preceded by discussion first of programmes to respond to needs, and second the personnel and institutions required to run the programmes.

Mobilizing and implementing the strategy – developing participatory approaches

Of great importance was achieving the commitment of health and social services leaders from district health authorities, family health service authorities, county social services, professional associations, educational institutions and voluntary bodies. To this end, the strategy was launched before 280 of these leaders in November 1989 in a highly engineered event. The view had been taken that the Welsh Health Planning Forum should develop its ideas without the pressure of publicity and in the most cogent way possible. But a very active roll-out programme was designed.

In succeeding months, presentations were given and discussions held with over 800 senior managers, clinicians, professionals and voluntary group board members throughout Wales in a series of cascade meetings. More importantly, many of those attending agreed to set up study groups within their own organization using a video recording of the November launch displayed in a news bulletin style to give a sense of immediacy, of having been there. About 2000 more people were involved this way. Anecdotally, a year later a junior nurse in a hospital was reported to have asked whether a particular action would bring health gain – one measure of the penetration!

By the time the Secretary of State for Wales endorsed the strategic intent and direction, most health authorities had already adopted the approach informally. A formal timetable was then set out in a Welsh Office circular that had the support of authorities; and in November 1990, the Chairman of District Health Authorities and Family Health Service Authorities agreed to form a new partnership across organizational boundaries (thereby creating an historical precedent), to develop local strategies for health. At the same time, the NHS Director emphasized the need to integrate existing strategic health promotion work and to develop other strategies concerned with personnel (5) and information management (6).

Fig. 2.10 displays the overall framework through which the strategy of the health for all type was forged into the management and clinical consciousness of the NHS and the attempt made to improve equity, create local community participation and begin intersectoral approaches that ultimately might address the need for health and social gain and to place the responsibility for producing health beyond the NHS alone.

Protocols for investment in health gain

The purpose of the protocols

For the past few years, approaches have been organized in the United Kingdom aimed at establishing an evidence base for various aspects of clinical practice: the Cochrane collaborations (7). Clinical effectiveness is a major policy issue and is linked to better utilization of health care expenditure.

The protocols, produced from 1990 to 1993 (8–19), preceded these activities in the United Kingdom. They identify where further NHS investment would bring worthwhile health gain and indicate where

Fig. 2.10. The framework for overall implementation of the strategic intent and direction

```
              ┌─────────────────────────────────┐
              │  Strategic intent and direction │
              └─────────────────────────────────┘
                              │
                              ▼
              ┌─────────────────────────────────┐
              │        Health gain areas        │
              └─────────────────────────────────┘
                              │
  ┌──────────────┐            ▼
  │ Health plan for│         ┌─────────────────────┐
  │     Wales     │         │      Protocols      │────┐
  └──────────────┘         └─────────────────────┘    │
         ▲                  ┌─────────────────────┐    │
         │                  │     Contracting     │    │
         │                  └─────────────────────┘    │
         │                         ▲ ◀─────────────────┘
         │                  ┌─────────────────────┐
         │                  │   Local strategies  │
         │                  └─────────────────────┘
         │                         ▲        "Commissioning"
         │                  ┌─────────────────────┐
         └──────────────────│    Assessment of    │
                            │   community needs   │
                            └─────────────────────┘
```

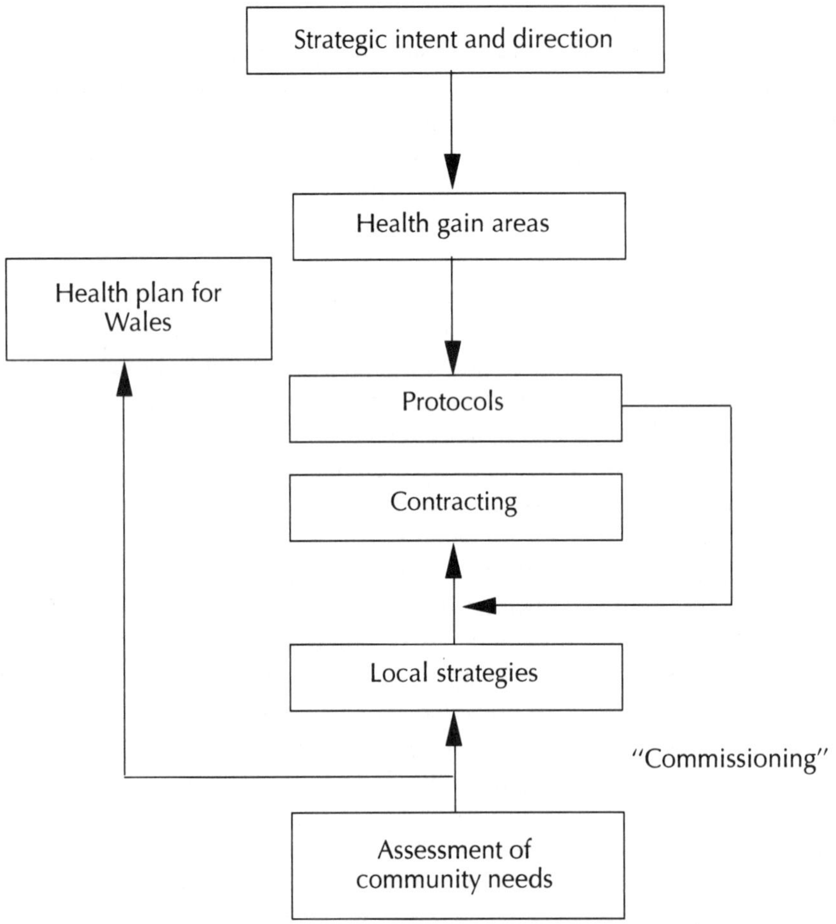

current practices are questionable and reinvestment might be considered. Of importance, many of the issues identified could be addressed at minimal cost, whereas others, over time, involved the reallocation of resources.

Engaging clinicians, managers and the voluntary sector
The approach used for the production of each protocol was important. Clinicians of all types, managers, self-help and voluntary groups, researchers and educators were brought together from across Wales to form three panels of review – for health gain, people centredness and resource effectiveness; they were assisted by internationally recognized experts. Thus, multidisciplinary expertise and wide geographical representation were combined to ensure broad ownership of the product. The panel members, as opinion

leaders, became ambassadors for implementation in their own districts; about 80 were working voluntarily with the Planning Forum at any one time.

The protocols were mainly addressed to the board members of the health authorities to assist them in developing their local strategies for health and a contracting process. Health care providers, local authorities, community health councils and the voluntary sector also found them of value in beginning to set priorities.

Protocols – the conceptual framework
Two sets of items delineated the final form of the protocols. First, it was recognized that a balance had to be struck between the three elements of the strategic intent and direction – health gain, people centredness and resource effectiveness. Second, all aspects of the NHS – prevention and promotion, diagnosis, treatment and care, and rehabilitation and monitoring – were considered. Both were represented in the final statement of goals, objectives and targets.

By design, no attempt was made at that stage to think intersectorally. Tactically, the view was taken that thinking broadly and in a way that would require action by several government departments would be likely to encourage inertia. In addition, territorial boundaries are jealously guarded; and beyond this, the NHS needed to put its own house in order first to achieve a strategic reorientation.

Protocols – assessment of health gain
Assessment of health gain was very central to the strategy implementation process, especially in the light of the emerging purchaser–provider arrangements. Commissioners had to decide what they would emphasize in their contracts. The difficulty of integrating health gain requirements into contracts for services is discussed below.

Table 2.7 illustrates three examples of health gain assessment made by the panels and their expert advisers, indicating the strength of the evidence. Health authorities and providers were expected to give high priority to items marked 1, though not neglecting those marked 2. No new resources were to be invested in interventions rated 3 and 4; where appropriate, disinvestment was to be made in these items.

Protocols – goals, objectives and targets
Overall goals were set in each of the protocols that recognized the two elements of health gain – quantity and quality of life. Hence, for cardiovascular diseases they were:

* to reduce premature deaths by 33% by the year 2002 compared with 1988; and
* to achieve continuing significant and measurable increases in the quality of life of those suffering the consequences of cardiovascular diseases.

The protocols also set out the priority planning messages or main objectives (Box 2.2). These identify current deficits and therefore demand attention.

Table 2.7. Examples of health gain assessment

Condition	Prevention and promotion	Diagnosis and assessment	Treatment and care	Rehabilitation and continuing care
Respiratory diseases: childhood asthma		• greater awareness of asthma in children (1) • more education of primary health care professionals (1)	• early therapy (1) • self-help groups (1) • attention to method of administration (2) • consistent approach (2) • nebulizers (2) • use of antibiotics (4) • inappropriate hospital referral (4) and hospital follow-up (4)	• good follow-up (1) • physical exercise (1) • education of patients, carers and other contacts, especially teachers (1)
Mental health: personality disorders	• promote adequate parenting (2) • reduce sexual abuse (3)	• promote greater awareness in primary care (2) • full multidisciplinary assessment (2)	• behaviour therapy (2) • dynamic psychotherapy (2) • long-term therapy (3) • judicious use of carbamazepine neuroleptics (3)	• long-term support and limit-setting (2) • inpatient milieu therapy (3)
Pain and discomfort: chest pain of oesophageal origin	• reduce smoking (1) • reduce alcohol intake (3)	• endoscopy (1) • barium swallow (2) • X-rays (2) • oesophageal manometry (3) • acid perfusion studies (3) • oesophageal radioisotope studies (3)	• weight reduction • stop smoking (1) • avoidance of alcohol (1) • sleeping position • drug therapy (2) • surgery (3)	• acid-suppressing agents (1)

Note: 1: interventions that increase health gain
2: interventions that appear promising but require further evaluation
3: interventions with uncertain effects that require further evaluation
4: interventions that should be abandoned in the light of the available evidence

---

Box 2.2. Cardiovascular disease: the main planning messages in Wales

- Ways of coordinating an intensive prevention and promotion programme must be agreed on.

- There should be a coordinated approach to opportunistic (that is, if and when possible) assessment in Wales.

- Rapid assessment must be available to people with suspected coronary heart disease.

- A rapid and effective response to a heart attack is vital.

- The service must be responsive to an individual's need for rehabilitation after a heart attack or heart surgery.

- Efforts must be made to improve treatment and secondary prevention for people after a stroke.

- Suitable rehabilitation and support must be available to all people after a stroke (see Box 2.3 for details).

- There must be a sensitive system of review for people with chronic disability resulting from cardiovascular disease.

Box 2.3 shows an example of health gain targets for one planning message – rehabilitation for people who have experienced a stroke. For achievement in the shorter term, service targets are suggested as marker points on the way to health gain: these become surrogates for the health gain targets. Managerial performance was to be measured against their achievement.

In addition, health promotion and disease prevention were the subject of major work by the Health Promotion Authority for Wales, and the reduction of risk factors (in this case for stroke and cardiovascular diseases) played a vital role in producing a balanced group of targets in both this and all other protocols.

Equity issues were also incorporated in the health gain targets. For example, the protocol concerned with oral health stated that "People do not at present have an equal opportunity for good oral health" and proceeded to set a health gain target: "Disparities in tooth decay both within and between counties should be reduced by 50% by 2002, through improving the status of the worst".

Box 2.3. Targeting cardiovascular disease in Wales: stroke rehabilitation

Health gain targets

- By 1995, to demonstrate a 10% improvement in the average physical functioning (as measured on the Bathel Scale or similar) of people six months after a stroke, compared with the average measured in 1992.

- By 1995, to demonstrate a 10% improvement in the average psychological functioning (using such measures as the Mini-Mental State Examination, the Wakefield Self-Assessment Depression Inventory or the General Health Questionnaire) of people six months after a stroke, compared with the average measured in 1992.

- By 1992, to ensure that all people with stroke and their families are given the opportunity to discuss the setting in which long-term care takes place.

Service targets

- By 1992, each district is to develop a comprehensive policy for the management of people with stroke.

- By 1992, the Welsh Office is to stimulate the development of proxy indicators related to physical, mental and social functioning to measure the quality of life of people who have suffered stroke.

- By 1993, the Welsh Office is to stimulate studies into the most effective methods of rehabilitating people with stroke.

Two main problems emerged in the target-setting process. First, for the two early protocols (cancers and cardiovascular diseases), insufficient attention was given to the criteria to be applied for a target to be included. Second, data insufficiency, if allowed to remain, would have jeopardized the requirement to set wide-ranging targets and also to monitor progress.

Criteria for the adoption of targets were thus developed to ensure that they were:

- credible
- selective
- quantifiable
- timely
- capable of being monitored
- balanced across all areas of care.

When four protocols had been completed, data availability was reviewed (Table 2.8). It was clear that considerable new investment would be required, and this has now been carried out in the form of morbidity and health survey data from general practitioners *(20)*. Fig. 2.11 summarizes the extent to which the targets could be measured in late 1996; those not practically measurable need to be revised, but important progress has been made in other ways.

Table 2.8. Protocol health gain targets – data availability

Health gain area	Number for which data are available	Number for which a survey and questionnaire are required	Number for which a new data set is required
Cancers			
• Overall goals (2)	1	1	0
• Health gain targets (16)	12	4	0
Cardiovascular diseases			
• Overall goals (2)	1	1	0
• Health gain targets (22)	7	8	7
Maternal and early child health			
• Overall goals (3)	2	1	0
• Health gain targets (13)	8	2	3
Physical and sensory disability			
• Overall goals (3)	0	0	3
• Health gain targets (9)	0	0	9

Targets continue to be a matter of considerable debate. Their value is acknowledged if they indicate reasonable aspirations for improving health and are based on logical, professional evaluation of potential advances. Targets become more complex, however, when quality of life and other people-centred issues are included. The arrival from the Rand Corporation of the short form of the Health Survey Questionnaire (SF-36) *(21)* and its development by the King's Fund is doing much to overcome the challenge of measuring these items, using a well validated instrument people can complete both before and after an episode of care.

Fig. 2.11. Evaluation of intervention by the Welsh Health Planning Forum

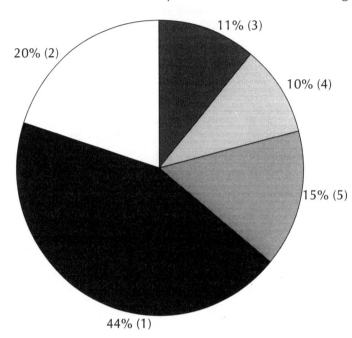

Key
1   Measurable from the outset.
2   Measurable from 1996 using the Welsh Health Survey.
3   Measurable from 1996 using the general practitioner morbidity database.
4   Measurement possible but not carried out.
5   Not practically measurable.

Source: Welsh Office *(20)*.

In summary, targets have more advantages than disadvantages; in particular, the first disadvantage listed in Box 2.4 is countered by the introduction of the service targets, which act as short-term surrogates for longer-term health gain objectives. Nevertheless, it is agreed that most health authorities would have preferred fewer targets and an indication of Welsh Office priorities, since resource constraints meant they could not pursue all the targets at one time *(22)*.

Local strategies for health and needs assessment
The policy development process had been quite top-down in its approach, even though the main strategic ideas had been widely disseminated and discussed and the protocol developments involved local clinicians, managers and voluntary workers.

Box 2.4. The advantages and disadvantages of targets as a measure of health gain

Advantages
- Quantifiable indicators of achievement
- Inspire action, commitment and purpose
- Stimulate debate
- Encourage rational purchasing

Disadvantages
- Overemphasize "destination" and distract "process"
- Encourage guesswork
- Overemphasize measurable items
- Excessive optimism leads to disillusionment

Fig. 2.10 shows another process – local strategy development and commissioning, which represent the bottom-up elements of policy implementation. This involved both assessing community needs and developing local strategies to allow informed contracting.

The main challenge for any strategy process is to produce strategic plans that can be carried out. Fig. 2.10 also shows the operational link between the strategic intent and direction and local strategies for health *(23)*. The process adopted to formulate a local or response strategy is illustrated in Fig. 2.12. The protocols were intended as guidance to assist in step 4 and beyond.

Each health district set up multidisciplinary health gain teams, variously under the leadership of public health medicine or planning personnel, which included typically the voluntary, social service and other local authority sectors such as education and housing, as well as clinicians from different backgrounds. In time all local strategies are planned to be brought together to form a health plan for Wales.

Some lessons about the development of local strategy and the groups that undertook the work can be learned from an evaluation undertaken in 1992 *(24)*.

Although the overall philosophical framework was valid, it was difficult to implement conceptually and operationally. Scientifically tested methods of assessing needs and measuring cost–effectiveness were lacking, which hampered managerial decision-making at all stages of the process of developing local strategies for health. At the same time, however, this stimulated innovation at the local level and required using research findings within a strategic framework.

Clear dimensions of people centredness were lacking, and many ad hoc tools were therefore developed with variable outcome. The roles of the voluntary organizations and community health councils remained

Fig. 2.12. Steps in formulating a response strategy

Step	Questions	Output
		Output
1	Where are we now? How are we doing?	Summary of current strengths and weaknesses
2	Where are we going?	Summary of future opportunities and threats
3	What are the key areas for attention?	Summary of areas for attention
4	What issues can be identified?	Summary of key issues and priorities
5	What aims can be developed?	Statement of health district aims
6	What are our objectives?	Local statement of direction
7	What are the service response options? What options exist or can be identified?	Summary of preferred response options
8	What are the preferred response options?	Preferred response strategy

Source: Welsh Office *(23)*.

more marginal than intended, and thus professional and clinical perceptions dominated the input of users and carers. Similarly, expert advice was poorly defined, which adversely affected approaches to improving resource efficiency.

Since the strategic intent and direction and the local strategies for health were leading the return process in the United Kingdom, there was considerable time pressure. Coupled with the other tasks resulting from the NHS reforms, such as business planning, districts were concerned about the tight time scales. They experienced difficulty in testing fully all the steps in developing local strategies for health and in using the all-Wales protocols optimally.

The three districts that were subjected to a pilot approach and evaluation developed three distinct approaches to local strategies for health, creating different structures and processes and consequently addressing different aspects of the local strategy process. Nevertheless, each district provided valuable insight, highlighting the various elements of local strategies for health that, taken together, help to reformulate parts of the framework. Further, examples of good practice were developed and important issues requiring further theoretical and operational work were revealed.

In summary, no ideal model for developing local strategies for health emerged in any one district, but components of a more flexible and locally adapted model can be identified, leading to an amended version of the framework for local strategies for health. In subsequent years the framework has been refined but more by way of fine tuning.

A later, more comprehensive, evaluation by the National Audit Office in 1996 *(22)* commented on an additional aspect.

> Health authorities have been successful in some instances in persuading organizations outside the National Health Service, such as local authorities, to take action likely to improve health. There have also been instances, such as with the major water supplier (relating to fluoridation), where health authorities have not been so successful.

People centredness

People centredness is discussed as a separate subject because of its importance within the strategic intent and direction and the considerable theoretical and operational confusion surrounding the concept. The strategic intent and direction document defines the clients of the health service in two ways:

• the total population who can take advantage of broad health care programmes; and
• the limited number who are patients at any one time.

The document goes on to define objectives for a people-centred service as follows:

- there should be participation in planning services;
- service delivery should be of high quality;
- facilities should be appropriate for the patient group;
- staff must be responsive to the needs of patients and carers; and
- patients and informal carers should be able to make informed choices about treatment.

These objectives focus on the interface between the NHS and individuals receiving services. Neverthe-less, the NHS plans strategically for populations and client groups, and yet these are collections of individuals with diverging, and sometime overlapping, needs. An overview of a pattern of needs has to be constructed, and a flexible pattern of response (both for client groups and individuals) has to be developed.

The evaluation *(24)* focused on the first objective of the people-centred approach, the participation in planning, because this was the key to achieving the other objectives. The strategic intent and direction stated very clearly that participation is sought to ensure that individuals and communities can influence the types of health services provided. The nature and extent of that influence, however, varied widely in the three prototype districts.

The districts tended to focus on how people should be involved, rather than on why and in relation to which issues. This led to participation taking the form of "being there", and the role and influence of the participants were not necessarily formulated. Thus, the three districts were willing to strengthen the people-centred approach but lacked a coherent methodological framework. In principle, the community health councils could play an important role and so could the voluntary organizations, but their capacity would have to be reinforced before they could fulfil this role. Apart from these two channels, other approaches had to be developed to systematically cover client groups and populations by applying specific research methods capable of measuring the perspectives of users and informal carers.

Precisely because the users' views were insufficiently underpinned with scientifically based findings, the professionally based assessment of need continued to dominate. There was little balancing of views: for example, in one authority the strong recommendation from the seminars on people centredness, that counselling for cancer patients should be a priority, was not adopted.

Thus, the three prototype districts referred to people-centred issues, which were articulated mainly in clinical terms. This is an inevitable consequence of the lack of validated methods for eliciting user and carer views, which can be used as a scientific basis for defining needs and deciding on priorities. The purpose of the local strategies for health, the appropriate methodological framework and the nature and extent of user influence must be defined clearly if people-centred issues are to be the main focus of the local strategies.

The experience gained from this early evaluation was disseminated to other district health authorities engaged in developing local strategies for health; but even four years on some of the fundamental methodological questions remain unresolved.

In the mean time, other approaches have been implemented at the national level across the United Kingdom as a whole, involving setting standards of service that patients can expect. These are embodied in patients' charters and are most often aimed at reducing waiting times for treatment. This makes sense politically, but the health gain tends to become secondary.

Intersectoral policy

Central and local arrangements
The strategic intent and direction emphasizes that the NHS must work together with others to achieve health gain.

Engendering intersectoral action at the level of the government department responsible for Wales – the Welsh Office – should be relatively easy. All the major departments are together under one roof, and they report to a common head. Nevertheless, although departments consult one another about individual department initiatives, active cooperation to implement integrated programmes is more difficult. Good progress has been made, however, in such areas as mental health and learning disabilities, in which intersectoral action is vital.

The development process for the protocol on injuries showed that the NHS had little role other than high-quality treatment, and most preventive action would be required of other sectors – education, social services, leisure services and public works. Central NHS leadership within the Welsh Office to convene meetings about concerted action was not highly successful, perhaps because various departments protected their territory vigorously; in addition, the broader health agenda, and its relevance to them, was incompletely framed.

Outside the regional administration, however, there has been considerable activity. The NHS is developing local strategies at the district level to coordinate activities across sectors. Local government is contributing through the involvement of social services, environmental health, education and public works. Schools, hospitals and communities have been active in the relevant WHO health-promoting programmes. All this has continued to the present.

Reviews in other sectors
The Health Promotion Authority for Wales led in reviewing work in other sectors. From 1985 to 1993, the Authority initiated intersectoral activity and review, particularly in the area of food policy, involving both the farming and retail industries *(25)*.

Mental illness and mental handicap were also the subject of policy reviews *(26,27)* led by the Welsh Office, involving all the bodies relevant to health, social services, housing and education. The same was the case for the new Children Act *(28)* and for developments in combating drug dependence *(29)*.

The Welsh Health Planning Forum produced two further protocols on both health and social gain for children and older people *(30,31)*. Again, representatives from the full range of agencies were involved.

Various policy instruments were proposed to assist change according to the area under consideration: gathering information and conducting research; building awareness; consultation and negotiation; changes in funding; human resource development, especially through an NHS Staff College project with a remit to cross organizational boundaries; and monitoring (across all areas). More recently, a white paper on primary care *(32)* has promoted recognition that joint action must be developed between health care and social care. During the early years of implementation, however, there were few changes in structure and management, although these were carried out for both health and local government in 1995–1996. (Legislation can be changed only for the entire United Kingdom, not just for Wales.)

Mechanisms

The National Health Service and Community Care Act 1990 *(1)*, *The health of the nation (4)* and the strategic intent and direction in Wales *(2)* have emphasized that community need must be assessed broadly. The approach to this activity has been subject to local discretion, although the output required has been uniform across Wales. Where appropriate, special study groups have been initiated and local interagency groups have been set up to promote health and social gain. The most appropriate agency has assumed leadership.

Alliances, which often existed before, have been strengthened, and new ones have been formed. Health gain has been a useful common language for discussion, and its very imprecision appears to be its strength: "adding years to life and adding life to years" can be interpreted slightly differently by different people working across the health and social care spectrum. Clarity would not necessarily be helpful in increasing support!

Health status orientation

Slowly, slowly

A major shift in thinking must accompany change in the culture or orientation of a large organization. As noted earlier, the NHS in Wales, and indeed across the United Kingdom, has focused on input and output for many years with scant attention to outcome, as related to improving health status or achieving health gains.

In 1990, relatively early in the process in Wales, it was recognized that strategic planning:

*   often hurts
*   narrows down the practical options for action

- forces tough choices:
  - can't do everything
  - can't serve everyone
  - can't go in too many directions at once
  - can't send too many messages
- promotes better targeting by:
  - geographical area
  - high-risk group
  - health gain pay-off
- focuses resources.

Somebody and something usually has to give, but win/win partnerships are the aim. This is very difficult!

As a consequence, a phased roll-out approach was used that could take five years or so to complete. The major activities from 1991 to 1993 are summarized in Table 2.9.

The process was interrupted in 1993 by the arrival of a new Secretary of State for Wales, with a personal agenda focused on reducing bureaucracy in the NHS and with an aggressive view opposing strategic activities and planning. This led to the end of the Welsh Health Planning Forum in 1995. The concept of health gain was also anathema, being considered an accounting term. At a time when a major new initiative on monitoring was considered vital, it was held up. But this is to step ahead!

Monitoring health status

Mortality data are much more routinely collected than are morbidity data. Since its inception, the NHS has collected a wide range of data on hospital activity and on deaths and discharges. General practice data banks are even less well developed and effort has been fragmented, much caused by the independent contractor status of general practitioners and the failure to develop information systems that can be integrated *(33)*.

The Health Promotion Authority for Wales conducted pioneering work on lifestyle and morbidity surveys in Wales *(34)* and established many useful baselines for 1988; their analysis included socioeconomic distinctions. The replication of this work was delayed to 1995, but the results are now available from the Welsh Health Survey *(20)*.

The main aim of the Welsh Health Survey was to collect aggregate information on representative samples of the population with a range of illnesses and disabilities, and information on comparable groups of healthy people, without using any medical records. Questionnaires were sent to 50 000 people living in Wales; over 28 000 were completed and returned (in line with the expected response rate). This resulted in large enough numbers of people with the targeted illnesses and disabilities that the data were statistically reliable. The questions solicited people's views of the NHS and the areas they would most

Table 2.9. Developing a health status orientation through local strategies for health

1991	1992	1993
Began the culture change.	Defined most pressing issues and necessary action.	Continued 1992 approaches, plus: • conducted comprehensive analysis of health gain decision-making in relation to:
Raised awareness of new concepts and approaches.	Balanced quantity and quality of services.	– pain, discomfort and palliative care
Identified existing strengths and weaknesses.	Avoided data overload.	– mental illness – healthy living
	Developed costing approaches.	– healthy environments;
Sharpened up ideas about roles and organizational development.	Enhanced community input.	• initiated a scenario approach to analysing the health system of the future.
Began development of a new agenda.	Avoided paralysis by analysis.	
Emphasized the change in gear.	Extended comprehensive health gain decision-making to: • physical and sensory disability • respiratory diseases • injuries.	
Developed health gain decision-making in relation to: • cancer • cardiovascular diseases • maternal and early child health.	Tackled the need for assessing the complexity of: • priority-setting • contracting for health gain.	
Developed initial health system analysis.	Developed further analysis of health system.	

like to see improved, illnesses diagnosed by a physician, their own assessment of any disability and how they lived their everyday lives. There were also questions about their socioeconomic circumstances and lifestyle. The questionnaire included the short form of the Health Survey Questionnaire (see Appendix 1). Further analysis is now to be carried out by an Equity Audit Group composed of academics from several universities in southern Wales.

Evaluation, review and revision
The Welsh Office carries out annual reviews of all district authorities. Each review begins with an assessment of the key public health issues and includes discussion of how authorities have tackled health

improvement initiatives included in their contract with the Welsh Office; these might total three or four health gain and other issues per year. The areas for assessment are selected following an analysis of the common data sets on public health for each authority. The main vehicle for reporting the overall state of health in Wales is the annual report of the Chief Medical Officer, which is structured around the health gain areas and notes actions requiring priority. It acts as a form of social conscience to the NHS and other services and to the Government as a whole.

Beyond this, two end-points were originally proposed (Fig. 2.9) – achieving the strategic intent and direction and developing an overall health plan for Wales. The first, yet to be attained as a whole, involves meeting, in time, the targets for service and health gain within each health gain protocol, and thus the objectives and overall goals. In total, if the targets are achieved, then the strategic intent and direction will be also. The second is scheduled for completion in the late 1990s.

The central review process has involved the use of health for all indicators. The position of Wales is compared, over time, with that of other countries across a range of health indicators. A relative change for the better is what is required – an attempt to move into the upper quartile of performance in health for all indicators in Europe.

Central reviews take place annually, but the health authorities are expected to maintain constant scrutiny. Although local target-setting can be revised relatively flexibly, translating targets into contracts based on health gain can be difficult, because providers have yet to fully adapt to the approach and because contracts are expected to run for only 1–2 years.

One special difficulty is linking the emerging and sometimes changing evidence base related to clinical intervention and the need to have quality-based contracts that maximized health gain. Greater flexibility is required in the purchaser–provider relationship with regard to contract setting, and issues need to be contested more openly, which can include public input.

Overall, in this area, Wales is in the same position as the rest of the United Kingdom. Much effort is being devoted to doing what is effective, but there is considerable debate and dissent about how effectiveness should be assessed. Disinvestment is a major political issue, but marginal analysis of shifts in investment could prove a powerful tool for change *(35)*.

Summary and conclusions

Table 2.10 brings together the items that have been key to the development of the approach towards health for all in Wales and could act as a checklist elsewhere. Most need little expansion, having been identified fully in earlier sections. Nevertheless, additional explanation might be helpful, especially where success has been less than might have been hoped for.

Table 2.10. Levels of success of health for all in Wales

Item	Level of success	Facilitating factors	Obstructing or inhibiting factors
1. Mobilization of strategy		Strategic documents *(2,3)*	
Early	High	Early action Protocol development Revenue neutrality Influencing the agenda in the entire United Kingdom	
Later	Moderate	Health and social care 2010 *(36)* Information management strategy Clinical effectiveness programme Building into research and development strategy	Revenue neutrality No development money; local strategy process de-emphasized (1993) Conflicting agendas Political dogma
2. Equity, targeting and monitoring	High	Getting targeting accepted Building equity into strategy and protocols Separating targets for health gain and health services	Early inability to be explicit about equity Early lack of admission criteria for targets Delay on investment in information systems Impact on health unclear
3. Intersectorality	Moderate	High local motivation Health Promotion Authority for Wales Linking health and social gain WHO activities – healthy schools, hospitals, cities, etc.	Central leadership Separation of local government and health service Reorganization of local government and health service
4. Wales within the United Kingdom	Moderate	Purchaser–provider split *Health of the nation* Contracting for health gain	Political dogma Conflicting agendas Downgrading of strategic approaches
5. Audit	High	External review of Welsh strategy Strategic intent and direction and local strategies become central to agenda again	

Mobilization of the strategy

The launch and much of the early and mid-term activity went very well, but some underlying tensions emerged.

Revenue neutrality, which acted as a useful discipline throughout the protocol development process, became a hindrance during strategy implementation at the local level; and no transition money was available from the Welsh Office.

Development of local strategies for health, which had been at the heart of the implementation process, was de-emphasized in 1993 because of central political changes. This, combined with new national agendas (such as patient's charters and waiting list initiatives), adversely affected the strategic intent and direction because the health authorities felt that there was ambiguity about the strategic path they should be following.

Some important items have moved on to the agenda to support the strategic developments: *Health and social care 2010 (36)*, which identified a future scenario for the supply side of the health service; information and communication *(6)*; research and development *(37)*; *Caring for the future (38)*, focusing on quality; and a clinical effectiveness initiative *(39)*, which will broaden the impact of the health gain analysis within the protocols.

Equity, targeting and monitoring

Equity proved to be difficult in the early phases of development, although it is now starting to blossom nationally.

Targeting was aided by distinguishing between targets for health gain and those for services; but the initial admission criteria were too relaxed. Debate still takes place about whether there should be fewer targets. The proponents suggest that this would allow better focusing; others say that motivation will improve if there are targets upon which everyone in the NHS (especially professional provider groups) can act.

Monitoring has been a constant source of concern and requires considerable resources. Political commitment has been difficult to achieve in the recent climate, which has emphasized maximizing the amount spent on direct patient care. This situation has been remedied recently and more balanced investment has been achieved. The impact of the strategy on health cannot be assessed yet, but it may affect the achievement of service targets.

Intersectorality

Local leadership, expressed through the vital processes of developing local strategies for health, has been of high quality, and intersectoral cooperation remains good at the local level. Local government and NHS reorganization, given the smaller geographical areas of local government and locality planning for the NHS, could enhance the situation further.

Central leadership has been less obvious and has not begun to deal, operationally, with the intersectoral relationships of the elements that comprise the social determinants of health.

Wales within the United Kingdom

The purchaser–provider split and contracting, introduced nationally in 1991, provided the key to putting into operation the concept of a service based on health gain and people centredness. Wales also benefited from the fact that *The health of the nation* supported the thinking behind health gain. Developing contracts explicitly oriented towards health and social gain still has a considerable way to go.

On the negative side, the political hierarchy in Wales changed to a Secretary of State for Wales with overt leadership ambitions on a broader level in the United Kingdom. This resulted in Wales being used as a showcase for the political dogma of the far right: notions of strategy and planning developments emanating from the centre were anathema.

Postscript

External audit

The United Kingdom has a National Audit Office that scrutinizes, on behalf of Parliament, how public money is spent and the results that accrue and recommends good practice.

The NHS in Wales and its strategic approaches had earlier been commended in a Treasury report, and the National Audit Office undertook a more detailed evaluation *(22)*. Its important and influential conclusions are broadly consonant with those detailed in the comments in Table 2.9 but are worth reproducing in full (Appendix 2).

As a result, the Welsh Office has agreed on an action plan to take the strategic intent and direction forward that includes an early relaunching of its principles and approaches. The local strategy process, emphasizing the need for a service led by primary care, is resulting in reinvigorated local strategies being submitted during 1997. A complete review of all the health gain targets will result in both a smaller number and revision, where appropriate. The new health authorities may be asked to focus on a number of key areas. Not everything can be done at once! Of great importance will be the concentration of implementation through contracting.

Most if of not all the factors that have inhibited progress for the past two years can be overcome, although intersectoral considerations remain difficult. During 1996, the Association of Local Government Authorities launched an important initiative, with the support of health authorities, to investigate how local government activities can best contribute to producing health in Wales. Health and social gain are moving to a wider agenda in the public sector!

Government change

On 1 May 1997, New Labour won an election after 18 years of Conservative government. A number of significant actions have already been undertaken that indicate changes for both the NHS and public health.

For the NHS in Wales, the new Secretary of State has asked the Welsh Office to consider some important issues "including breaking down barriers, being more responsive to local needs, reducing variations in health, improving efficiency and providing the best possible level of care". New targets for health and health services have been set, noting explicitly the foundation of the idea in the strategic intent and direction strategy. The two Ministers appointed to Wales have been given overall responsibility for economic development and quality of life – the latter identified earlier as an essential component of health gain.

At the United Kingdom level, a Minister for Public Health has taken office – the first ever with this specific responsibility. Recently she said: "Our new Government was elected on a dual pledge to rebuild the National Health Service to tackle the root causes of illness. We are committed to reducing inequalities in health and we shall do so with a clear sense of our priorities".

The Minister announced:

- an autumn 1997 green paper for health strategy in England;
- an independent review of health inequalities by Sir Donald Acheson;
- *Our healthier nation* – a new approach to health targets across government; and
- plans to promote healthy schools and workplaces.

She said: "We want to attack the underlying causes of ill health and to break the cycle of social and economic deprivation and social exclusion. This signals a major change in the nation's policy, to maximize good health, as well as treating sickness. You might call it being tough on the causes of ill health.

Health gain investment is back on the agenda.

References

1. *National Health Service and Community Care Act 1990.* London, H.M. Stationery Office, 1990.
2. *Strategic intent and direction for the NHS in Wales.* Cardiff, Welsh Office, NHS Directorate and Welsh Health Planning Forum, 1989.
3. *Local strategies for health: a new approach to strategic planning.* Cardiff, Welsh Office NHS Directorate and Welsh Health Planning Forum, 1989.
4. *The health of the nation: a strategy for health in England.* London, H.M. Stationery Office, 1991.
5. *Management development strategy.* Cardiff, Welsh Office, NHS Directorate, 1993.
6. *Information and information technology: strategic direction for the NHS in Wales.* Cardiff, Welsh Office, NHS Directorate, 1989.
7. CHALMERS, I. & ALTMAN, D., ed. *Systematic reviews.* London, BMJ Publishing Group, 1995.

8. *Protocol for investment in health gain: cancers.* Cardiff, Welsh Office, NHS Directorate and Welsh Health Planning Forum, 1992.

9. *Protocol for investment in health gain: cardiovascular diseases.* Cardiff, Welsh Office, NHS Directorate and Welsh Health Planning Forum, 1991.

10. *Protocol for investment in health gain: maternal and early child health.* Cardiff, Welsh Office, NHS Directorate and Welsh Health Planning Forum, 1991.

11. *Protocol for investment in health gain: physical and sensory disability.* Cardiff, Welsh Office, NHS Directorate and Welsh Health Planning Forum, 1991.

12. *Protocol for investment in health gain: respiratory diseases.* Cardiff, Welsh Office, NHS Directorate and Welsh Health Planning Forum, 1992.

13. *Protocol for investment in health gain: injuries.* Cardiff, Welsh Office, NHS Directorate and Welsh Health Planning Forum, 1992.

14. *Protocol for investment in health gain: mental handicap (learning disabilities).* Cardiff, Welsh Office, NHS Directorate and Welsh Health Planning Forum, 1992.

15. *Protocol for investment in health gain: pain discomfort & palliative care.* Cardiff, Welsh Office, NHS Directorate and Welsh Health Planning Forum, 1992.

16. *Protocol for investment in health gain: oral health.* Cardiff, Welsh Office, NHS Directorate and Welsh Health Planning Forum, 1992.

17. *Protocol for investment in health gain: mental health.* Cardiff, Welsh Office, NHS Directorate and Welsh Health Planning Forum, 1993.

18. *Protocol for investment in health gain: healthy living.* Cardiff, Welsh Office, NHS Directorate and Welsh Health Planning Forum, 1993.

19. *Protocol for investment in health gain: healthy environments.* Cardiff, Welsh Office, NHS Directorate and Welsh Health Planning Forum, 1993.

20. WELSH OFFICE. *Welsh Health Survey, 1995.* London, H.M. Stationery Office, 1996.

21. GARRATT, A. ET AL. The SF-36 Health Survey Questionnaire: an outcome measure suitable for routine use within the NHS. *British medical journal*, **306**: 1440–1444 (1993).

22. NATIONAL AUDIT OFFICE. *Improving health in Wales.* London, H.M. Stationery Office, 1996.

23. *Local strategies for health: a new approach to strategic planning.* Cardiff, Welsh Office, NHS Directorate and Welsh Health Planning Forum, 1989.

24. ONG, B.N. *An evaluation of local strategies for health Nuffield prototypes.* Cardiff, Welsh Health Planning Forum, 1992.

25. CATFORD, F. & NUTBEAM, D. Heartbeat Wales. *In*: William, K, ed. *The community prevention of coronary heart disease.* London, H.M. Stationery Office, 1992, pp. 164–172.

26. *Mental illness services: a strategy for Wales.* Cardiff, Welsh Office, NHS Directorate, 1989.

27. *All Wales mental handicap strategy.* Cardiff, Welsh Office, NHS Directorate, 1992.

28. *Children Act.* London, H.M. Stationery Office, 1989.

29. *Drug misuse & dependence: guidelines on clinical management: a report of a medical working group.* Cardiff, Welsh Office, NHS Directorate/Department of Health/Scottish Home & Health Department, 1991.

30. *Health & social gain for older people: guidance to inform local strategies for health.* Cardiff, Welsh Health Planning Forum, 1993.

31. *Health & social gain for children: guidance to inform local strategies for health.* Cardiff, Welsh Health Planning Forum, 1993.

32. DEPARTMENT OF HEALTH, WELSH OFFICE AND SCOTTISH OFFICE. *Primary care: the future, choice and opportunity.* London, H.M. Stationery Office, 1996.

33. WARNER, M.M. ET AL., ED. *Primary care information policy: into the next century.* Cardiff, Welsh Health Planning Forum, 1995.

34. *Health-related behaviours in Wales 1985–1993: findings from the Health in Wales Survey.* Cardiff, Health Promotion Wales, 1994 (Health Promotion Wales Technical Report, No. 8).

35. COHEN, D. Marginal analysis in practice: an alternative to needs assessment for contracting health care. *British medical journal,* **309**: 781–785 (1994).

36. *Health and social care 2010 – a report on phase one.* Cardiff, Welsh Health Planning Forum, 1994.

37. *Sharpening the focus: a research & development framework for the NHS in Wales.* Cardiff, Welsh Office, NHS Directorate, 1992.

38. *Caring for the future.* Cardiff, Welsh Office, NHS Directorate, 1994.

39. *Towards evidence based practice: a clinical effectiveness initiative for Wales.* Cardiff, Welsh Office, NHS Directorate, 1993.

Appendix 1. A note on the short form of the Health Survey Questionnaire (SF-36)[a]

Three areas of health are measured by the SF-36 (functional status, wellbeing and health perceptions) using eight components, together with a measurement of the change in health. These are shown in the following table.

Health concept	Description
Functional status	
Physical functioning	Extent to which health limits physical activities
Role functioning – physical	Extent to which physical health interferes with work
Role functioning – emotional	Extent to which emotional problems interfere with work
Social functioning	Extent to which normal social activities are limited
Wellbeing	
Bodily pain	Effect of pain on normal activities
Mental health	General mental health including depression and anxiety
Vitality	Feeling energetic rather than weary
General health – perceptions	Personal evaluation of health
Change in health	Current health compared with one year ago

Each component of the SF-36 has a scale that ranges from 0 to 100, where 0 and 100 represent the worst and best possible states, respectively. Recent research has shown that factor analyses of the eight SF-36 scales have consistently identified two summary components: the Physical Component Summary (PCS) and the Mental Component Summary (MCS) scores. On the strength of their correlations with the eight scales, they have been interpreted as the physical and mental dimensions of health status.

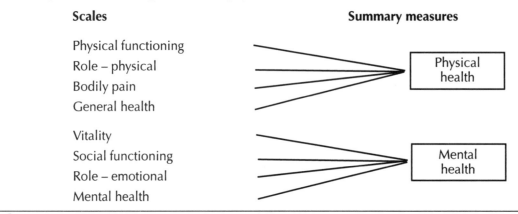

Scales

Physical functioning
Role – physical
Bodily pain
General health

Vitality
Social functioning
Role – emotional
Mental health

Summary measures

Physical health

Mental health

[a] *Source: Welsh Health Survey*. London, Stationery Office, 1996.

Appendix 2. Summary and conclusions of the National Audit Office evaluation[a]

1. In 1989, the Welsh Office announced an initiative, the Strategic Intent and Direction, which aimed to "take the people of Wales into the 21st Century with a level of health on course to compare with the best in Europe" (paragraph 1.1).

2. The initiative covers 10 areas where health could be improved. Together, the areas account for about 80 per cent of the health service expenditure in Wales, which in 1994–95 amounted to some £2.1 billion. Three strands run through each area (paragraphs 1.2 to 1.6):

- Health Gain, focusing on improving health by, for example, shifting resources to more effective treatments;
- Making services more responsive to people's needs and preferences, for example considering the total effects of services on people's lives rather than narrower clinical perspectives;
- Effective Use of Resources, for example providing an appropriate balance between prevention and promotion; diagnosis and assessment; treatment and care; and rehabilitation and monitoring.

3. The Strategic Intent and Direction has co-existed with a number of other developments in the National Health Service as a whole, such as the establishment of the internal market. It has also been followed by developments specific to Wales, principally the publication of "Caring for the Future" – the NHS in Wales plan for improving the quality of services (paragraph 1.9).

4. The cumulative cost in the years 1990–91 to 1993–94 of establishing the initiative was about £65 million, 0.1 per cent of the total spend of the NHS in Wales over the same period. Of this, £4.7 million represents the estimated cost of the work of existing staff rather than additional expenditure. In addition, health authorities assessed the cost of changes to services needed to make progress towards – but not to achieve all – health gain and service targets at £112 million between 1994–95 and 2000–2001 (paragraph 1.10).

5. This report examines how well the initiative was designed and implemented, and what impact it has had so far.

(i) On how well the initiative was designed and implemented

6. The Welsh Office set objectives which developed the strategic intent into more specific aims and overall goals. The Welsh Office issued guidance to overcome the difficulties created by the various approaches to defining health gain, but some areas of overlap remained (paragraphs 2.2 to 2.5).

---

[a] *Source: Improving health in Wales.* London, Stationery Office, 1996.

7. The Welsh Office communicated their objectives to NHS bodies effectively. But the publication in 1994 of Caring for the Future – a document which emphasised more heavily than previous ones the need to improve the quality of services – raised doubts as to the status of the Strategic Intent and Direction, even though the Welsh Office had undertaken extensive consultation with the NHS. Most health authorities saw the greater emphasis on making services more responsive to the needs and preferences of individuals as a sign that the Patient's Charter has assumed a more influential role in the planning of services (paragraphs 2.6 to 2.8).

8. The Welsh Health Planning Forum proposed, and the Welsh Office set, a large number of targets for improving health and services, covering a wide range of health issues. They did so to avoid causing health authorities to concentrate their efforts on too narrow a range of services. In June 1993, the Welsh Office signalled their intention to rationalise the targets when they had completed a survey of the health status of the population of Wales. The complexity of the exercise and the need to validate questions delayed the survey, and the process of reviewing the targets has only recently begun. The original targets had clear dates for achievement and were relevant to achieving the objectives of the initiative (paragraphs 2.9 to 2.15).

9. At the outset, progress towards more than half of the health gain targets could not be measured. This reduced the value of targets in the eyes of clinicians and hindered health authorities' efforts to identify areas for local action. The lack of historical data also makes it unclear whether some targets are achievable, or whether they call for improvements over existing trends (paragraphs 2.16 to 2.21).

10. Most health authorities would have preferred a smaller number of targets and an indication of Welsh Office priorities, since resource constraints – on funds and staff time – meant that they could not pursue all of the targets at once (paragraph 2.23).

11. Each health authority developed long term plans – called local strategies for health – for implementing the initiative. The Welsh Office approved the current strategies in 1994. These documents reflected properly the objectives of the initiative. The five new health authorities established in April 1996 are to submit new strategic plans in 1997 (paragraph 2.24).

12. Health authorities generally used the targets as one of a number of starting points for identifying options for local action. The Welsh Office intended health authorities to prioritise and recalibrate targets in the light of local needs. In the event, the extent to which health authorities explicitly prioritised targets varied, and they recalibrated few. Some authorities evaluated a large number of potential service developments, of which only a limited number could proceed (paragraphs 2.25 to 2.28).

13. The Welsh Office conveyed advice on the initiative through "Protocols for Investment in Health Gain" which health authorities found generally useful. Because summaries of clinical effectiveness can get out of date as further evidence becomes available, the Welsh Office have now commissioned

health authority directors of public health to review those included in the documents and to publish updated assessments (paragraphs 2.29 to 2.32).

14. In drawing up their plans all health authorities consulted their populations and liaised with clinicians and other agencies – especially local authorities and voluntary bodies. Targeted consultation of patients and carers was more informative than less specific methods such as public meetings. Health authorities closely involved senior hospital health care professionals in the development of local strategies for health. But they found it difficult to obtain representative views of general practitioners (paragraphs 2.33 to 2.37).

15. The Welsh Office's capacity to monitor progress towards all the health gain targets was limited by a lack of data. Nonetheless they did not use all the data available to them; and called health authorities to account for only a small number of targets (paragraphs 2.38 and 2.39).

16. Health authorities' monitoring of progress towards the health gain targets is often limited by lack of data. And for service targets, their monitoring tends to be restricted to those which have been incorporated in contract specifications (paragraphs 2.40 and 2.41).

17. The Welsh Health Survey will result in a significant improvement in the availability of data. But more than a quarter of the original targets will remain unmeasured. The Welsh Office are content that the data now available will enable them to agree an appropriate range of health targets (paragraphs 2.42 to 2.44).

(ii) On the impact achieved

18. Insufficient time has passed for changes in trends to be identified with any degree of certainty, even where data are available. The report therefore examines a proxy: the extent to which the changes to services and activities identified by health authorities as necessary to make progress in improving health have occurred (paragraphs 3.2 and 3.3).

19. The impact of the initiative on services has been marginal so far. The Welsh Office and health authorities expected, however, that change would be evolutionary rather than rapid. Health authorities' actual expenditure in 1994–95 on changes fell short of the level planned. The Welsh Office consider this shortfall can be attributed to the fact that they did not approve the local strategies until July 1994. They expect a similar shortfall in 1995–96, owing to the pressure on authorities imposed by the sharp increase in emergency admissions (paragraphs 3.4 to 3.6).

20. The Welsh Office have a policy of minimising the top-slicing of NHS resources and did not allocate specific funds for this initiative. Most health authorities planned to generate funds for new or enhanced services by discontinuing or reducing existing, less effective, services. However, they had

difficulty in realising savings from reductions in services before embarking on service developments (paragraphs 3.7 to 3.12).

21. Most of the service developments were community or primary care-based. In some cases, they may be in part attributable to other initiatives, such as "Effective Health Care Bulletins". But health authorities considered that the Strategic Intent and Direction had created a climate which was conducive to change. Authorities gave effect to service targets by adopting them as specifications in contracts with health care providers (paragraphs 3.13 to 3.16).

22. The majority of hospitals and community health services indicated that they had made changes in response to the initiative. These changes were mainly in terms of ways of planning services: relatively few identified specific service developments. About one half of clinical directors reported that they had made changes. One in three of the general practitioner fundholders responding to a National Audit Office survey had made changes to their contracts with providers of health care services; and just under half of all general practitioners responding had made some change in the services they provide (paragraphs 3.17 to 3.20).

23. Health authorities considered that the initiative had changed the way in which they evaluate service developments. It also prompted them to consult more widely about the services they commission, thus improving the co-ordination and delivery of some services to patients (paragraphs 3.21 to 3.23).

24. Health authorities have been successful in some instances in persuading organisations outside the National Health Service, such as local authorities, to take action likely to improve health. There have also been instances, such as with the major water supplier, where health authorities have not been so successful (paragraphs 3.24 to 3.27).

General conclusions

25. The Strategic Intent and Direction was a pioneering response to the World Health Organisation's strategy for "Health for All by the year 2000", and therefore lacked models to follow. It is too early to judge the impact on the health of the Welsh population. So far, though, its impact on the direct delivery of health services to patients has been relatively limited. The initiative has had a more substantial effect on the way in which the NHS in Wales plans service developments.

26. While changes in services might be expected to be marginal in the early years of the initiative, progress has been inhibited because not all health authorities were clear as to the present status of the initiative; there were some weaknesses in the way that targets were set and the arrangements for monitoring progress towards them; and health authorities had difficulty in realising savings from relatively ineffective services before embarking on service improvements.

In taking forward their work the Welsh Office should:

- **clarify and communicate the status and priority of the Strategic Intent and Direction**

In May 1996, the Welsh Office confirmed that the broad thrust of the initiative continued to be relevant to the planning of NHS services and the establishment of priorities. The five health authorities established in April 1996 are to submit new strategic plans in 1997.

To support the development of revised local strategies for health the Welsh Office have established a project board, including NHS representatives, chaired by the Director of the Welsh Office Health Department. This will have two working groups focusing respectively on priorities and targets, and on the best approach to the review and revision of existing local strategies.

- **review the targets, in the light of information now available, to focus on a small number of national priorities**
- **devise measurable key targets for those aspects of health which are still considered to be important, but for which no measurable targets currently exist**

The priorities and targets working group, chaired by the Chief Medical Officer and including NHS representatives, will develop a set of national targets for improving the health of the population. This group will draw on information from the Welsh Health Survey and other sources. It is expected to report by the end of 1996.

- **work with health authorities to agree local targets and priorities which, while remaining broadly consistent with national objectives, ensure that resources are directed at those areas which are important locally and offer the greatest scope for impact**

The Welsh Office have confirmed its earlier advice that local strategies should be sensitive to local needs and circumstances. In doing so, it recognises that the focus on a smaller set of national priorities will allow more scope for local initiatives based on health care interventions of proven value.

- **consult health authorities and other interested parties to ensure that guidance on implementing the initiative is clear and meets their needs**

The working group addressing the revision of local strategies comprises mainly NHS representatives. It will develop practical guidance for health authorities on how best to approach the review and the revision of existing local strategies, including making services more responsive to individual users. The Welsh Office have asked it to work to the same timetable as the group on priorities and targets.

- **publicise best practice in consulting interested parties about local strategies, and encourage health authorities to find ways of securing greater input from general practitioners**

The Welsh Office have asked the working group on implementation issues to review existing guidance on the involvement of local communities and to recommend changes, if necessary. The working group will also propose ways in which health authorities can secure the ownership of those in primary care for the revised strategies.

- **hold health authorities to account for carrying out the action specified in their plans aimed at achieving national and local targets**

The Welsh Office are committed to close monitoring of the national targets to be agreed in the autumn and will hold health authorities to account for performance against those that relate closely to healthcare interventions by the NHS.

Progress towards national and local objectives will feature in the annual Accountability Reviews with the Welsh Office. The emphasis in the reviews will be on agreeing the action needed to address areas where performance falls short of expectations.

Health authorities will be asked to publicise their performance against both national and local targets in their annual reports. They will also be required to include service action judged to be of particular importance in achieving national and local priorities in their shorter term health plans and in their annual performance agreements with the Welsh Office.

3

An overview of experience in the European Region

Anna Ritsatakis, Ruth Barnes & Patsy Harrington

The countries and their policy environments

The countries of the WHO European Region are extremely diverse in geography, population, socioeconomic situation and health status. This section explores the implications of this diversity for the development of health policy.

The European Region has 51 Member States with about 870 million inhabitants. It stretches from Greenland and the Atlantic seaboard of western Europe to the Pacific in the far east of the Russian Federation, and from the Arctic Ocean in the north to the shores of the Mediterranean Sea in the south. The Region encompasses the 15 countries of the European Union, Israel, Malta and Turkey as well as the newly independent central Asian republics of the former USSR – an intriguing mix of diverse histories and cultures.

The very diverse physical and geographical characteristics and the different climates prevalent in the countries in the Region influence patterns of agriculture and population distribution and even family and social interaction. The colder climates tend to persuade people to remain indoors in the warmth and relative seclusion of the home environment, whereas the warmer climates encourage more social interaction in streets and squares. The contrasting images of older people sitting alone with their televisions or sitting outside watching the world going by in warmer climates, and of children in rural areas able to play safely outside without fear of the traffic or crime prevalent in some urban areas, indicate the complex effects on health of climatic and geographical differences.

Population size and distribution

A Region of mainly small countries
About half the Member States in the European Region are small countries, with 6 million or fewer inhabitants. These include the city-states of Monaco and San Marino as well as Andorra, Iceland, Luxembourg and

Malta with less than 1 million inhabitants, and such countries as Albania, Armenia, Bosnia and Herzegovina, Croatia, Denmark, Ireland, Norway, the Republic of Moldova, Slovenia and the Baltic countries. Nine countries have between 8 and 11 million inhabitants, four are between 15 and 25 million, with Poland, Spain and the Ukraine having about 40–50 million. France, Italy, Turkey and the United Kingdom have about 60 million people each. Germany is the second largest country with 82 million inhabitants, and the 147 million people in the Russian Federation, which is the largest country, alone account for 17% of the Region's total population. Although the population size of a country is not necessarily related to economic prosperity, population affects the available pool of human resources and expertise and the feasibility, for example, of carrying out certain kinds of basic research or providing high-technology services at the country level. Small can also be beautiful when this leads to close interaction and cooperation for health. The governments of each of these countries have the same responsibility for the health and wellbeing of their people regardless of the size of their population and the resources available.

A largely urban population in many countries

Almost 90% of the population lives in urban areas in Germany, the Netherlands and the United Kingdom and 97% in Belgium. The population is more rural than this in many countries in the eastern part of the Region, where many people still work in agriculture. For example, in Albania just 37% of the population lives in urban areas, in Azerbaijan and Georgia 55–60% and in Hungary about 65%. With the exception of Kazakhstan, the Asian countries in the Region are mainly rural, with only about 40% of the population living in urban areas.

In much of western Europe, many inhabitants of the urban areas that developed in response to the growth of industry in the nineteenth century or early part of the twentieth century have only known city life. In the urban areas that expanded in the mid-twentieth century in southern Europe and parts of central and eastern Europe, many inhabitants spent their childhood and youth in a rural environment and still keep links with their villages. Most of western Europe became urbanized much sooner, and this process is proceeding at varying rates in different countries. For example, the United Kingdom experienced relatively early urbanization, and city populations have not increased greatly over the last two decades. The urban population in other western European countries such as Germany and Greece has increased by up to 10 percentage points over the last two decades, and by up to 20 percentage points in some countries in the eastern part of the region such as Hungary. The speed of urbanization and the density of urban settlements have important implications for health policy in terms of the quality of living and working environments, problems of pollution and waste disposal, changing lifestyles and also the potential for introducing options in service delivery that a more densely populated urban area allows.

Problems of access to services in rural areas

Regardless of the size of their rural population, all countries experience some challenges in achieving equal access to services and opportunities. This can become acute in some remote rural areas. The situation is exacerbated when an exodus of young people from rural areas results in an imbalance in population age distribution, and a declining available labour force in these areas makes providing certain services even less viable. This can become a vicious circle, as the lack of employment opportunities and of a wide range of services influences further population outflow and endangers the economic and social sustainability of regions. For some rural areas, one of the most important ways of maintaining health and providing adequate health services may be to reconsider social infrastructure, patterns of production and job opportunities to influence the distribution of population *(1)*.

Demographic trends

An aging population in many countries in the Region
In the 15 European Union countries, the proportion of the population 65 years or older ranges from about 11% in Ireland to over 17% in Sweden. The average for the countries of central and eastern Europe is about 12%, whereas in the central Asian republics the population is much younger, with only about 5% being older than 65 years. The positive picture of more people enjoying a longer life is tempered by some of the challenges presented by an aging population. For example, the European Commission says that, by 2000, an estimated 8 million people in the European Union will have Alzheimer's disease *(2)*.

A continued decline in birth rates
The birth rates in most European countries have declined during the period of this study (early 1980s to 1996), more so in the eastern part of the Region than in western Europe, and there is wide variation in the Region. In the European Union countries, live births per 1000 population range from about 9 in Italy and Spain to over 13 in Denmark, whereas they are over 25 in some of the central Asian republics. Overall fertility rates in the Region have fallen to well below replacement levels.

The number of births and the proportion of children, old people, and especially very old people in the population strongly influences the demand for certain types of health, social and other services.

Human resources for development
The implications for health and development policy are much wider, however, since the age structure of the population largely determines who is available to participate in the labour force and contribute to the national income and who needs to be supported. The dependency ratio (the ratio of the number of people 0–14 years old plus the number 65 years and older to those 15–64 years old *(3)*) indicates this relationship to some extent. This ratio does not account for people 15–64 years old who are not actually working for a variety of reasons such as health problems, unemployment or participation in full-time education. Nevertheless, the dependency ratio indicates roughly a country's capacity to meet the demands for goods and services of all kinds. The recent experience of high unemployment rates can make it easy to forget that the size of the labour force constrained economic growth in the not too distant past in a number of countries. In Finland, for example, stress and fatigue are causing many people to retire early. A shortage of labour is therefore expected as the cohort from the baby boom years approaches 60 years of age *(4)*. In addition, in some countries the health and welfare services do not have a comparative advantage in

attracting job seekers, and a shrinking labour force could worsen this problem. Keeping people healthy and happy will result in economic and health benefits.

The dependency ratio is not clearly different in the eastern and western parts of the Region, since the large proportion of children in some eastern countries is offset by a small proportion of older people. The dependency ratio of the European Region as a whole was 51% in 1995. About half the Member States have a dependency ratio of about 45–50%, and these countries are evenly divided between east and west. Some countries with the lowest dependency ratios have high per capita income (Andorra, Germany, Luxembourg, the Netherlands and Switzerland), and some are located in southern Europe (Croatia, Italy, Slovenia and Spain). The very high dependency ratios in some countries seem to be determined more by the proportion of children in the population than the proportion of elderly people.

Economic growth and resources for health care
In 1995, average gross national product (GNP) per capita ranged from US $340 in Tajikistan to US $41 210 in Luxembourg (Fig. 3.1).

More than half the Member States, 12 countries in central and eastern Europe and 15 newly independent states, are in transition from centrally planned to market economies. In many of these countries, which tend to have lower GNP than those in western Europe, the problem of low average incomes and

Fig. 3.1. GNP per capita in 44 countries of the WHO European Region, 1995

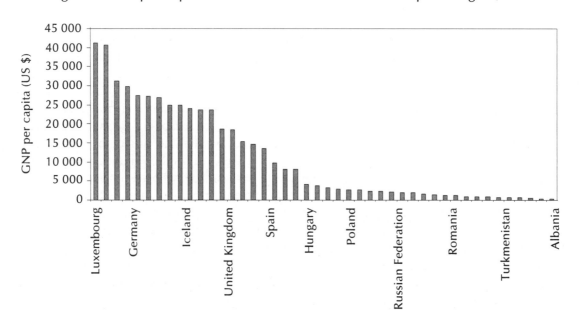

purchasing power is compounded by high annual rates of inflation. These rates were about 130–150% in 1996 in some newly independent states, compared with rates as low as 1–2% in some Scandinavian countries, for example.

Economic restructuring and the political and economic transition in the eastern part of the Region have resulted in increased unemployment across the Region, with rates reaching as high as 20% in a number of countries. Parts of the former Yugoslav republics have the highest levels of unemployment in the Region (over 30%). The average for the European Union in 1995 was just over 12%, but was 23% in Spain and 17% in Finland, for example. The people in the countries in the eastern part of the Region had not previously been exposed to the stress and uncertainty of unemployment. The picture within countries is even bleaker, with some areas of cities exhibiting unemployment rates of up to 80% *(5)*. A 1996 report of the European Commission *(6)*, for example, stated that, although the 15 countries seemed to be converging economically and socially, economic and social cohesion within most of the 15 countries seemed to have declined during the 1990s in the form of widening disparity in income and unemployment. In 1995, the ten most disadvantaged regions in the European Union had an average unemployment rate of 26.4%, nearly seven times the average rate (just under 4%) in the ten most affluent regions.

The trends in unemployment are of serious concern to policy-makers, given the implications of employment for people's health and wellbeing. Those in work tend to live longer than those without jobs. In the United Kingdom, a middle-aged man who loses his job is twice as likely to die within the following five years as one still employed *(7)*.

Poverty has increased very sharply in most countries in the eastern part of the Region. For example in Lithuania, the Russian Federation and Ukraine, real wages declined to as low as about 40% of the 1989 levels. In some countries in western Europe, the traditional benefits of the welfare state have been restricted because of pressure to reduce public spending, and poverty has increased considerably *(5)*. However, the most serious repercussions of the economic transition in eastern Europe appear to be over, and prospects are good for nearly all countries, given the relatively productive and skilled workforce and extensive basic infrastructure *(5)*.

Health care structures vary across the European Region, from pluralistic systems such as those in Germany and the Netherlands to national health service systems of the type in the United Kingdom and Scandinavia. In parallel with their political and economic systems, many countries in the eastern part of the Region are currently going through a period of transition and reform in health care *(8)*. The way health care services are structured, and especially whether public responsibility for health care lies at the central or local level of government, can influence the process of developing health policy. Nevertheless, since this study deals with policy for health care as just one part of wider health policy, the framework for analysis did not distinguish between countries or groups of countries with different health care systems.

All countries in the European Region have economic constraints to health care expenditure. In 1996, the proportion of gross domestic product (GDP) spent on health care ranged from 10.5% in Germany to less than 3% in some newly independent states. The European Union average was 8.4% and that for the Nordic countries 7.2%, while that for the countries of central and eastern Europe and the newly independent states was 5.1% and 3.1%, respectively. As the countries in the eastern part of the Region have low total income, the differences in the money spent on health care are enormous, even when differences in purchasing power are taken into account. For example, in 1995 the amount per capita spent on health care in the European Union was about three times that spent in Hungary. Patterns of expenditure relative to national income have varied widely over the last three decades. For example, the proportion of GDP spent on health in Germany increased from 5.7% in 1970 to 8.1% in 1980, to 8.2% in 1990 and to more than 10% from 1992. In contrast, the average proportion for the Nordic countries has largely stagnated since 1980; Sweden's spending increased from 7.1% in 1970 to 9.4% in 1980 and then declined again to 7.2% in 1995.

Most countries in the Region believe that containing current levels of expenditure and coping with new issues such as the rising number of elderly and chronically ill people are among the most important challenges for the future. There are burdens on the welfare purse other than health. Meeting the costs of violence and crime associated with income inequality *(9)* – the costs of supporting victims and of preventing and controlling criminal activity – is a major challenge for health and social services in all European countries. Some countries have also had to cope with the adverse consequences of political and economic upheaval, which can result in forced migration. Countries receiving migrants and refugees face particular challenges: a sudden influx of people can exacerbate existing problems of substandard housing and homelessness, which are already a feature of many European cities.

Health status in the European Region

The European Region has a relatively high level of health status compared with many other parts of the world, but inequity in health is substantial. The average life expectancy at birth in the Region in 1995 was 68 years for men and 77 years for women. These figures, however, do not reveal the decline in recent years in some countries, and the stark reality is considerable inequity both between and within countries. The subregional averages and trends show a steady increase in the east–west gap in mortality and life expectancy, starting about three decades ago. In about 1970, the difference between the average life expectancy for the European Union countries and that for the countries of central and eastern Europe and the newly independent states was approximately 2.5 years. By 1995, this gap had increased to 11 years for the newly independent states and 6 years for the countries of central and eastern Europe. The differences are especially large for men. In 1995, the gap in life expectancy for men between Sweden (76 years) and Latvia (60 years) was 16 years; for women the gap was 9 years (82 years in Sweden versus 73 years in Latvia).

The gaps in mortality between different socioeconomic and geographical groups within countries have been remarkably persistent. In many countries such inequity has continued to widen *(10)*.

Infant mortality has declined steadily in nearly all parts of the Region, but the health of infants and young children in the eastern part of the Region continues to be of concern. In 1995, the average infant mortality rate in the Nordic countries was 4.3 per 1000 live births, whereas that for the countries of central and eastern Europe and the newly independent states was was 14.4 and 22.3, respectively (Fig. 3.2). Not surprisingly, countries with the lowest average incomes (Fig. 3.1) have the highest infant mortality rates.

Within countries, infant mortality also varies between social classes, in some countries quite considerably *(11)*.

The process of formulating health policy

Initiating a process for health for all in countries

The development of health policy based on health for all principles began in earnest in the 1980s after the European strategy and targets for health for all were adopted. As the health for all policy is complex and a wide variety of partners need to work together, the type of political and administrative system in a country might be expected to be an important driving force or negative factor in health for all development. Health for all policies have been formulated since the mid-1980s in all types of political and administrative systems, including centralized, decentralized and federal ones.

Fig. 3.2. Infant mortality per 1000 live births in 35 countries of the European Region, 1995

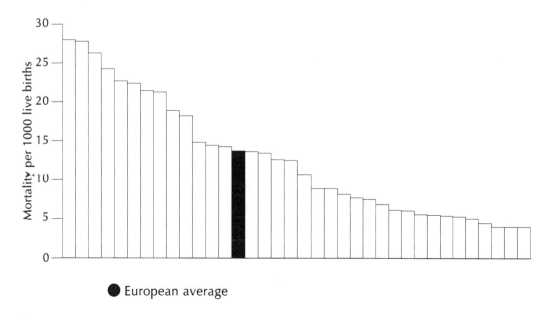

● European average

Some of the countries in which the health for all approach has persisted have a more centralized decision-making process (such as Finland), a national health care system or a strong tradition of searching for consensus in a pluralistic system. The countries with a strong public sector may have found it easier to initiate a policy based on health for all. The information available, however, does not clearly indicate the extent to which the system, administrative structure or size of a country makes a difference to the potential for success.

The influence of the administrative structure on the feasibility of adopting a health for all approach in a country would be worth exploring in future studies.

An ongoing process

In some countries, the health for all process has reflected trends that had been evident for some time. Finland and the Netherlands were two such examples: because of their considerable experience, WHO asked them to act as pioneers in developing national health for all policies. A number of countries in central and eastern Europe also formulated health for all policy documents at an early stage, including Bulgaria *(12)*, Hungary *(13)* and Poland *(14)*. The German Democratic Republic formulated a document *(15)* in 1987 that took the 38 European targets for health for all and indicated for each target the provisions already being implemented that would enable the targets to be achieved. By 1989, 17 of the 32 Member States had, at least on paper, initiated a process of developing a health for all policy *(16)*. Most of these were in central and eastern Europe and seemed comfortable with the target-setting approach given their centrally planned systems.

The two pilot countries, Finland and the Netherlands, have persevered in trying to implement, revise and further develop this approach. Some countries in central and eastern Europe also have a long involvement with the health for all framework, but so many of the policies they had formulated in the early part of the period were then superseded by the political events following the fall of the Berlin Wall in 1989. It is therefore difficult to say whether these policies would have remained a paper exercise or if they would have led to concrete action if the policy environment had not been affected by the upheaval of transition to a market economy. Even when formulating a policy does not lead to action, the process of formulating an intersectoral policy can have lasting effects on how future decisions are taken if a serious attempt is made to more broadly assess the factors influencing health and if the policy has been formulated by reaching out to new partners.

Assessing the secondary impact of the process of formulating comprehensive policies for health in selected countries would be valuable, even when this appeared to have been little more than a paper exercise.

Economic austerity

In the first years of economic transition, the countries of central and eastern Europe abandoned the health for all policy documents developed under the old regimes and were reluctant to engage in planning for health, which seemed too much like the previous system. There was, however, a very strong movement to reform health care systems prompted by general economic trends towards privatization, declining economic growth and the desire to cut the cost of health care. The eastern part of the Region began to look to the western part to find a solution to the problems.

In western Europe, containing the cost of health care had become an urgent priority, and some Member States turned to the process of setting targets for health as a way of measuring progress and allocating resources for health more effectively. In England, *The health of the nation (17)* emphasized that clear priorities should be established so that action and resources can be directed to the best effect: "if everything is regarded as a 'priority' then there is, in effect, no priority at all". The Government proposed that the strategy for health should be based on selected key areas, each with specific objectives and targets. Parallel to this, the National Health Service in England had been creating internal markets characterized by differentiating between the purchasers and providers of health care services and had been promoting work with contracts. These developments in health care in England were the first that attracted attention and imitators, but *The health of the nation* played a role in WHO reassessing the need for developing more comprehensive health policies in the eastern part of the Region, and others set out to use the experience of England in this area also.

Soon a number of countries in the eastern part of the Region were developing overall policies for health alongside moves to reform health care systems. Albania and Bulgaria, for example, seemed to focus on health care reform first and broader policies for health second, in what appeared to be a two-stage process. Other countries, such as Estonia, Lithuania and Slovakia, were trying to develop documents on health care reform parallel to or as part of wider health policies.

In the early 1980s, the pioneer countries had been developing health for all policies in a favourable economic climate. Finland, for example, had enjoyed strong economic growth at that time, and the necessary resources for developing primary health care and health promotion programmes could be obtained without necessarily reducing secondary and tertiary health care; the less painful decision was made to reduce the growth rate of these services. In the 1990s, many countries were presented with a quite different fiscal climate. Many countries apparently hope that the health for all approach might reduce health care costs, but substantial anecdotal evidence indicates that, when the going gets tough economically, the tough focus on saving the health care services at the expense of health promotion activities. In some countries in central and eastern Europe, not just health promotion activities were under attack but international loans were at stake unless they agreed to reduce hospital beds as instructed by lenders. It is hardly surprising, therefore, that these countries mainly focused on health care services and were slow to refocus on health for all.

Apart from economic reasons, however, the reassessment of health policy development can be linked to part of an overall process of economic, social and political reconstruction, such as in Lithuania following independence. Re-establishment of a medical association and parliamentary health committee, restructuring of the Ministry of Health and development of a health policy were seen to be important markers of regained independence in Lithuania.

Political commitment – at various levels

As governments change, many new ministers do not support the long-term visions of their predecessors, with the result that the number of valid national and regional health for all policies is constantly changing. Currently, 22 of the 51 Member States in Europe have valid documents on national health policy. Some countries have documents that are in draft or consultation form or are awaiting government approval. Many more have begun the process at the national, regional or local level or at a number of levels simultaneously.

National-level policies for health are inappropriate in a number of countries, since another level of government is responsible for developing policy. For example, in Austria and Germany, the *Länder* are responsible for formulating, financing and implementing policy; in Belgium the regions are also responsible for health policy; in Switzerland the cantons formulate health policy. Nevertheless, these federal countries do have strong mechanisms for discussing issues related to policy at the national level, in addition to their national legislative bodies, and the regions meet regularly, both formally and informally, and develop joint projects. In Switzerland, for example, the cantons of Berne, Tessin and Vaud began working together in 1987 to develop indicators related to the WHO European health for all policy *(18)*.

The national and subnational levels are synchronized to various degrees. For example, all the autonomous regions in Spain developed their own health policy at some time in recent years, but an attempt was also made to formulate a national integrated health plan bringing subnational policies together under a common umbrella (this was presented to Parliament but not formally approved). The United Kingdom does not have an overall health policy. Departments of health in each of the four constituent countries (England, Wales, Scotland and Northern Ireland) have separate responsibilities for health policy. Each developed its own policy in the early 1990s, and all have been revised in the light of the vision and objectives of the new Labour Government *(7, 19–21)*. In Sweden, a number of counties developed health for all policies some years ago, and the formulation of national targets for health is being discussed.

This study has primarily examined published national or regional health policy documents and some documents from cities. Halfway through the period under examination enormous changes took place, with a large number of new countries emerging from the USSR. In this period of discontinuity and change, it is difficult to say whether a top-down (national government leading) or bottom-up (led by regions, local authorities and potentially grassroots movements) approach to developing health policy has been most common in countries in the Region as a whole. In western Europe, the different administrative systems have led to a relatively balanced mix of the top-down and bottom-up approaches. In the countries in the eastern part of the Region, the approach was certainly top-down when the health for all process began in the 1980s. In the present situation of increasing pluralism in these countries, the process is much less top-down, but since the role and responsibility of regions in these countries (under whatever name) is still being clarified, they have not yet had a chance to try a bottom-up approach. In Poland, for example, substantial regions were first being delineated in 1998 by combining a number of voivodships. In the coming years, it will be interesting to see whether regions make use of opportunities presented by the fact that their roles have not yet been circumscribed and move strongly ahead, or whether a tradition of relying on central guidance will slow them down if such guidance is not forthcoming.

The role and potential of the subnational level in policy-making for health and the influence of national, regional and local relationships is a potentially valuable area for analysis, especially as decentralization is continuing and opportunities are increasing for regions in different countries to link directly for information exchange and collaboration.

The effect of WHO

After the health for all framework for Europe was formally adopted in 1984, the WHO Regional Office for Europe appears to have been an important catalyst for the development of health policy in many countries. Many national-, regional- and city-level policy documents clearly refer to the European health for all policy, the health promotion movement and the Ottawa Charter for Health Promotion *(22)* in which WHO has been strongly involved. The Regional Office has also played a role in actively encouraging and supporting health for all policy development, as demonstrated by the replies to the questionnaire sent out for this study. Countries have continued to consult the Regional Office on policy development.

Over the years, 12 countries and 2 regions within countries have formally requested comments from WHO on their draft documents on health for all policy as part of their consultation process. A number have worked closely with the Regional Office, using WHO to advise them when formulating their own policies. The health for all policy in Finland materialized in response to policy trends that were already apparent in Finland. Nevertheless, following the first four years of attempts to implement the policy, Finland requested that WHO review their progress, partly to revitalize the process of developing health policy within Finland and also to provide a test case that other countries might then consider following *(23)*.

WHO networks have also played a strong role in initiating or formulating health for all policies in some countries. Policy-makers and health professionals working with such WHO European networks as Healthy Cities *(24)*, the Regions for Health Network *(25)* and the countrywide integrated noncommunicable diseases intervention (CINDI) programme *(26)*, for example, appear to have been influential in the process of developing health policy in their respective countries. These people have acted as advisers to national, regional or city authorities and used their knowledge of the European experience to influence local politicians. The European Healthy Cities network, in particular, makes a strong attempt to involve city mayors in its annual meetings so that they gain personal experience of innovations for health gain.

Other organizations

In recent years, countries in the eastern part of the Region have been working with international organizations such as the European Union (for example, Poland), the United Nations Development Programme, other United Nations agencies and the World Bank to develop overall policies for health. The approach taken frequently appears to be influenced by health for all. This trend in the countries of central and eastern Europe has been especially apparent since the 1993 *World development report (27)*, which focused "primarily on the relation between policy choices, both inside and outside the health sector, and health outcomes, especially for the poor".

Legitimizing the process of developing health policy

The process of developing health policy can be legitimized in a number of ways: through a transparent process of formulating policy, clearly indicating who gets involved and on what terms; the style of the debate and criteria for decision-making; the form of the policy; and the process for monitoring and evaluation. (Public participation is discussed in a later section.) The way health for all policy documents (the main focus of this study) are finalized and legitimized differs according to the normal political or administrative practice in every country or region. The 1991 European health for all policy *(28)* suggests that commitment should be "affirmed at the highest level". The following examples indicate the variety of approaches to this.

In some countries, health for all policy documents were presented to parliament, either to be approved, such as in Slovakia, or, more usually, simply for discussion and to disseminate information and build support across party lines, such as in England, Finland, Iceland and the Netherlands. Elsewhere, for example in the regions in Spain, policy documents sometimes need to be discussed in parliaments of the autonomous regions in order to then introduce legislation that will underpin the health policy. Lithuania involved the Parliamentary Health Committee very closely throughout the process of developing health policy, organizing national health policy conferences with the participation of parliamentarians, health professionals, local authorities and nongovernmental organizations, to further expose the policy and win support across parties. In the Czech Republic, the health policy was discussed in the parliamentary Committee for Social Policy and Health, which recommended that the Government accept it. Legitimation through the parliamentary system seems to have played a key role in keeping health for all on the political agenda in a number of countries, since this generated support from several political parties, ensuring that the approach survived in some form even following a change of government.

The potential role of parliamentarians in developing health for all policy and how this could be strengthened and expanded would be worth investigating further.

In other countries, such as Estonia and Latvia, the policy is legitimized through discussion and approval by the cabinet or is simply presented under the auspices of the ministry of health, but this reduces the potential for cross-party and multisectoral support. In many countries, the minister for health may not have the authority to achieve the collaboration with his or her colleagues that is essential to implement a health for all policy. Only recently in the Russian Federation, for example, have ministers been given the right to approach each other directly to seek collaboration. Bringing the policy to the cabinet can give it greater political weight, achieve wider ownership and promote better collaboration between cabinet members for its implementation.

Countries with a more federal system have their own specific ways of legitimizing a national-level process. In Spain, for example, the Interterritorial Council of the National Health System discussed the national policy; the Council is chaired by the Minister for Health, and all the autonomous regions are represented. Germany and Switzerland have a similar process. In Turkmenistan, although the health policy documents are discussed in the Halk Maslahaty (People's Council), which is the highest representative body and meets at least once a year, the president has the final responsibility.

The transparency of the process for policy formulation, monitoring and evaluation inherently confers legitimacy. This is discussed further in the section on public participation (page 301).

The content and form of the policy presentation

This section provides examples of the content and format of health for all policy documents to highlight the diversity of the approaches used in countries. Although the content of the general health policy documents varies, they have common features.

Stating the purpose

Most health for all policy documents start with a statement of purpose or a vision of the future. For example, Tajikistan's vision is of "a country in which the policy of health for all allows people to be in harmony with nature, in which individuals value health and realize that health is the most indispensable feature of the quality of life, and in which health providers work in adequate conditions." *(29)*. That for Scotland states: "our goal is a healthier Scotland, with less ill-health and higher levels of well-being and fitness across the nation and social spectrum" *(20)*.

Clarifying the process

Although the transparency of the process confers legitimacy, few of the policy documents examined actually explain how the document was formulated or how it will be monitored and revised in the future. Including such information on the process itself would alert people to the points at which they might intervene and would encourage the kind of feedback that is essential if the policy is to be evaluated and adjusted.

Defining the challenges

All the overall health policy documents available to us analysed the current situation and stated the problem. The extent of the situation analysis depended partly on whether or not the policy document had been preceded by a more extensive public health report or issue-specific reports. The Bulgarian document *Health for the nation (30)*, for example, analysed the situation quite extensively, whereas the

Lithuanian health programme (31) gives a much briefer analysis since it was preceded by an extensive public health report *Lithuanian health report – 1990's (11)*. The document from Malta takes a middle road: analysing the situation in user-friendly language. This document is also interesting, as it places the development of a policy for health within a broader challenge, that of preparing for Malta's entry into the European Union.

Selecting priorities

Almost all the documents state the overall objectives, supported by quantitative or qualitative targets. The documents issued in recent years differ from earlier documents in two main ways. First, most of them are more selective, focusing on a smaller number of areas of concern or key issues than did the first national documents to be formulated, many of which covered most of the 38 European targets for health for all. Second, the criteria used to select these priorities are made more explicit, making the process more transparent. For example, all four country documents from the United Kingdom circulated for discussion in 1998 *(7, 19–21)* state why certain issues are given priority and discuss somewhat why other issues have not been selected as priorities.

The most common criteria for selecting priorities and targets are:

- the extent of the health problem as a major cause of mortality or morbidity;
- the scope for improvement through effective and acceptable intervention;
- public and professional opinion of whether the health problem is a major concern;
- whether progress towards achieving the targets can be measured through available data or data that can be easily collected, and whether reliable indicators exist to monitor progress;
- whether solving a health problem would reduce inequity in health; and
- other constraints imposed by policy or societal characteristics, including cost constraints (for example, substantial sick leave).

Setting targets

In the earlier part of the period under review, most countries in the eastern part of the Region favoured setting quantified targets, whereas some western countries were reluctant to set targets. The first policy document from Finland *(32)*, for example, opted for qualitative policy statements that indicated the general policy directions, and the first document from the Netherlands *(33)* showed similar reluctance, also relying on qualitative statements.

More recently, however, the value of setting targets has been much more widely recognized. The main reasons for setting targets are as follows *(34)*.

- The process of setting targets requires an assessment of the present situation and expected future trends, on as scientific a basis as possible.
- Monitoring the targets offers an excellent learning experience through discussion of what had been hoped for, how far this was achieved and why.

- Targets provide a powerful communication tool.
- Targets indicate to potential partners what must happen, and what their role might be in making this happen.
- Targets can provide a rallying call for groups at the grassroots level to demand action.
- Targets can be an excellent tool for strengthening accountability for health (which is one reason why some groups would like to avoid them).
- Certain targets can provide a reference point for assessing the advisability of day-to-day actions.
- Involving people in the process of setting targets raises awareness and can be the first step in implementing health policy.

The main reasons deterring some countries from setting quantified targets include:

- the difficulty in providing scientifically credible evidence for some targets;
- the reluctance of politicians and health professionals to set targets for which they will be held accountable, especially in areas in which they have little or no influence; and
- the danger of appearing to give priority to issues for which targets can be easily quantified, when other issues that are less easy to quantify might be considered equally or even more important.

Examples of the different types of target used are set out in Box 3.1.

The recent trend is to set fewer targets. *Working together for a healthier Scotland (20)*, for example, states that: "In considering the need for indicators and targets, the government believe it important that these should be kept to the minimum necessary for the proper assessment of improvement in Scotland's health". At the regional level, during the meeting of the Regional Committee for Europe in 1997, Member States requested that the number of regional targets for health for all be limited. This position was reinforced in the consultation process for the renewal of the European health for all policy, leading to a reduction from 38 to 21 targets in HEALTH21 *(34)*.

The earlier policy documents tended to set targets related to one time horizon, such as the year 2000. As long-term targets must be seen in relation to more medium- and short-term efforts, and achieving certain intermediate targets may be required to achieve long-term targets, more recent policy documents specify targets with varying time horizons.

Setting short- and medium-term targets allows politicians to show progress within the time during which they expect to be in office. The mix of time horizons probably also relates, however, to the different types of target set in the more recent documents. The earlier documents seemed to try to focus mainly on outcome targets. Experience has shown that this is not sufficient and that it is also important to set targets for strategic steps or action in the implementation process. The case study for Catalonia, for example, shows that the health policy included many input and process targets as well as outcome targets.

Box 3.1. Examples of different types of target

Countries, regions and cities that have emphasized formulating quantified targets have used various types of target.

- **Outcome (or primary) targets**

"By the year 2005, to reduce infant mortality rate by 25%"
Lithuanian health programme (31), 1998.

- **Intermediate targets**

Intermediate targets are related to risk factors and must be achieved in order to reach the primary target. These can be grouped into three subtypes.

i) Health conditions or symptoms

"To reduce mean systolic blood pressure in the adult population by at least 5 mmHg by 2005"
The health of the nation: a consultative document for health in England (17), 1991.

ii) Exposure to risks or hazards

"Carbon dioxide emissions should be reduced to the 1990 level by the year 2000"
Health for all by the year 2000. Revised strategy for cooperation (35), Finland, 1993.

iii) Behaviour

"By the year 2000, to increase the number of pregnant women who stop smoking at the start of their pregnancy and subsequently, by 75% of the 1996 figure"
Health vision 2000. A national health policy (36), Malta, 1996.

- **Input and output targets**

Input and output targets relate to the resources or services that must be available to achieve the primary and/or intermediate targets.

"Providing eight small-scale nursing units in the community by the end of 1997 to replace unsuitable accommodation and to meet the needs of the expanding population of old people"
Shaping a healthier future (37), Ireland, 1993.

"By the year 2000 at the latest, all pensioners-to-be should have the opportunity of participating in the programmes preparing them for retirement"
[Better health for all in Östergötland] (38), Sweden, 1990.

Box 3.1. (contd)

• **Process or action targets**

Process or action targets relate to action that must be taken to reach the primary targets.

"During 1995–96, the Ministry of Agriculture should develop standards for the use of pesticides in agriculture"
Strategy of Tajikistan for future health by 2005 (29), 1995.

"By 1994, the use of the protocol for the early detection of gestational diabetes will be general"
Health plan for Catalonia 1993–1995 (39), Spain, 1993.

• **Targets related to underlying causes**

Targets related to the underlying causes of health are quite rare.

"… it is the investment of time and resources such as the £5 billion Welfare to Work programme, the establishment of the National Minimum Wage and the reform of our welfare system to help support people back to independence which will make the most significant contributions to the strategy."
Our healthier nation: a contract for health. A consultative document (7), England, 1998.

Perhaps because general policies fail to reach some vulnerable groups, there are also increasing examples of separate targets being set both for the whole population and for specific groups based on age, gender, socioeconomic status or geography.

The international literature does not offer much insight into the advantages and possible disadvantages of working with quantified targets in this complex field or on the methods appropriate for selecting targets of the various types discussed. This would be an area of interest for an international exchange of views and experience.

Concern with diseases or with groups of people?
The various national and local health policy documents approach target-setting from different vantage points. Some focus more on dealing with diseases or with health risks; others give more weight to dealing with the needs of population groups and the means of tackling the health challenges. For example, the first health policy document for England *The health of the nation (17)*, took this approach, as did the health plan for Catalonia *(39)*, although it also included many process-related targets. Others combine the focus on diseases and risk factors with targets related to changing health services, management, research, information or other aspects of health policy. Malta's *Health vision 2000 (36)* and the ten priority health targets for North Rhine–Westphalia (see case study on p. 41) are examples of this approach. Most

documents strongly focus on health care services, although they do not all include targets related to changes in the organization and delivery of services. The targets included in the policy for the Östergötland County in Sweden *(38)* focus strongly on changing unhealthy behaviour such as smoking, promoting healthy behaviour such as physical exercise and changing people's knowledge, but also the availability of information and support, such as access to study circles, and outcome targets related to functional capacity. Different age groups have different targets, with specific emphasis on older people.

Other policies that focus on diseases and health risks also target specific groups such as children, disabled people and elderly people. The documents from Bulgaria *(30)* and Turkey *(40)* are examples of this approach. In Ireland, in addition to the overall approach *(37)*, a separate policy for women's health has been developed, dealing with: health issues that are particular to women, predominantly affect women and affect women differently to men; and access to health care by disadvantaged women *(41)*.

The increased focus on people in a number of policy documents has brought with it greater attention to the importance of dealing with people's needs and using the opportunities presented at different stages in life to promote and protect health. Scotland's present consultation document *(20)* refers to the influence of parenting on young people's health and social behaviour. The strategy for Northern Ireland *(21)* refers to the long-term benefits of investing in the childhood years: strategies that promote the health and wellbeing of children.

Working in settings where health is created or at risk

An increasing number of policy documents examine health challenges in relation to various settings such as the family, schools and the workplace. The current consultation document in England *(7)* strongly focuses on schools, workplaces and neighbourhoods to tackle inequity in health, and financial resources have already been designated for health development in disadvantaged areas through integrated action by multiple agencies in health action zones *(42)*. The health plan for the City of Copenhagen *(43)* strongly focuses on settings and also on social networks, which should be encouraged and supported for three main strategic reasons: developing social relations, support in connection with certain life events and support for people in vulnerable positions.

Although all countries use a mix of approaches, most are still oriented towards disease and, to some extent, risks to health, and most have a strong component related to health care. One reason for this traditional approach could be that it is easily recognized and understood both within and outside the health sector and therefore might be more easily accepted. The disease-oriented approach, however, presents an inherent danger of encouraging a vertical, compartmentalized way of working. In recent years, however, the focus has shifted somewhat towards dealing with specific population groups and settings, which should encourage a more horizontal or integrated approach.

Examples of foci in national policy documents are given in Box 3.2.

Box 3.2. Focus on disease, risks to health, people and settings

- **Focus on disease**

"… reduce the death rate from heart disease and stroke and related illnesses amongst people under 65 years by at least a further third (33%) by 2010 from a baseline at 1996"
Our healthier nation: a contract for health. A consultative document (7), England, 1998.

- **Focus on risk factors**

"By the year 2000, the number of school children who take up smoking should be reduced by 50% of the rate established in the 1995 census."
Health vision 2000. A national health policy (36), Malta, 1996.

- **Focus on people**

"By the year 2000, under 5 mortality will be reduced to 50 per thousand and infant mortality will be reduced to 30 per thousand."
National health policy of Turkey (40), 1993.

"By 1997 carers should be offered a separate assessment of their own needs."
Health and wellbeing: into the next millennium (44), Northern Ireland, 1998.

- **Focus on settings**

Homes
"During the period of this strategy the target remains that at least 88% of people aged 75 and over will be supported in their own homes."
Health and wellbeing: into the next millennium (44), Northern Ireland, 1998.

Workplaces
"To reduce by 15% exclusion from working life in the form of early retirement due to functional impairment in the neck/shoulders/lower back by the year 2000"
[*Better health for all in Östergötland*] *(38)*, Sweden, 1990.

Strategies to achieve the objectives and targets
A number of the currently valid policy documents are still at the consultation stage, so that detailed strategies for carrying them out, including plans for monitoring, evaluation, review and revision, have not yet been clearly articulated. In other cases the general statement of policy is underpinned by links to issue-specific documents or legislation. Malta's policy *Health vision 2000 (36)* summarized in annexes

its policies and strategies for controlling drug and alcohol abuse and for improving nutrition. The recent document for Northern Ireland *(21)* and a supporting strategic document *(44)* are prime examples of overall policy documents linked closely to issue-specific policies, some of which are in other sectors. On the whole, however, issues traditionally outside the domain of the health service sector, such as employment, housing and the environment (as potential indicators of social cohesion), are not covered well, and the issue-specific policies usually refer to combating particular diseases or providing care for certain groups. Malta's policy is one of the exceptions, since it also deals with the possible health impact of its main economic sector, tourism. The region of Valencia in Spain also attempted some years ago to develop a policy for public health in conjunction with the two main economic sectors, agriculture and tourism *(1)*.

Implementing the principles of health for all

The main aim of this study was to provide a broad overview of how Member States approach health policy and how countries have tried to achieve the health for all principles.

Fig. 3.3 summarizes the extent to which countries are using various policy instruments (past, present or future plans) to address various principles for health for all. The darker the shading, the more countries are using a particular category of policy instrument; the lighter the shading the less common is the use of such tools. In this section of the study we will examine each of the health for all characteristics in turn, exploring the types of policy instrument reported as being used to implement them, and then try to draw some general conclusions. It will be seen that countries use a range of policy instruments, but the combination of tools used varies between the principles.

The following sections discuss each health for all principle in turn, explore whether the various types of policy instruments were used, and give examples of their use.

Promoting equity in health

Target 1 of the 38 European health for all targets approved in 1984 and 1991 and targets 1 and 2 of the 21 targets approved in 1998 relate to equity in health. Unfortunately, however, inequity in health between countries has been growing rather than diminishing. The increasing gap in health status is mainly caused by a deterioration in the situation in the eastern part of the Region.

In 1995, the difference between the countries with the lowest and the highest life expectancy in the Region was about 15 years versus about 7 years in 1970, and the east–west gap in mortality is present in all age groups (Fig. 3.4) *(5)*. Indicators related to life expectancy free of disability and/or chronic disease demonstrate that social inequality in health expectancy may be even greater than the inequality in life expectancy *(5)*.

Poverty, one of the main causes of these disappointing trends, remains a main focus of the health for all policy in the 21st century. The 1998 *World health report* defines public health as being "the art of

Fig. 3.3. Use of policy instruments in relation to the health for all policy principles

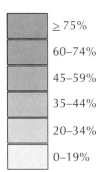

	Equity	Public participation	Intersectoral action			Reorienting primary health care	Out-come orientation
			life-styles	environ-ment	health care		
Research and information							
Health education and awareness							
Consultation and negotiation							
Structural, administrative and management							
Financial							
Legislation and regulation							
Human resource development							
Monitoring and evaluation							
Other							

≥ 75%

60–74%

45–59%

35–44%

20–34%

0–19%

Percentage of countries (45 = 100%)

applying science in the context of politics so as to reduce inequalities in health while ensuring the best health for the greatest number" *(45).* This section examines how art and science were combined in Europe to promote equity in health.

Fig. 3.4. Life expectancy at birth in subregional groups of countries
in the European Region, 1970–1996

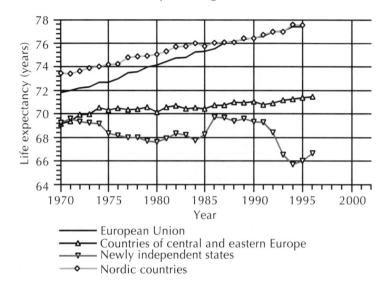

Research and information

After the health for all policy for Europe was adopted in 1984, two documents were prepared to encourage research supporting health for all development *(46,47)*. The priority topics included improving official health statistics so that they reflect differences in health, and investigating the causes of inequity in health.

The amount of research on inequity in health and its causes has increased vastly in the last two decades. Similarly, the WHO European health for all monitoring exercises show that most countries continue to provide information on geographical or urban versus rural differences in health status, but in more recent years almost one third also refer to differences between occupational groups, the health of poor people and unemployed people, indicating that Member States better understand the causes of inequity in health *(48)*.

Considerable effort has been made, mainly in countries in western Europe, to ensure that national statistics link health data with socioeconomic variables such as income, occupation and education in order to reflect possible inequity. The Nordic countries have a tradition of working together to prepare joint reports on inequality in their countries, dating back to 1980 *(49)*. More recently, a study funded by the European Union *(50)* covering 12 countries involved considerable efforts by national statistical services to provide comparable data. In the last few years, a number of countries in central and eastern Europe have also started to map out inequity, including Albania, Hungary and Lithuania.

The United Kingdom has perhaps the most sophisticated information on inequity, in part because these data have been collected since the 1860s and refined over many years. In relation to *The health of the nation*, a Variations Subgroup was set up, which reported *(51)* on the inequality existing in the early 1990s and what the Department of Health should do about it. When the Labour Party came into power in 1997, they immediately set up the Independent Inquiry into Inequalities in Health chaired by a former chief medical officer, Sir Donald Acheson, with a mandate to investigate the situation further and to propose specific strategies to deal with inequity in health. The Inquiry published its report in November 1998 *(52)*, and its findings should feed into *Our healthier nation (7)*, which will be finalized at the same time. Such research and reports have also been carried out in the United Kingdom at the level of regions *(53)* and in some cities. Spain also set up a special commission, chaired by Vincente Navarro, which published an extensive report *(54)* on inequality in health in 1996.

In recent years, there has been considerable interest in research to investigate the effects on health of adverse socioeconomic circumstances and experiences accumulated over the life course. Denmark is one of the countries where considerable research is being carried out on this *(55)*.

One of the most concerted research efforts comes from the Netherlands; in 1987, the Ministry of Welfare, Health and Cultural Affairs established a programme committee on socioeconomic health differences *(56)*. Since then, one five-year research programme has been completed (1989–1994) and a second is under way (1995–2000). Efforts have included measuring inequity, trying to assess the causes, and evaluating various types of intervention to promote equity in health. It is especially interesting that the Netherlands Parliament has been kept informed of progress, and members of all the main political parties have participated in conferences held to discuss the results.

As most countries in the Region have focused so strongly on health care reform in recent years, countries might have been expected to maintain research to assess the impact of the changing organization and provision of health care on equity in access to care, especially in the eastern part of the Region. Although anecdotal evidence suggests concern about possible unintentional effects in compounding inequity, there is less evidence of anything being done about it. Finland, Spain and Turkey were reported to be undertaking relevant research and, in the eastern part of the Region, Armenia, Hungary, Kyrgyzstan, Poland and Slovenia reported being involved in similar research. This is still a relatively small number of countries, given the scope of reforms, especially in the eastern part of the Region, but this issue may actually be given more attention than indicated in the replies to our questionnaire. A number of countries were also undertaking research on the uptake of health screening and on people who are reluctant to access preventive services. Even a brief examination of some of the main health journals indicates that academic departments are doing substantial work on this issue; it is less clear whether this influences policy.

On the whole, most countries still appear to emphasize measuring health status, which is essential if health policies are to be oriented towards outcome. A few countries reported monitoring the health status of ethnic minorities, and in Hungary, Ireland and Slovakia, for example, changes in the health status of gypsies and travellers were being examined.

Gender and the health of women was of particular concern for countries as disparate as France, Norway, the Republic of Moldova, Sweden and Tajikistan. Whereas in the Republic of Moldova and Tajikistan the issue of women's health was very much considered to be linked to their reproductive health, Sweden took a much broader view, stressing the importance of integrating information on gender and socioeconomic variables in health research.

This study focuses on what countries do to develop policies for health. Their actions may be influenced, however, by external factors such as the availability of funding for research. In this respect, the European Union has funded a number of international studies such as one dealing with inequality in health status (50), and a review of current studies in 18 European countries (57). Funding has also been provided for research in related areas. The European Commission established an observatory on national policies to combat social exclusion, which reported for several years on issues related to social integration and integration in the labour market that are relevant to equity in health (58).

Although the availability of information reflecting inequity in health improved in almost half the Member States and the research community is increasingly interested, as shown by the international literature, research activities are not yet strongly linked to policy formulation, implementation and evaluation. Efforts are being made to change this situation. Finland and Slovenia, for example, stated that the results of the research would contribute to the development of guidelines and standards; Malta, the Netherlands and the United Kingdom specifically linked improvement in information on inequity to the development of their national health policies. The efforts involved in the two five-year programmes of research being carried out in the Netherlands indicate the time and commitment needed for such a process.

Raising awareness of equity
Given that promoting equity in health means offering a fair chance to all, one would hope that everyone would embrace this ethical principle. This has not been the case, however. One of the best documented cases is that of the United Kingdom (59,60), where the availability of relevant data on the growing socioeconomic inequity in health created considerable concern among health professionals in the late 1970s. The Secretary of State for Social Services of the Labour Government appointed a working group to assess the national and international evidence and draw some policy implications. The working group, chaired by Sir Douglas Black, submitted its report in April 1980. By that time, however, there was a new Conservative administration. The new Government did not print and publish the report. Instead, only 260 duplicated copies of the typescript were made available. There was no press release or press conference. A few copies were sent to a number of journalists on a Friday afternoon at the start of the long holiday weekend in August. As was suggested in *The Lancet (61)*, there appeared to be a clear attempt to "reduce the report's impact to a minimum". Citing the cost of carrying out the report's recommendations, the Secretary of State said that he could not endorse the recommendations. Considerable efforts were

made by other groups to raise awareness of the report's findings, including a special conference organized by the Association of Community Health Councils for England and Wales.

In January 1986, the Director-General of the Health Education Council commissioned an update of the evidence since 1980 and an assessment of the progress made on the recommendations of the Black Report. Margaret Whitehead *(60)*, who carried out the update, reported back later in 1986. Again political events overtook the process of launching the report. This time, prepublication copies had been sent out to health authorities and a briefing involving a panel of distinguished experts had been arranged for 24 March 1988. A general election was imminent, however, and political sensitivities were high. One hour before the planned meeting was due to take place, the chairman of the Health Education Authority cancelled the briefing. This had perhaps the opposite effect of that intended, creating enormous press interest so that *The health divide* was probably read by many more people than would otherwise have been the case. These events are described in detail in Whitehead *(60)*. Under the recent Conservative Government, *The health of the nation* in England did not use the word inequity, referring instead to variations, and it is only with the change to a Labour Government in 1997 that high visibility is now being given to inequity and how to deal with it (see Box 3.3).

Reports from Spain suggest that the work of the Navarro Commission has not been as widely disseminated as had been hoped. In the eastern part of the Region, prior to the political changes, inequity was not discussed because the political system prevailing at the time was not considered to allow inequity. After the political changes there was some brief difficulty with the word equity, since this was one term used to describe the communist system and was thus discredited together with the previous regime. But where there is a will there is a way, and just as in England, in which the word "variations" was used when "inequity" was politically unacceptable, some countries in the eastern part of the Region repackaged the concept under the term "human rights"; the Czech Republic, for example used the term "solidarity". More recently, the issue of inequity appears to be gaining increasing recognition in the countries in the eastern part of the Region.

These examples very clearly indicate that equity in health is a highly political issue. Sound research and reliable information are not in themselves sufficient to ensure action. Political support is a prerequisite for initiating the type of policies and programmes necessary to promote equity in health. Lithuania and the Netherlands are good examples of the health sector making efforts from the beginning to engage the support of all major political parties (Box 3.3). In the Netherlands, careful attention was paid to obtaining a political balance on the committee overseeing the five year research programmes and on the public panels organized at the conferences to discuss the results. The approach was to carry out a careful analysis over a number of years, reporting back regularly and publicly, with the aim of keeping all the main parties on board and preparing the basis to translate research into action *(62)*. In Lithuania, the Parliamentary Health Committee, on which all the main parties are represented, has been continually and comprehensively briefed not only on the situation in Lithuania but also on the findings from other countries, in order to strengthen the evidence that equity in health is a persistent and widespread challenge that concerns policy-makers across Europe.

Box 3.3. Promoting equity in health:
examples of actions to inform the process and raise awareness

The Netherlands – long-term commitment with cross-party support

In 1987 a Programme Committee on Socioeconomic Health Differences was set up. The main political parties participated. The task was to report on the magnitude of the problem, relevant explanations and possible intervention that could close the gaps. Action included two five-year research programmes involving research institutions throughout the country, regular and public reporting on progress, strong links to similar action in other countries and attempts to assess what works.

Lithuania – link to an international programme strengthens the process and provides a test case for other countries

In 1996 Lithuania was invited to join the global initiative on equity in health and health care launched by WHO and the Swedish International Development Agency. More than 20 existing sources of health and socioeconomic indicators have been identified that can be used to map out inequity in health *(34, 63)*. The action comprised:

- phase 1 – examining existing data sources for possible use;

- phase 2 – working groups processing information and preparing a public report; and

- phase 3 – presenting the report in a public forum for health, discussing the intervention in the framework of the health for all policy approved by Parliament in 1998.

Experience has been shared through WHO networks and with countries in other WHO regions.

The United Kingdom – adapting to shifts in the policy environment

The health of the nation (17) noted the need to identify the variation that occurs in specific health problems in order to concentrate efforts on people at risk and adopt different strategies for different groups. The Chief Medical Officer established a group to report on the variation and on what the Department of Health and the National Health Service can do about it. Prior to the 1997 general election, the Labour Party announced that tackling inequity would be a major part of its political programme and that it intended to establish a commission (the Independent Inquiry into Inequalities in Health *(52)*) to go deeper into this issue. *Our healthier nation (7)* highlights tackling the root causes of avoidable illness such as poverty, low wages, unemployment, housing and air pollution. Pilot intervention projects are being launched to tackle inequity in disadvantaged areas.

Health education

Fig. 3.3 shows that a number of countries report using health education to change people's behaviour. Nevertheless, better educated and more affluent people are more receptive to health education messages, assimilating them faster than do less advantaged groups *(64)*. Some countries did report having introduced special health education programmes targeting vulnerable groups. The groups most often mentioned were ethnic minorities, migrants, travellers and gypsies. It was not clear, however, how far these efforts went beyond preparing information material in ethnic minority languages and, more importantly, whether health education was accompanied by measures to reduce some of the stressors such as inadequate income or social support that can cause disadvantaged people to turn to smoking and drinking in order to cope with their lives.

Consultation and negotiation

Although equity is a sensitive issue, between 35% and 44% of the countries responding to the question-naire reported having used consultation and negotiation as a means of implementing their objective of promoting equity in health (Fig. 3.3). The countries that did had four main categories of action related to negotiation for resource allocation, for collaborative action, with the health professions and with voluntary organizations.

Resource allocation, both between the central level and regions and between particular institutions. Spain, for example, reported negotiating with scientific associations and the regions to agree on the criteria for equitable resource allocation, and Switzerland negotiated to reach agreement between the cantons on criteria for allocating care that is necessarily limited, such as organ transplants.

Collaborative action from other sectors in support of vulnerable groups. Bulgaria reported negotiations with the Ministries of Education, Labour and Social Affairs for the implementation of the United Nations Convention on the Rights of the Child. Slovakia negotiated to agree on the needs of vulnerable people for special transport and Tajikistan to find a means of integrating mentally disabled people into in the workforce.

Negotiation with the health professions. Numerous countries referred to negotiations with the health professions. For example, in Turkey negotiations were conducted with the health professions on changes in the insurance system to benefit vulnerable people; in Poland discussions were held on the regional allocation of staff positions; and in Slovakia consultation was instigated to secure mobile vaccination teams to reach out to people who were being missed.

Consultation with voluntary organizations.   The United Kingdom reported that regional health authorities had been required to consult local groups on the development of health care in their area. Countries from both the eastern and western parts of the Region negotiated with representative associations of disabled people.

Structural, administrative and management measures

Most of the action related to structural, administrative and management measures focuses on equity in access to health care and, in particular, on decentralizing health care services or expanding primary health care. This includes such measures as expanding the package of services covered by national health insurance. For example, in Austria the range of services was expanded to include psychotherapy and home nursing. Bulgaria published regulations regarding the right to reimbursement. Italy applied uniform rules and standards throughout the country. Ireland reduced the time spent on waiting lists. In Portugal, when health care provision was decentralized to five regions, the regions were given the right to set their own user charges, subject to minimum and maximum levels set by the Ministry of Health; the Government later found this ruling to be inequitable, however, and this right was again reserved for the national level.

Structural changes included specific actions to support vulnerable people, such as financial incentives for general practitioners to work in disadvantaged areas in the United Kingdom, primary health care initiatives targeted specifically at homeless people, travellers and refugees in Ireland, providing screening services for Moroccan women in the Netherlands at times when their husbands can be present and, in Uzbekistan, providing separate entrances for pregnant women in rural medical centres.

The few types of structural action not related to health care included access to safe drinking-water in Albania, extension of nutrition programmes in Ireland and the establishment of a Commission for the Advancement of Women in Malta.

Financial measures
Countries most frequently mentioned financial measures as a tool to reduce inequity (Fig. 3.3). These measures generally did not focus on the root causes of inequity such as income and poverty, however, but were mainly restricted to equity in health care, including:

- the geographical distribution of financial resources for health care;
- exempting vulnerable groups from out-of-pocket payments; and
- introducing special packages of health care benefits for vulnerable families and various subsidies and allowances for vulnerable groups.

One innovative exception was in Sweden, where interest in examining and improving conditions of work has long been keen. Following research to identify where the worst working conditions were, a special levy on business was used to create a Working Life Fund *(65)*.

Geographical distribution of financial resources for health care. In the United Kingdom, for example, the Resource Allocation Working Party recommended that financial allocations for regional authorities account for population-, age- and gender-specific rates of hospital utilization, standardized mortality ratios, the regional flow of patients and the high cost of health care in London and south-east England. Methods for allocating resources were further refined in the late 1980s and early 1990s, especially to account for differences between small areas within regions. Several countries, including those in the eastern part of the Region restructuring health care services, refer to developing a similar formula to try and bring the allocation of resources more in line with need. In some Scandinavian countries, block grant allocations are used to offset regional differences in local revenue. Some countries in the eastern part of the Region have set up an equalization fund to adjust the regional distribution of funds and ameliorate geographical inequity. A common practice is to give priority to applications from disadvantaged areas when funds for a specified purpose are to be allocated. In the European Union, regions have been classified according to their level of development, and the European Commission allocates considerable funding to the most disadvantaged regions (Objective I regions).

Exempting vulnerable groups from out-of-pocket payments. A number of countries in the eastern part of the Region are moving to establish basic benefit packages for everyone. The cost of certain aspects of health care, such as pharmaceuticals, is also partially reimbursed in some countries as a means of supporting vulnerable groups. When this relates to certain age groups, such as children or elderly people being exempt from payment, or to an easily identifiable condition such as pregnancy or large family size, little problem is encountered in implementing such measures. Defining and assessing who is poor or needy, however, creates problems in most countries; in some this opens the door to corruption, such as when the designation of being vulnerable requires simply the signature of a political figure such as the local mayor or community leader.

Various subsidies and allowances for vulnerable groups. Several eastern European countries mentioned subsidies for housing. A number also mentioned subsidies for food, specifically for bread in Georgia, reflecting the severe economic situation in some countries. Countries in both the east and west were worried about the effects on health of reducing certain subsidies or benefits, such as disability pensions in Norway and housing subsidies in Belarus.

Huge resource transfers that are not assessed for health effects. Although the study has been concerned with what individual countries have included in their policies and strategies to tackle inequity in health, two European Union programmes are important. The European Union poverty programmes and the European Social Fund, which stimulates infrastructure improvement and economic regeneration in disadvantaged regions, were not designed to improve health. The substantial money these programmes distribute, and the fact that they focus on relatively limited geographical areas rather than whole countries, must considerably influence the determinants of health positively or negatively, but comparatively little attention appears to have been given to assessing the health effects of these activities.

Interest in health impact assessment is growing rapidly in the Netherlands, Sweden and the United Kingdom. The Government of the Netherlands has funded research into both qualitative approaches and adapting quantified models for health impact assessment, and guidelines for policy appraisal were prepared in connection with *The health of the nation* in England (66). Improved methods of health impact assessment are supported by developments related to the environment; there have been some tentative attempts to prepare environmental accounts so that they reflect not only changes in income but costs such as environmental damage and depletion of resources (67). In Sweden, leading politicians in municipalities and counties have been analysing the health impact of proposed policy decisions at the local and regional levels. A number of tools for carrying out this assessment are being tested in a sample of county councils and municipalities *(68)*.

Legislation and regulation

Legislation and regulation can provide a powerful tool to ensure that people are at least not formally barred from obtaining an equal chance in life. Again, this study shows that the use of legislation mostly tends to be restricted to measures designed to ensure access to health care. Most countries mentioned that equal access to health care is guaranteed by law. The document from Bulgaria, *Health for the nation (30)*, for example, begins with the relevant excerpts from the constitution. A number of countries in the eastern part of the Region also stated that, in practice, moves to insurance-based health care and, in some cases, the introduction of co-payments are thought to have increased inequity. Some countries said they had taken precautions against this by exempting certain groups, such as children and elderly people, from co-payments.

Human resource development

Efforts are under way in a number of countries, including Armenia, Finland, Ireland, Norway, Poland, Romania, Spain and the United Kingdom, to raise health professionals' awareness of the health needs of various population groups, such as children and older people, and especially of the importance of socioeconomic status in health. Some countries have taken specific steps in planning human resources to meet health care needs. For example, in Iceland, human resources for health are being managed partly on the basis of demographic trends; in France, the health care sector is trying to achieve a more equitable geographical distribution of resources. A couple of countries have also tried reaching out to vulnerable groups by training people from those groups as health care workers. In the Netherlands, for example, the number of people working in the health care sector who are not citizens of the country has been raised to increase participation of ethnic minorities in the labour market and to promote better understanding of ethnic cultures and perceptions. In Slovakia, special efforts are under way to support women from the gypsy community in studying nursing, so as to promote health among the gypsy population. Tajikistan is one of the few countries reporting on attempts to sensitize workers outside the health sector to the health needs of disadvantaged groups. Initiatives are being taken to train the people who prepare food in schools, hospitals and other institutions for disadvantaged groups and for the general public about specific customs relating to food.

Monitoring and evaluation

The process of implementing policies to promote equity in health is monitored and evaluated less often than changes in health status are monitored. This is probably explained in part by the fact that less policy action has been explicitly designed to reduce inequity and partly because the methods for evaluating such action are comparatively underdeveloped. Some of the methods accepted in other areas of evaluation, such as randomized controlled trials, are not easy to use here. Social benefits cannot ethically be given to some groups and withheld from others in order to evaluate the results. Certain research circles appear to be reluctant to accept that research methods are needed that differ from those used in evaluating medical intervention. This can have implications when applications are made for funding and the funds provided for such research appear to be inadequate.

Gepkens & Gunning-Schepers *(69)* have reviewed the international literature to identify evaluations of intervention projects tackling aspects of inequality in health. They identified 98 evaluated studies; most related to interventions dealing with individuals rather than broad policies aimed at groups or communities. In the United Kingdom, a database of good practice is being set up in the framework of *Our healthier nation*. If such information could become available, and especially at the international level, more attention could be focused on evaluation.

A few countries in both the east and west of the Region referred to evaluation of the impact of health care reforms. Spain, for example, was trying to identify barriers to the utilization of health services. When countries mentioned broader social issues such as long-term unemployment or participation in the labour force according to gender, the focus was on monitoring and evaluating what was happening in society rather than evaluating interventions designed to tackle such risk factors.

Evaluating intervention to promote equity in health needs to be given much greater attention in the future. Policy interventions need to provide for evaluation right from the planning stage. The development of databases of current or planned evaluation should help in developing this field.

Facilitating public participation in decision-making

Public participation in decision-making is one of the underlying principles of the health for all policy. Chapter 1 clarified that people have the right to participate in decisions that affect their health and that of the society in which they live and that they should be enabled to do this in a well functioning civic society. But public participation in decision-making also makes practical sense in policy terms, since a health for all policy can only be implemented with the involvement of people from many walks of life *(22)*.

Agreeing to the need for and having the right to participate is one thing; each country's unique institutional and political history very much affects, however, the reality of public participation. In federal and pluralistic countries, for example, many groups share decision-making *(70)*, which is not concentrated in the hands of the government or one institution or group. In Germany, Luxembourg and the Netherlands, for example, the trade unions, sickness funds (many of which are private non-profit organizations) and the local authorities have traditionally played a strong role in consultation and negotiation. Until recently, Finland had a centralized system of public administration, but there was also strong participation at the local level and a long tradition of participating in nongovernmental organizations. In Denmark, Norway and Sweden, responsibility for health is decentralized and the municipal and county administrative systems facilitate participatory decision-making and consensus-building.

In contrast, under the Soviet system, people were not encouraged to participate in decision-making. Anecdotal evidence suggests that the disempowering effect of this still has important implications for the achievement of participation. The number of nongovernmental organizations in these countries has increased tremendously in recent years, but because these organizations are comparatively young, people still have to learn how to make the best use of these mechanisms *(71)*. The countries of central and eastern Europe have a longer and stronger history of participation in decision-making than do the newly independent states, and have made the transition to democracy more rapidly. In particular, countries that experienced large-scale public demonstrations and strikes prior to transition, such as Bulgaria and Poland, exhibit a higher level of public participation and a relatively more stable political situation than do others. In some newly independent states, the institutional and legislative framework for democracy has yet to be established.

Some countries apparently may even decide that moving to a more democratic model is not in the best national interest. For example, in Turkmenistan at the time of this study the Government decided that moving from a centrally planned economy to a market economy required maintaining strong state power to create the socioeconomic conditions necessary to achieve reforms *(72)*.

Other countries in the eastern part of the Region have begun to clearly initiate a move towards a more democratic model. Efforts to further democracy include establishment of a multi-party state, trade unions, nongovernmental organizations and development of the legislative framework. Paradoxically, intense pressure to develop a legislative framework has somewhat inhibited the development of a wider consultation process. Although there are many new actors, such as new political parties, nongovernmental organizations and trade unions, parliaments are under such tremendous pressure to develop a wide array of legislation that there is often little time for real consultation. This means that new bodies are not always participating in policy decisions as had been originally anticipated: for example, nongovernmental organizations may be more involved in implementing rather than formulating policy and as charities rather than as representatives of consumer interests. The source of funding may also unduly influence the organization and operation of some nongovernmental organizations. In some countries, because of the relatively weak relationship between nongovernmental organizations and the state, the organizations have survived and developed largely as a result of foreign aid. In some exceptional cases, deep-seated mistrust of the state system has resulted in more credibility for nongovernmental organizations *(72)*. In Albania, for example, organizations dealing with human rights and democratization generally appear to be well organized and enjoy considerable support from western governments.

Many countries experiencing severe economic problems do not consider health to be one of the more pressing issues, and it can prove more difficult to mobilize the public in poor economic times. Severe economic problems, such as the situation in Georgia, can prevent people from participating in normal life and carrying out their usual social activities, including attending family celebrations and buying gifts.

Evidence from the United Kingdom suggests that most people are reluctant to be involved in setting health priorities and prefer that decisions be left to the medical profession. When the public is involved, the process of consultation can not only elicit opinions on policy issues but also change them, as in the Netherlands following consultation on choices in health care that took place over 5 years *(8)*.

This study examined two main aspects: the process in countries for allowing public participation in the formulation of written health policy documents, and the instruments used to facilitate public participation. From this, we hoped to gain some understanding of whether broad participation is easier to achieve in some countries or under certain conditions and what might be some of the implications for strengthening public participation in the future. Following the general pattern for this chapter, we examined how various policy instruments were used to facilitate public participation.

Participation in policy formulation

A review undertaken in 1989 *(16)* of how 17 national health for all policies had been formulated explored how far a horizontal process involving sectors other than health, nongovernmental organizations, politicians, the mass media and the general public had been established and how far there had been an attempt to make vertical links engaging the national, regional and local levels. The results of this survey showed that formulating health policy groups in the 1980s appeared to have suffered from the "3-M syndrome" – they were monosectoral, largely medical and mainly male. Those who took part in the 1989 consultation were reluctant to consider that non-experts might have a role to play in defining the problems to be addressed, although they did feel that non-experts could usefully comment on a draft policy after it had been formulated by experts. There was little sign of any vertical links, and one of the recommendations from the consultation was that subnational levels should be involved in the process from the early stages. The failure to involve the subnational level was also one of the main criticisms of Finland's first health for all policy process, for example *(23)*.

Still too little, too late?

In 1996, the situation of the groups formulating policy was assessed in the framework of this study. The disciplines involved in the process appear to have widened somewhat and the gender balance has improved, but sectors other than health are still not normally involved in the process of formulating policy.

Attempts to find ways of ensuring links between different levels of decision-making seem to be more common. Examples include the national or regional conferences to discuss draft policies organized in England, France, Lithuania and Wales. As the case study shows, cascade meetings were organized in Wales, with those taking part at one level disseminating the knowledge they gained and stimulating discussion at the next level down, and so forth. Nevertheless, the case studies show that the process of making the vertical links often begins after a health policy has already been formulated, whereas involving the different levels in deciding on a process and in defining the challenges to be addressed might secure wider ownership.

Although the number and type of participatory mechanisms has increased, the process of formulating health for all policy in the 1990s continued to be led by experts and largely dominated by the health sector. The strong role of the experts can give credibility to the process, such as in Finland and Lithuania, but if the experts are almost exclusively from the health professions, which they seem to be in most cases, this can lead to excessive medicalization and difficulty in moving later to a more social health policy dealing with the underlying determinants of health rather than their symptoms. Malta is one of the few countries that tried to involve other government departments, political parties, professional organizations, unions and other nongovernmental organizations at a comparatively early stage.

Not only is a wider public usually involved only after a health policy has been formulated (at least in draft form), but from the examples available, the final policy documents rarely differ substantially from the consultation documents. The perception of different groups as to which specific as well as society-wide challenges should be tackled can differ according to their life situation. Unemployed men, older people, low-income women, mothers of young children and young professionals can be expected to have different priorities *(73)* and different perceptions of what would improve the health and quality of life of their group and other social groups.

Achieving broader participation might be easier at the regional or subnational level. Östergötland County in Sweden established strong links with politicians at an early stage, ensuring a broad base of political support for the policy. The public was not involved at that point but was still involved relatively early in the process, when their participation was facilitated by setting up study groups. The involvement of the public in setting targets was regarded as the first stage in the implementation process in Östergötland (Box 3.4).

Awareness-building, consultation and negotiation
There have been innovative attempts to raise awareness among politicians and the general public at different stages of the process of developing policy and to consult with various groups.

Policy formulation stage. Although non-expert participation at the earliest stage of policy development is still relatively weak, awareness appears to be growing of the need to establish the views of the general public and patients. The general public has been surveyed to establish their perceptions of health risks, their views on the adequacy of health care services (Hungary) or satisfaction with health care reforms (Kyrgyzstan). What is not as clear is how this information is being used to inform policy decisions, especially if public opinion contradicts the current position taken in public policy.

One critical issue in policy-making is defining the criteria for decision-making. In Sweden, a parliamentary commission *(74)* laid out principles that should form the basis for health care priorities: human dignity, need and solidarity and cost–efficiency. In discussing the rank order of these principles, the commission tried to create awareness of the need for transparency in setting such criteria by demonstrating the practical implications of such ranking. For example, if human dignity is the top priority, the commission felt that the cost–efficiency principle could not justify impairing the quality of care given to people who are dying, to older people or to people with dementia. Some years previously, in a similar exercise in the Netherlands, the Government Committee on Choices in Health Care *(75)* laid out a system of criteria that could be used to decide which types of health care should be excluded from the basic

---

Box 3.4. Involving the public in policy development – selected examples

Policy formulation – Östergötland County, Sweden
The County Council organized meetings and study groups in which professionals from the health care, social, educational and other sectors, together with representatives from voluntary organizations and the general public, discussed the possible content of a health for all policy for Östergötland County. In addition, in four pilot areas health facilitators were employed to link the local community and the local services, to develop a local health profile and to plan health interventions.

Copenhagen, Denmark – a health plan for the city
Through a survey in 1991, 26 000 people were asked for their ideas on their own state of health. This information was used to prepare health profiles for the 14 districts of Copenhagen. Groups from schools, churches, sports associations, trade unions, libraries and day care centres were invited to participate in citizens' meetings to discuss the profiles and make proposals for a city health plan.

Using the Internet in the United Kingdom
The consultation document *Our healthier nation (7)* in England was put on the World Wide Web. NHSnet and other Web sites also harness the advances in modern information technology to involve citizens in comment and discussion of policy issues. *Better health, better Wales (19)* was also put on the Web in May 1998 and included a four-page questionnaire requesting citizens' views, which are to be taken into account in developing an action plan for health.

---

package to be covered by social insurance. This "funnel" technique was later considered by some to be impractical, and the Scientific Council for Government Policy *(76)* suggested an alternative approach based on what is included in, instead of not excluded from, the package. Whether one agrees with the criteria proposed in either case, these were efforts to create greater transparency in decision-making and to make a wider public aware of the implications.

Some countries have made specific efforts to raise awareness among politicians and the general public about health challenges, using parliamentary discussions to provide the focus. Lithuania organized a parliamentary health day to discuss general health issues, and this discussion was broadcast on television and radio, giving interested citizens the opportunity to be informed.

Consulting on a draft policy. Consultation and negotiation on draft policy documents with the main interest groups and other partners generally appears to be more common now than it was two decades ago. In England, following the usual process of first launching a consultation or green paper, the first draft of *The health of the nation* was taken around the country in road-shows, with high-ranking officials leading discussions on the new policy with the general public. The new Labour Government has put its consultation document, *Our healthier nation,* on the World Wide Web to elicit comments, with very specific questions posed, for example, on the priorities and the level of the targets set (see Box 3.4).

Turkey used large national conferences, with participation from all over the country, to consult on possible policy directions. Turkey also followed an unusual path of publishing all the comments made to the consultation health policy document, including comments from public services, nongovernmental organizations and private individuals. When the consultation document was revised, one could see how far the various comments had been incorporated.

Östergötland County paid special attention to soliciting views from vulnerable groups, including young people and old people. Children were encouraged to present their views through pictures and elderly people at locally organized hearings and seminars, and broader public discussions were organized through local newspapers.

It would be interesting to explore how far substantive changes are made to policy documents as a result of the consultation process and what reasons are given, if any, for accepting or not accepting suggested revisions to a draft policy.

Policy implementation stage. In the Netherlands, when the first health for all policy had been finalized in a weighty scientific document, popular versions were produced, written by a journalist and using cartoons to express some of the messages. In addition to the popularized version of the first English document (*The health of the nation, The Chief Medical Officer's challenge*), a leaflet suggesting how people can change their health-related behaviour in simple ways during their daily life was widely distributed and was even included, for example, in Manchester United's football programme for one of their FA Cup games. It would be interesting to learn what practical impact these efforts had on changing behaviour. Although this might be difficult to measure, it should be well worth the effort to try to assess which strategies for reaching and influencing the public on policy-related issues are most effective.

More recently, policy-makers in the Netherlands sought to raise awareness among the general public regarding the critical health policy choices that must be made on a daily basis. The medium used to do this was a television programme whereby the public phoned in decisions on who should receive medical treatment given limited resources, such as a bypass operation for a 60-year-old man or a hip replacement for a 75-year-old woman.

Consulting with health professionals. Health professionals are the one group all countries consulted, although in most countries this usually means physicians rather than nurses or other professionals. An interesting example comes from Romania before 1989, when the achievement of targets influenced physicians' remuneration. In that case, physicians accepted working with targets they felt they could control, such as increasing the coverage of immunization, but not with targets they felt to be beyond their control, such as reducing the prevalence of smoking. Some countries in the eastern part of the Region, such as Armenia, Romania, Slovakia and Slovenia, have taken special care in recent years to consult health professionals, many of whom are frustrated with poor salaries and working conditions. Their support is crucial to the success of the reforms taking place in any country.

Media for health. Many countries, regions and local communities broadcast television and radio programmes that aim to promote and protect health. As watching television, listening to the radio and reading newspapers and magazines is a major leisure activity for many people of all ages, the mass media is a potentially powerful channel for encouraging greater public participation. In the countries in the eastern part of the Region, a substantial amount of time on television and radio is still available for public service at little or no cost. In England and Catalonia, for example, newsletters and progress reports on policy implementation have been produced on a regular basis.

Financial measures to promote participation
Funding patient or consumer groups dealing with health and health-related matters is a well established practice in western Europe and appears to be becoming more common in the eastern part of the Region. In Finland, national nongovernmental organizations have been given more control over certain discretionary funds for public health and health promotion. Subsidies have also been made available to consumer groups in the Netherlands, Norway, Slovakia and Switzerland. Some countries in the eastern part of the Region plan to introduce subsidies in the near future. Countries did not indicate, however, what the criteria might be for subsidizing such organizations.

Examples of how countries ensure that financial incentives encourage the participation of patient or consumer groups in accordance with policy objectives, without allowing this to stifle differing opinions and objectives, would be valuable for the countries with rapidly increasing numbers of nongovernmental organizations.

Legislation and regulation
Legislation can be an effective tool in safeguarding people's right to participation in the policy process. Many countries are developing legislation to protect patients, particularly with regard to confidentiality and rights to services and information. Some countries have developed patients' charters, such as France, Ireland and the United Kingdom; other countries such as Finland, Israel, Lithuania and the Netherlands have opted for more binding legislation. In Italy this has been very much a bottom-up process built by the activities of a broad democratic movement, which the public sector then supported.

In Denmark a Patients' Board of Complaints, including members from professions other than health, has been set up to examine patients' complaints, express criticism and, in especially serious cases, recommend prosecution. In the eastern part of the Region, legislation on patients' rights continues to be weak, although policy documents are increasingly referring to the need for strengthening this area. When Slovakia introduced legislation on patients' rights, the law was published in the newspapers and given high visibility.

Legislative and financial measures may be combined. In the United Kingdom, the Department of Health has a statutory duty to financially support community health councils. In Poland, a national fund for services for disabled people has been established and is financed through fines imposed on firms who do not employ disabled people.

Countries provided few examples of legislation being changed as a result of public pressure; where this has happened it has largely been in relation to the environment. For example, in Italy public referenda resulted in changes in laws on nuclear power and pesticides.

Under the Soviet system, some countries had laws to promote public participation in decision-making, such as a law on local administration and self-rule in Belarus and, in Poland, the People's Councils and Territorial Self Government Act of 1983. The old system sometimes provided an overtone of enforced public participation or simply of formal participation in youth or women's associations, which were linked to the party system. Following the recent political changes, there was therefore an initial lack of interest in public participation in such formal mechanisms linked to the public sector. More recently, voluntary organizations have rapidly grown, and efforts are being made to involve people more informally and to strengthen social support and support to family networks.

Structural, administrative and management tools

Some countries have established interagency consultation committees or councils, involving not only health-related sectors but also representatives from other government departments, voluntary organizations, professional associations and trade unions. In Portugal the regional health councils have representatives from regional health services, local authorities and social organizations and have served a similar purpose. The main purpose of the councils is to develop consensus on planning and budgetary measures. In Östergötland County, Sweden, health facilitators *(77)* were appointed in some districts to involve local communities in developing local health plans born out of the concerns specific to that community. This example is also related to human resource development, since the health facilitators were a new type of staff.

Monitoring and evaluation

Establishing the mechanisms for consultation and negotiation is necessary but not always sufficient. Despite determined attempts in Wales to involve local communities, the case study from Wales indicates that users' views were not always taken seriously, and clinical perceptions dominated. Public participation in such a situation can take the form of "being there" rather than "being heard". Ensuring that individuals and communities are really heard is one of the challenges of the new millennium. Already, there is a growing body of research on the participation of local communities, ranging from their awareness of health issues and satisfaction with services to the greater potential for involving different groups and using specific settings to achieve wider participation.

We did not receive much information on how the participatory process was monitored and evaluated. Information was available in the Regional Office from informal papers, travel reports and presentations in working groups. For example, in 1992 the Netherlands organized a seminar in Bilthoven for top-level administrators from England and the Netherlands to frankly discuss progress in implementing policies based on health for all in both countries. The discussions showed that sufficient enthusiasm had been generated in England for *The health of the nation* approach to ensure that at least small steps were being taken towards implementation throughout England, whereas enthusiasm appeared to be running low in the Netherlands at that time. This could be partly explained by the fact that the approach was new in England in 1992 and many people in the health sector had been waiting for it, whereas in the Netherlands, in the usual roller-coaster progress of policy development, by the time this seminar took place, people in the Netherlands were probably at the stage where motivation was flagging.

Implications for the future

As in other areas, well trodden paths are being taken to encourage public participation in national health policy development. Signs are positive that the public, and their representatives, have increasing input into important discussions about priorities and rationing. Nevertheless, more consultation and public involvement is still needed in wider health programmes and projects, at all levels, outside the traditional health (care) sector. The spin-off benefits of such initiatives would include greater public ownership of health issues and, in the longer term perhaps, greater social inclusiveness and cohesion. The Healthy Cities movement, countrywide integrated noncommunicable disease intervention (CINDI) initiatives and other locally based programmes and projects may offer examples of how such public involvement can take off.

More research could usefully be carried out in this area to develop examples of good practice. This may involve considering whether countries with similar cultural and political backgrounds have clear patterns of similar action to identify how the advantages of specific policy environments have been maximized. How, for example, can municipal models of administration be harnessed to foster participation, and how can the problem of their subdivision into sectors of responsibility and budget-holding be overcome? By contrast, in pluralistic systems the question arises of how overarching structures can be established to bring together a wide range of interest groups under the umbrella of a common set of aims and objectives and how commitment to health can be assured so that health issues are given adequate attention and funding. According to the health for all philosophy, one way of doing this is by clearly defining objectives and targets and presenting them in a written policy document.

Settings are being increasingly used to promote health: for example, the family, schools and workplaces, in other words places where people are living, learning and working. Health promotion in schools has become a particularly strong movement in recent years. The Health Promoting Schools project of WHO, the European Union and the Council of Europe promotes informed decision-making at a young age. Each school has the opportunity to develop its own health policy in collaboration with parents, teachers and pupils. In addition to educating pupils in health, the aim is to instil young people with decision-making skills and train them in participatory processes and consensus-building. Coupled with this, traditional methods of health education are increasingly being dropped in favour of more innovative methods such as peer-led education.

Working with other sectors

The whole philosophy of health for all is based on the fact that health can only be improved and maintained when prerequisites such as peace, adequate nutrition, income, education, housing, a rewarding occupation and fulfilling social relationships are in place. This is why working with many sectors is basic to health for all. The current policy document in the Netherlands *(78)*, for example, includes an interesting table showing what are considered to be the main diseases and their determinants. It indicates the potential effectiveness of preventive measures in departments other than health and the effectiveness of three types of action that are usually part of the policy of the Ministry of Health, Welfare and Sport. These include legislation and education, which is usually carried out by social organizations, and detecting disease early, which is usually carried out by the municipal health services or general practitioners.

Attempting to promote and protect health through collaboration across many sectors that links different levels of authority can be extremely complex. Some excellent initiatives since the health for all policy was launched have created a win-win situation for the sectors and actors involved. In these cases, other sectors and organizations were convinced that they can also gain from promoting health. For example, in the early 1980s, the Heartbeat Wales project showed that farmers, meat-packing companies, butchers, supermarkets and consumers can gain from the production and consumption of leaner meat. Even when there has been political will to take such an approach, some of the challenges may be underestimated. There has not always been sufficient expertise to carry it through and to deal with possible apparent conflicts of interest and competing struggles for power and resources (see Box 3.5) *(79)*.

In the questionnaire used for this study, countries were asked what type of policy tools had been used to achieve intersectoral action in relation to lifestyles, the environment and health care. The responses to these three areas have been consolidated here in one analysis. By examining whether or not countries adopted an intersectoral approach in formulating and implementing health policies, what measures they have taken to facilitate and promote intersectoral action for health, and whether they are monitoring and evaluating the processes and action designed to achieve intersectoral action, we hoped to begin to sort out the reality from the rhetoric. As in all the sections in this chapter, we examined the kinds of policy measures that had been used. We also hoped to explore whether there were identifiable patterns and trends associated with success as well as the implications for the future.

Research and information

Countries in Europe have been increasing research and information to support intersectoral action in the areas of lifestyles, the environment and health care. The principal areas of research have concerned health risks arising in people's living, working and physical environments. Much of this has been carried out in university departments of occupational and environmental medicine. Other bodies such as the National Food Administration in Sweden carry out such research, and institutes run by industry in some countries have carried out valuable health-related research *(80)*.

Box 3.5. Obstacles to intersectoral collaboration

- Awareness and understanding of the determinants of health are inadequate.

- Political will and leadership are lacking.

- The stakeholders appear to have competing interests, which prevents them from recognizing their interdependence.

- The distribution of national and local powers is such that it frustrates intersectoral collaboration. Implicit tension between top-down and bottom-up approaches may hinder effective collaboration.

- Existing mechanisms and processes do not facilitate and strengthen public participation.

- The role of the mass media may not be supportive or conducive of intersectoral action.

- A lack of experience and essential expertise leads organizations to stick to the status quo.

Source: Pederson et al. *(79).*

There is a growing bank of information on a range of health issues for which action by sectors other than health is required to promote and protect health. This has focused greater attention on the development of new tools and methods such as health impact assessment, although this still seems to be in its infancy.

The areas that have been given most attention appear to be those in which intersectoral collaboration has long been established: home and road accidents, occupational health risks and pollution of the environment. Although the assessment of the health impact of these areas still needs to be improved, these areas of concern offer relatively concrete things to measure such as levels of pollution, numbers of cars on the road, kilometres driven and deaths and injuries from accidents. For such challenges as reducing the impact of crime or mental stress, for which intersectoral action is equally important but valid indicators are less easily defined, fewer countries report attempting to provide the evidence for the effects on health.

Research on the process of achieving intersectoral action tends to be less common. Early on in the health for all approach, the Netherlands made strong efforts to place intersectoral action within a research and development framework, holding a preliminary workshop on making partners and undertaking studies on the dynamics of intersectoral decision-making *(81).* The Netherlands was also among the first countries in the Region to carry out research on the development of new policy tools such as scenarios. A number of scenarios were made and used in the process of formulating policy. Rather than simply extrapolating present trends into the future, the Netherlands allowed different policy options to be considered by forecasting what might happen under different assumptions about the future and by applying different patterns of allocating resources in response to a complex and rapidly changing society *(82)*. Finland was another country that carried out research in this area.

Health education and awareness-building

More resources and new methods. More resources are being allocated to health education, especially in the eastern part of the Region. Seven countries reported establishing new institutes dealing with health education and health promotion between 1980 and 1996. In some countries, health education has changed over the years in favour of new approaches such as peer-led education and more interactive teaching methods. The Health Adventure at Linköping, in Östergötland County, Sweden, for example, is an interactive way of teaching children at a young age how they can promote or damage health through everyday choices, by allowing them to carry out a wide variety of practical experiments.

Wider use of the mass media. Building awareness of the need for intersectoral action has been strongly facilitated by an explosion in mass media. In all countries, the mass media are being used far more to promote health and raise awareness about lifestyle: tobacco, alcohol, diet, nutrition and sexuality, including HIV and AIDS. As most Europeans spend substantial time watching television and, more recently for some, surfing the Web, mass media channels are probably still vastly underexploited.

Using the settings approach. Based on countries' replies and the available policy documents, the health care sector more strongly emphasizes health education and awareness-building in various settings, most often homes, schools and workplaces. In a few cases, newer settings for health promotion are also mentioned, including universities, prisons and nightclubs. Using a settings approach seems to make the complex health for all approach more manageable by identifying the boundaries of action and the potential partners or possible antagonists operating within these boundaries. It provides an opportunity to observe and measure the impact of intervention for health gain and, unlike action aimed at the country level, offers the potential for pilot testing.

In the examples given, the range of partners involved in local intersectoral projects also seems to be increasing. Frequently, multiple partners rather than just two departments or sectors work together. In Bulgaria, for example, the Ministries of Education, Internal Affairs and Sports worked with the health sector to devise health and fitness programmes for children.

Using parliamentary support. Parliaments are naturally intersectoral bodies, dealing with legislation across the full span of social, economic, cultural and political activity. All parliamentarians, and not only those serving on parliamentary health committees, could therefore be potential allies for intersectoral action for health, both in national legislative bodies and in their capacity as representatives of their local constituency *(83)*. Some countries have engaged the parliament early on in their process of developing health for all policy as a way of building support for intersectoral action. Finland and the Netherlands, for example, engaged their parliaments as part of their process of formulating policy, and Lithuania organized a national conference involving the parliamentary health committees and ministers responsible for social security, labour, economy and finance, education, science and culture to discuss its national public health report *(11)*. A number of countries used the parliament to ratify their health for all policies, thus bringing the issue of intersectoral action to the fore. In the Russian Federation, a subgroup of the health committee of the Duma is charged with examining all draft legislation to assess the possible impact on health. Other countries may follow a similar process but we did not have information on this.

Consultation and negotiation

When should consultation begin? To ensure intersectoral ownership of health policy, all relevant sectors should be involved at the very earliest stages of the consultation process. This means involving all economic sectors and all the key players in these sectors: the public services with their responsibility as guardians of people's right to health, the private sector as a facilitator of economic growth, non-profit organizations as a catalyst for change and, as far as possible, the general public and the people directly affected by the problems. The evidence available did not allow us to draw firm conclusions on how far this is happening across Europe, but consultation with other sectors, beginning with defining the problems and before a draft policy document has already been produced, appears to be comparatively rare.

Consulting with colleagues. Most consultation is undertaken with sectors that already have a high degree of contact. Social welfare and health care services have a long tradition of working together, especially in caring for specific groups such as elderly and disabled people. The education and health sectors have traditionally worked together to promote and protect the health of young people. The transport and health sectors have the mutual objective of reducing the number of accidents. Eleven countries cited consultation with these sectors as an example of intersectoral collaboration. Two countries cited negotiations between the health and agricultural sectors in relation to food policy, and six referred to the health sector consulting and negotiating with other sectors in banning the advertising of harmful substances such as alcohol and tobacco. Consultation between two sectors can sometimes be hindered by internal power struggles, as indicated in the case study from Wales. Fortunately, in that situation, Health Promotion Wales was able to forge a successful partnership between the health sector, the agricultural sector and those responsible for food processing and commerce. As pointed out in the case study from the Netherlands (p. 110), opposing and parallel policy agenda can be distinguished in different sectors. For example, the interests of a ministry of health in higher alcohol and tobacco prices sometimes seem to conflict with those of a ministry of finance. In contrast, the interests of a ministry of labour often coincide with those of a ministry of health in matters of occupational safety and health policy at the workplace. The possibility of conflicting interests between sectors makes it essential to start the consultation and negotiation process early.

Environment and health – old allies. In the European Region, one of the most successful areas of intersectoral action has been between the sectors dealing with environment and health. Of the 51 WHO European Member States, 46 have developed national environmental health action plans. These plans collectively comprise a strategy to prevent and control hazards to environmental health in Europe. Each country writes its own plan with its own set of priority actions. Through their plans, European countries are bringing to life the Environmental Health Action Plan for Europe endorsed at the Second European Conference on Environment and Health in Helsinki in 1994 *(84)*. Explanations for the relatively smooth interface between environment and health could include the similarities of the two sectors. Both are often somewhat on the periphery of government agenda, ministers responsible for these sectors are not usually very high in the pecking order, and the sectors often share converging interests and objectives. Protecting the environment has now been recognized as a major global challenge, precipitating a worldwide reaction. As the health and environmental sectors are natural partners, many countries mention the possibility of sharing resources, especially in terms of expertise and information.

Health in the workplace – changing perceptions. In preparation for the Third Ministerial Conference on Environment and Health in London in 1999, Member States were asked to indicate their priority concerns in relation to exposure to environmental risks. Industry and the workplace was identified as a priority area (in addition to water and transport). This concern was reflected in the countries' responses in the present study.

Many large multinational companies have for some time been interested in and active in promoting health in the workplace, ensuring that their products are not harmful to health and promoting health in the community. Their representatives have been actively involved in working groups developing health for all policy in several countries. Countries report considerable problems but also good examples of health-minded companies and enterprises. In Wales, for example, the corporate health activity *(85)* aims to promote healthier workplaces and to encourage a consultative approach towards employees' needs. Solutions to reach those employed in small and medium-sized firms are, however, still far from being found.

In countries in the eastern part of the Region under the old system, some health care services were provided at the workplace. The emphasis was more on disease surveillance and prevention rather than health promotion. More recently, some of these countries have established committees involving regional and local health centres, professional organizations, employees and trade unions to develop initiatives related to health at the workplace. The changes in the last decade in the eastern part of the Region and the high unemployment rates in most countries in the Region tend to foster insecure employment, and many workers across Europe therefore feel that they have little choice but to accept harsh and hazardous conditions. Many trade unions have focused on protecting jobs and wages rather than demanding health-promoting conditions of work.

The number of small enterprises in the Region is mushrooming. Most have not even considered a health policy, and some even expose workers to serious occupational risks *(86)*. Trade union membership has declined in many countries, and membership in such representative organizations is especially low among those employed in small firms. The informal economy accounts for a sizeable proportion of employment in some countries, which also makes reaching large numbers of workers difficult.

Structural changes and administrative and management tools
Structures and mechanisms. An impressive number of countries have set up structures and mechanisms to support and facilitate intersectoral collaboration. When *The health of the nation* was developed in England, for example, a cabinet subcommittee including members from most government departments was established to oversee the process of implementing policy. A wider health working group drew members from a wide range of organizations, including public and voluntary groups, private enterprise and sports councils. For *Our healthier nation*, this has been taken further: a Minister for Public Health has been appointed for the first time to ensure coordination of health policy across the Government. A cabinet committee from 12 different departments will ensure implementation across sectors.

Finland, France, Germany, Hungary, Iceland, Malta and the Netherlands have also established intersectoral bodies to deal with: overall health policy issues; specific concerns such as tobacco control, accidents, chemical products and safe water; or the health needs of specific groups, such as elderly people and children. In Malta, multisectoral teams drew up strategic plans for each key area, and the interministerial committee was asked to appoint an intersectoral task force to implement the strategic plan. In the Netherlands, an advisory body was set up to deal specifically with what was called the "facet policy" and to develop the interface between health and other areas of policy. In countries that established intersectoral mechanisms at an early stage, such as Denmark and Israel, one of the challenges appears to have been in sustaining interest in the long term and maintaining the functions in the way originally intended.

An intersectoral committee can act as a mechanism for harnessing support and energy if the key actors are genuinely committed to change. Nancy Milio *(87)* criticized what she called the tradition of "democratic corporativism in Finland"; although parties with contradictory interests sit in the same council, state their views and argue about the formulation of documents, all return essentially unchanged to their home bases, with little net change to the action taken.

Creating something new or adapting something old? In Catalonia, an intersectoral involvement agency was set up in the initial stages of the policy development but is no longer active. It was believed that, in the longer term, cooperation can best be achieved through several other mechanisms that already exist in Catalonia, such as interprofessional committees, advisory boards and task forces. In Turkey, new mechanisms were established in the Ministry of Health, including a special project coordination unit, but existing mechanisms were also used. Turkey offers a specific example: the State Planning Organization still formulates regular five-year development plans, and health is one of the components included in the development plans. Nevertheless, the extent of collaboration between the two mechanisms and the extent to which the State Planning Organization tried to get health on the agenda of other sectors, dealing with possible common or conflicting objectives, is not clear.

The Netherlands was the only country known to create a special unit inside the Ministry to implement the health for all policy; this was later abolished.

Working at subnational levels. In the federal countries, the subnational level is the natural level for establishing mechanisms to promote intersectoral collaboration. The state health conferences established in 1992 in North Rhine–Westphalia played this role at the level of the *Land*, but similar mechanisms were also established at lower levels, including the 16 counties and more than 30% of major cities that had set up work groups for health promotion by that time *(88)*. Mechanisms for intersectoral action can be particularly effective at the local level, such as the local health groups set up in Östergötland County, Sweden. Special efforts have been made to encourage intersectoral action at the local level in the United Kingdom. The Healthy Alliance awards were designed to encourage innovative partnerships for promoting good health in each of the five key areas in *The health of the nation*. In the first year, the competition attracted over 300 entries and recognized the value of such alliances.

No country mentioned any management tool to promote intersectoral collaboration.

How mechanisms and structures to promote intersectoral action are established, who participates, how they operate, their success or lack thereof and the reasons for this would be a valuable area for investigation in the future.

Financial tools

Countries do not seem to have considered shifting a proportion of the health care budget to finance action to promote health in other sectors. Some instances of joint planning of existing budgets were cited. For example, the Ministries of Health and Education jointly financed health education programmes in Hungary, and the Ministries of Health and of Welfare together finance care of elderly people in Latvia. In some cases the use of joint or block budgets was reported, mainly between the health and welfare sectors, but it is not clear the extent to which this will ensure that equity in health is promoted.

Major structural changes, such as the move towards financing local authorities in Finland through block grants, can also facilitate intersectoral action. This mechanism ensures that the health and social sectors have nothing to gain by transferring costs to other sectors but are encouraged to work together in a more integrated way. The Netherlands plans to finance innovative labour market policy or specific issues such as reducing tobacco consumption. In Östergötland County, one incentive used has been to give intersectoral projects priority over monosectoral projects in funding decisions.

Although environment and health have not always been linked directly, the environment is one area of concern in which financial measures have been used as incentives for action. The polluter-pays principle has been applied for a number of years in Sweden, for example, and economic subsidies of various kinds are used to develop more environmentally sound solutions *(89)*.

Few countries allocate funds directly to intersectoral work, although the consultation health policy documents for England, Northern Ireland, Scotland and Wales *(7,19–21)* do suggest such direct funding for intersectoral action in deprived areas and communities. The new ideas include health action zones *(42)*, which are intended to bring together all those who may contribute to health at the local level to implement a locally agreed strategy. By August 1998, 26 such health action zones covering both rural and inner city areas were being set up, in an attempt to "improve the health of the worst off at a faster rate than the general population" *(90)*. The overall funding for this initiative is about £50 million in the fiscal year 1999/2000 and £60 million in 2000/2001. An attempt will be made to link the regional health authorities to the regional development councils, which should foster intersectoral action.

On the whole, however, investment in intersectoral action is very underdeveloped in most countries. One explanation might be the lack of convincing evidence on where investing in health provides the greatest return and the disappointing lack of interest from economists, as a quick glance at the international literature shows, on assessing the economic benefits of investing in health.

Economists can provide solid economic data on the possible benefits of shifting resources to invest in health. This could provide some of the evidence that is missing in the advocacy of intersectoral action.

Legislation and regulation

Our healthier nation (7) states that legislation and regulation should be a last resort in bringing about change. Legal and regulatory tools are, however, frequently necessary intersectoral action to protect and promote people's health. An example is legislation controlling pollution of air and water. It is interesting that, on the whole, the countries in the eastern part of the Region refer more frequently to legislation as a useful tool than do western European countries. This relates in part to the differences between countries as to measures that require a law for legitimacy and those that can be effected through administrative decisions. Lithuania, for example, introduced legislation aimed at strengthening intersectoral action and collaboration through the Law of the Health System (1994), which established a National Board of Health reporting to Parliament. The Law defines which sectors and agencies should be involved and how the Board should operate.

Most of the legislation that countries mentioned related to lifestyles, especially tobacco control and the environment, mainly the working environment. The most frequent examples of legislation were including health warnings on cigarette packs and banning the advertising of tobacco and alcohol. The more frequently cited environmental legislation aims to reinforce occupational health standards and regulatory controls on environmental pollution, such as limits on motor vehicle emissions, guidelines on the quality of the drinking-water supply and controls on sewage collection and treatment.

Legislation originating in other sectors, such as ministries of transport, frequently protects health. It is not clear, however, to what extent the health sector has played a role in initiating legislation such as that imposing speed limits for road traffic, controlling drinking and driving and requiring the use of seatbelts. Such legislation can certainly reinforce positive health behaviour.

More research is needed on understanding what triggers other sectors to initiate health-promoting legislation and how health impact assessment might be brought into the legislative process, so that the health sector can encourage and reinforce such health-enhancing action.

In their replies, many countries claim to have taken legal measures to promote social support and cohesion through social security benefits, control of the housing market and maternity benefits. These are important, since they relate to providing the prerequisites for health. Although legislation may be necessary, however, it is not sufficient in ensuring that people who have a right to certain things can actually exercise that right *(91)*.

Human resource development

Preparing for intersectoral action. Material was produced to complement *The health of the nation*, most notably *Working together for better health (92)*. This document explains why healthy alliances are necessary, how to set them up and who to involve, and is a good example of developing human resources in the widest sense. The need to build capacity for intersectoral action for health is quite pressing throughout Europe, even in countries that have been trying to take this approach for some time.

Education and training. The links made between sectors are first and foremost links between people who are open to working with other sectors. A systematic approach for ensuring a supply of people who are educated and trained to work in this way is therefore an essential part of any health for all policy. A number of countries reported transforming the content of medical curricula to embrace a broader approach to health; others are distributing information packages on health for all policy to nurses, physicians or other health professionals.

One of the most promising indicators for the strengthening of education and training for intersectoral action is the increase in the number of graduate and postgraduate institutes offering programmes in health promotion or occupational health and for community health workers. The Netherlands has innovatively linked such training with an active labour market policy; one objective is to increase the recruitment of people from specific target groups to work in the health sector, such as women who are rejoining the workforce and people of foreign origin. In an attempt to rapidly increase the numbers of trained staff, many countries have introduced programmes for training trainers in specific areas, such as preventing HIV infection and AIDS.

Nevertheless, training physicians and nurses to think intersectorally is not sufficient. A shift towards intersectoral action requires new skills and approaches in public administration at all levels, in many disciplines dealing with the development of the economic, social, cultural and physical environments.

Joint training programmes. Some sectors share similar objectives with others, for example, the health and social sectors. A number of countries reported running joint training programmes for staff to strengthen coordination and to redesign the interface between health care and social care. This tactic might be worth emulating in other sectors.

Monitoring and evaluation

Many countries have established systems to monitor changes in people's behaviour as a result of intersectoral action, such as in relation to diet or the consumption of alcohol or tobacco. Surveillance of such environmental risks as air and water pollutants has also increased in most countries, and recently in the countries in the eastern part of the Region, which experience much higher levels of environmental pollution than do western European countries. Some countries are evaluating health education policies or the effects of health promotion policies (Hungary) or of home care policies (Denmark and many other western European countries).

No country referred to evaluating the process of striving for intersectoral action: that is, how successful the health sector was in reaching out to partners in other sectors to encourage joint action. Were many new alliances made as a result of health for all initiatives? Were some approaches to other sectors rejected and, if so, why?

Such examples of success or failure in the process of reaching out to other sectors would be of interest for future study, in order to gather a body of experience to inform similar attempts to develop partnerships in the future. The methods for carrying out such policy analysis also need to be developed further.

Implications for the future

Countries are becoming increasingly familiar with the concept of and terms associated with intersectoral action, as shown by the increased references in overall and issue-specific health policy documents.

Taking account of the policy environment. Intersectoral action, like public participation in decision-making, is determined by each country's unique political and institutional legacy. The prevailing policy environment provides opportunities and constraints for intersectoral action. Some countries, including the early health for all pioneers Finland and the Netherlands, have a strong tradition of consulting interests outside the public sector, because of how health care is organized or the existence of strong nongovernmental organizations. Under the Soviet system, for example, establishing consultation and negotiation processes was difficult. A public sector that feels threatened by other groups will not be likely to reach out to them. In Turkey, one attempt to establish an intersectoral council consisting of representatives from sectors dealing with health, social services, education, food and agriculture failed because the Ministry of Health at that time feared that the council would weaken the Ministry's power.

Changing socioeconomic conditions. Escalating health care and welfare costs have forced policy-makers to reappraise existing policies and to contain expenditure. This reassessment could provide the opportunity to reposition health at the centre of economic and social development but it could also encourage strong competition between sectoral interests and retrenchment to familiar positions and action. In a number of cases, poor socioeconomic conditions have been used as an excuse for postponing intersectoral action, while the "real business" of providing health care is handled first. Most decision-makers have not realized that both can be done simultaneously and that intersectoral action does not necessarily require more resources, although it may entail a different way of using existing resources.

References to some of the broad socioeconomic changes, including globalization, may indicate that some of the barriers between sectors might become less rigid in a world where technical change, the Internet, migration, capital flows and international trade facilitate rapid connections between countries. Supranational structures such as the World Trade Organization, the European Union and other international trade organizations are increasingly influencing patterns of development and therefore creating either opportunities for health gain or the potential to harm health. One potentially extremely powerful opportunity for the future is presented by the fact that the Maastricht and Amsterdam Treaties have given the European Union new competence in health matters and an explicit mandate to explore the effects on health of policies in other sectors. If this challenge is taken up strongly, it could have a wide-ranging and long-term effect on health. The frameworks established by other international agencies also continue to guide national governments in promoting health and safety through intersectoral action. For example, in reply to the questionnaire, a number of countries said they had already ratified the International Labour Organization's conventions on occupational health. Council of Europe conventions that take a strong human rights stance can also significantly influence action in countries to promote equity in health through intersectoral action.

Heavy legacies from the past will also determine the shape of intersectoral action, at least in the immediate future. In the countries in the eastern part of the Region, the natural environment has been extensively damaged as a result of industrial activity, leading to unsafe drinking-water supplies and severe industrial pollution, especially in cities and large towns. In addition, new environmental problems are arising from increasing prosperity: for example, more widespread car ownership is already being reflected in higher levels of air pollution and more road accidents in some places. In some areas the ravages of war have left a legacy of serious environmental problems. Nevertheless, new opportunities have been created. For example, the number of telephones has already increased four-fold in some countries in the eastern part of the Region, providing opportunities for communicating with people who live alone and for developing telemedicine in remote areas. As many societal conditions are changing rapidly, it is to be hoped that efforts to address the challenges and make use of the opportunities will be intensified; otherwise, the potential for substantial health gain might be lost.

The health care system itself represents an important determinant of whether intersectoral action happens. Back in the nineteenth century, physicians themselves did not provide clean drinking-water, but they played a crucial role in publicizing the social cost of not providing such basic public health services. Today health professions can still advocate for public health. Countries that have an excessive supply of medical personnel might consider how their energy could be redirected towards advocating and supporting intersectoral action for health.

Further information on how countries have developed public health management to meet the needs of a health for all approach, and thoughts on how this could be developed in the future, need to be made available and shared.

Focusing on health outcome

Health for all aims to achieve optimal health gain by orienting health policies towards focusing on changes in the state of health of individuals and populations. This is assessed through morbidity, mortality, healthy life expectancy and quality of life and measured against accepted standards using agreed indicators. This section explores how countries are using health outcome to inform policy decisions and are supporting outcome-based research and ensuring that it becomes an established part of policy-making, and whether or not they are monitoring the use of a health outcome approach. We were interested to see whether there are identifiable patterns and trends across countries and what some of the implications for the future might be.

The European health for all policy calls for the issue of quality to be addressed more systematically than previously. Traditionally, quality has been the domain of health care professionals, confining the discussion somewhat to the quality of health care. The movement towards an outcome-based approach entails a broader view of health and draws on a variety of professionals, including statisticians, sociologists and economists as well as clinicians. This multidisciplinary approach has broadened the discussion so that health outcome is increasingly, although not yet widely, being viewed in terms of the quality of life and the broad determinants of health.

The quality of health care incorporates several different elements, including equity, effectiveness, efficiency, appropriateness of care, patient satisfaction and health outcome (8). In recent years, evidence of widespread variation in the types of treatment offered and their effectiveness (both within and between countries) has led to increased investment in the use of health outcome as a means of assessing quality.

Since change in health results from a combination of many different factors, it can be difficult to draw causal conclusions between health outcome and any one factor, especially the factors termed psychosocial. Even at a clinical level, concluding whether a poor health outcome results from a specific disease or the type of medical treatment provided can be difficult. Such issues were not the concern of this study; our aim was to assess the extent to which countries had shifted from their past approach of planning for inputs to health care to one of aiming to influence outcome and produce health gain.

The health policies formulated in European countries are diverse. Some are more oriented towards disease; some focus more closely on risk factors, others on services and still others on clients, community groups or settings. Most countries try to focus on a mix of these.

The focus on health outcomes in the development of health for all policy has improved vastly but still appears to be limited in Europe. Most countries emphasize outcome related to health care. Within the health care setting, an outcome focus is most evident in such specialties as perinatal and obstetric care and diabetes.

Setting outcome targets, either in overall or in issue-specific health policies, is one strong way of focusing on outcome. How this approach can be translated into action on a day-to-day basis is not clear.

Substitution *(93)* or the regrouping of resources, moving the location at which care is given, introducing new technologies and changing the mix of staff to improve the outcome of health care are slowly becoming more prevalent. It is less evident how an outcome-oriented approach influences daily management decisions in relation to lifestyles and the environment.

Research and information

Outcome-based research aims to collect and disseminate evidence on types of treatment and intervention known to be effective in certain circumstances. This usually relates to individuals. In relation to developing health for all policy, evidence on the outcome of policy processes needs to be collected and disseminated. This also aims to develop a research agenda to fill some of the gaps and to create a research infrastructure: ensuring a supply of trained researchers in outcome-based research and validated research instruments.

Collecting information related to health status has developed considerably in the last two decades, and research assessing what does or does not work in health care has increased. More resources are being given to epidemiological studies, as shown by the complex monitoring systems and sets of health indicators in most European countries. Most research remains centred, however, on traditional epidemiological studies and models focusing on individual risk factors, such as consumption of alcohol and tobacco, nutrition or local environmental risks. Most national data sets still do not include routine information to facilitate economic evaluation or quality assurance of health care.

There has been some shift towards a broader analysis of health determinants, with many more countries linking socioeconomic information to that related to mortality and morbidity. Countries are, however, at different stages of information development. In some countries in the eastern part of the Region, the recent changes disrupted the previous systems for data collection before effective new systems could take their place. The changes under way are wide ranging and varied. Georgia, for example, is now at a preliminary stage of registering all medical institutions. Others, such as Hungary, have recently established committees responsible for technology assessment. The United Kingdom, where information on socioeconomic differences in health has been compiled since 1860, is continuing to fine-tune such information and to ensure that this is available for small geographical areas.

Within the international research community, considerable work is being undertaken on the relationship between health and socioeconomic inequity, and this is expected to grow in the future.

In addition to official research and monitoring conducted by the ministry of health, other government departments very often carry out surveys that may be useful for guiding the development of health policy. In the United Kingdom, for example, the Department of Health and the Ministry of Agriculture, Fisheries and Food organized a joint survey on population nutrition and diet. Similarly, a regular survey by the Health Education Authority on the health and lifestyles of ethnic minorities can help define priorities and provide information useful in developing health policy. Information from the public also serves as a useful indicator, and many countries organize population surveys to get feedback on a wide range of health issues. Much of this information is used to establish how satisfied patients are with health care, an important indicator of quality. For cultural reasons, population surveys work better in some countries than others; the response rates are often higher in Scandinavian countries than in other European countries.

Finland has a strong tradition of monitoring health status and morbidity using information from a combination of various national statistics and registers, and the response rates to surveys are high. In recent years, Finland has focused on developing new mapping techniques to depict the use of health services, a health for all research policy, and an information system on healthy lifestyles. A framework for quality assessment in health care is due to be developed; feedback from clients will indicate how health care management systems should be reoriented. Overall, Finland is one of the most experienced countries in using an outcome-oriented approach.

At the subnational level, several countries are attempting to ensure that data are more comparable between regions. France, Ireland and Switzerland all report efforts to ensure that information systems on health outcome are established at the subnational level as a basis for national policy decisions and setting priorities. A number of countries reported having initiated improved information systems for hospitals. Spain, for example, has established a minimum basic data set to record and compare cases of hospitalization, diagnosis, the procedures carried out and discharge destination according to age, sex and socioeconomic status.

Although indications of the development of an outcome-oriented approach in certain areas of concern are promising, there are gaps in assessing how these various monitoring threads could be woven together to provide a more complete picture of a very complex system. There is a tendency to look at the parts without considering them in relation to the whole. Disease tends to be the main focus in examining health outcomes; less attention is paid to how disease affects functional capacity and much less attention to how it affects wellbeing. Much of the evidence that could be provided by political analysis of the impact of the socioeconomic environment on health outcome is ignored. Finally, although moving from research to action is frequently discussed, relatively little work has been done to provide the evidence for how this link could be achieved in practice.

One of the purposes of outcome-based research is to identify the gaps in research and to establish a research agenda that addresses these gaps. Most countries have adequate mortality data, but both eastern and western European countries complain about the lack of indicators to measure morbidity; Hungary, Malta and Wales mentioned this. There are also considerable gaps in data on healthy life expectancy and the quality of life. Although many new tools and methods are being developed to fill some of these gaps, such as disability-free life expectancy measures, new types of randomized controlled trial and health impact assessment, countries differ substantially in how much they use these methods.

Some countries mentioned assessing the cost–effectiveness of emerging and existing health care technology. France, Germany, Hungary, the Netherlands and the United Kingdom have established special agencies with the specific function of assessing new types of health care technology. International collaboration in this area would be valuable.

In conclusion, outcome-based research has become more systematic but is still conducted on an ad hoc basis, with few clear links between clinical databases and managerial statistical operations at different levels. This study provides little evidence of strong links between the research community and policy-makers. One reason is that many countries still have a poorly defined research agenda, as an initial attempt to develop research policies for health for all seems to have largely fizzled out and the appropriate research infrastructure is lacking. A more positive trend is that many countries are trying to establish mechanisms for ensuring more synergy between the national, regional and local levels and institutions in harmonizing data collection.

Health education and raising awareness

Publishing the results of relevant research indicates that countries are taking the outcome-oriented approach seriously. From this viewpoint, the outlook in the Region is more promising. Many countries now produce a national public health report each year that summarizes information and evidence in public health. Public health reporting is an important prerequisite for policy-making and has expanded vastly in recent years.

Publishing the evidence is only one step in building awareness. The health sector must take the first step in producing the information, but the broader determinants of health can only be tackled if other sectors are convinced by the information. Links on two levels are required: between the research community and policy-makers, and between policy-makers and other groups and sectors.

Hungary, Ireland, Kyrgyzstan, Slovakia, Slovenia and Uzbekistan mentioned plans or current initiatives to make health educators aware of the importance of health outcome. This study indicates, however, that the health sector needs much stronger efforts to build links to other sectors and to use health outcome more forcefully as a means of directing attention to health and putting health higher on the political agenda. The policy documents examined do not generally refer to the need for formally establishing these mechanisms, which might take the form of special task forces including researchers and policy-makers or intersectoral research bodies or programmes.

Consultation and negotiation

After information on health outcome is disseminated, this information needs to be used as an incentive to affect change in practice or procedures. Several countries report auditing nosocomial infection rates and pharmaceutical prescribing, and disseminating the results among peers. Countries also report developing clinical guidelines or treatment protocols based on assessing the outcome of various procedures. Disseminating such information does not automatically mean that health professionals will act upon it, but sharing such information confidentially influences health outcome more strongly. Some hospitals have experimented with peer review and clinical auditing, but this practice is far from widespread and requires that physicians be very open.

In the long term, however, working in this collaborative way can ensure a feeling of ownership. For example, one of the prerequisites for ensuring that clinical guidelines are adopted more widely is to involve the future users in developing the guidelines from the start. This study provides little evidence that countries are finding the most innovative means of dissemination and feedback mechanisms either between providers or with other sectors, to promote the wider use of an outcome-oriented approach.

Structural, administrative and management changes

Which strategies and structures support the use of health outcome in policy-making? For example, have countries established bodies to carry out research on health outcome? What mechanisms have been established to ensure feedback from regions and institutions?

Most countries have a national health research body. Some have more than one; for example, the Netherlands has established several bodies, including Statistics Netherlands (CBS), the National Institute of Public Health and the Environment (RIVM) and the Netherlands Organization for Applied Scientific Research (TNO) *(78)*. A sound research infrastructure is essential for the development of an outcome-oriented approach, and some countries reported the lack of such infrastructure to be an obstacle to measuring health outcome systematically and coherently. In Turkey, for example, where no single organization or body is responsible for monitoring health status, the lack of a coordinated infrastructure was considered to be an important obstacle.

Evidence is lacking on how the bodies or agencies responsible for monitoring health outcome link this outcome with other sectors and how they disseminate information. Apart from national agencies, many other bodies, including universities, hospitals, industry and research agencies at the regional and local levels, also carry out research on health outcomes. Although the national government will be aware of and more likely to use information collected at the national level for policy purposes, a mechanism should ensure that clinical and local research feeds into this process. Ways must also be found of disseminating information among clinicians. This is not always easy. It requires a specific set of social relationships and values, but experience from several countries shows that it can be done.

Most countries have established national systems to monitor health. In some cases, increasing decentralization of health care systems has required effective monitoring systems at the regional or local levels. In the United Kingdom, the development of a public health common data set allows regions to compare their progress with other regions. In Italy, central funds are allocated to the regional level based on performance indicators. Finland is attempting to integrate regional statistics into a central system and to link local decision-makers to the central system, not only giving them access to comparative data but also providing support in the use of comparative data for local decision-making. Some cities have begun to develop their own health information systems. In France, a national public health network has been set up to monitor infectious diseases and environmental risks and to provide information on which to base policy decisions.

Few countries have developed geographical information systems or information systems on hospitals or primary health care. At the local level, even more rigorous assessment and better links to other levels of care and policy-making need to be established at the level of general practice.

The Netherlands is an advanced country in public health reporting, making innovative use of public health status and forecasts and multi-criterion analysis *(94)*.

Financial measures

Health outcome can be used to promote quality in health care, but many countries are also increasingly interested in using health outcome to rationalize the financing of health care. Research funds on health outcome are therefore being increased. A broader range of research methods, including randomized controlled trials, has resulted in a new outcome vocabulary. Such terms can be a powerful platform for winning political and thus financial support for investing in specific areas of health. This situation has both positive and negative aspects; demonstrating the results of intervening in some areas may be relatively easy, such as clinical trials on the use and impact of certain drugs, whereas other areas present problems. Thus, health promotion and investing in health are vastly underfunded because of methodological difficulty in demonstrating their effects compared with those of health care, thereby continuing the vicious circle.

The countries that replied included those that intended to give more financial support to health outcome research (Croatia, Finland, Ireland, Israel and Turkey) and those that planned to reorient or were already reorienting resources to specific health issues based on such research (Austria, Hungary, Italy, Norway, Poland and Slovakia).

Legislation

Few countries referred to legislation on health outcome. In some countries, health care professionals are legally obliged to participate in quality assurance activities. A health outcome orientation does not seem to be legally enshrined as part of the planning process in any country; in fact, some believe that legislation should best be restricted to areas not suited to professional self-regulation, such as formal complaint procedures, patients' rights or appropriate technology *(8)*.

Human resource development

Creating a solid research infrastructure means ensuring a supply of researchers trained in outcome-based research and validated research instruments. Epidemiological education and training is becoming more common throughout Europe. A number of countries (Bulgaria, Estonia, Hungary, Ireland, Kyrgyzstan, Slovakia, Slovenia, Spain, Turkey and Uzbekistan) reported that they are investing in training in the use of health outcome by including this in medical curricula or postgraduate training for health care managers or workers. Less or negligible attention is paid to other professionals, such as policy analysts, who are needed to consider the outcomes of processes.

Work on developing validated research instruments has also been progressing. Especially in some of the European Union countries, new tools, such as those to measure disability-free life expectancy, health expectancy and health impact assessment, are being tested but are not used to the same degree in countries throughout the Region.

Monitoring and evaluation

Where countries have set quantified targets, this influences the development of their monitoring and evaluation systems, since they need to have the information necessary for measuring progress on the specific targets. Commitment to participate in the monitoring of the European health for all policy has had a similar effect in several countries, as they needed to collect specific data so that it could be included in the Regional Office's health for all database, which contains several hundred indicators.

Malta plans to establish a monitoring committee and to revise targets based on its recommendations. In the United Kingdom, the Central Health Monitoring Unit includes a unit dealing with health outcome. Turkey has poor data and virtually no mechanism to ensure effective monitoring. Turkey has, however, initiated the process by introducing epidemiological training, which is an important prerequisite for monitoring. Although Finland has not set targets, the progress and revision of the health policy still undergo rigorous scientific evaluation.

The responses to the questionnaire show that, although countries have strongly emphasized mechanisms to support monitoring and evaluation as well as epidemiological training, few monitor these processes themselves.

Conclusions and implications for the future

Effective use of health outcome requires a well functioning information system. Most countries in the Region have good information systems.

Information systems in the countries in the eastern part of the Region are being reassessed and restructured. Although the transition process has created some problems, the need to restructure puts these countries in a position to create systems that feed the decision-making process and incorporate a focus on health outcome. More bodies are being set up to supervise the development of the information systems. Two important areas of research in the eastern part of the Region are health systems and studies on cost–effectiveness.

Countries in western Europe and, recently, countries in central and eastern Europe such as the Czech Republic, Hungary, Poland and Slovenia are strongly emphasizing:

- registering inequity in health;
- promoting research on health and health services;
- developing practice guidelines and systematically reviewing evidence-based medicine;

- assessing cost–effectiveness;
- developing information systems on hospital services; and
- establishing national disease registries to provide evidence to define priorities and focus action.

The study reveals that countries have made tremendous headway in collecting information and expanding the research agenda to look at a wider range of determinants of health. Countries do not seem to have been as successful in using this information to manage change. There is little evidence that information on health outcome influences policy planning. Similarly, little evidence suggests that the information is substantially influencing other sectors. In some cases, the people responsible for producing and acting on the information have failed to communicate; sometimes other sectors simply do not listen. In any case the task of building awareness needs to be tackled more systematically. The evidence can be disseminated much better and used more effectively to strengthen health policy within and outside the health sector.

Nevertheless, there are signs of progress in some countries. Managers and health care workers are being trained to compile information on health outcome and to use such data in informing their decisions. Indicators to measure progress in health outcome are being developed. Health educators are becoming more aware of how to use health outcome. As the use of health outcome provides a strong tool for using resources more rationally, health outcome research has a strong position in competing for funding.

The European Union and a number of international organizations, including the World Bank and WHO, are promoting and supporting outcome-based research. In Hungary, for example, the World Bank is supporting the development of epidemiological analysis, the monitoring and evaluation of health policy, and epidemiological training. The European Union and WHO have established common indicator sets that most countries have adopted. The research community has considerable opportunity for international collaboration on health outcome.

Reorienting towards primary health care

What is primary health care?
According to the work carried for the International Conference on Primary Health Care in Alma-Ata in 1978 *(95)*, primary health care can be defined as:

> … essential health care based on practical, scientifically sound and socially acceptable methods and technology made universally accessible to individuals and families in the community through their full participation and at a cost that the community and country can afford to maintain at every stage of their development in the spirit of self-reliance and self-determination.

The Declaration of Alma-Ata takes the position that primary health care should be at the core of the health care system. Through attention to appropriate technology and cost–effectiveness, including the efficient allocation of resources, such a system should ensure that resources are redistributed away from hospitals and towards primary health care, so that secondary and tertiary care effectively support primary health care. This implies that primary health care should meet the basic health care needs of the population, providing a wide range of easily accessible services through locally organized delivery systems and ensuring a high degree of cooperation and coordination between providers of health care. The Declaration also advocates the active participation of the public individually and collectively, both in the decision-making process and in taking responsibility for one's own health. For primary health care to operate effectively, then, one might expect to see an integrated, multiprofessional team including general medical practitioners, community nurses and other health professionals such as dentists, chiropodists, physiotherapists, care assistants and social workers delivering health care in a holistic way to meet the needs of the individual, with the public playing a role in planning and influencing service developments.

Difficulties arise with this definition, depending on whether primary health care refers to the nature or type of services provided or to the access to and structure of services. For example, France does not have general practitioners in a gatekeeping role, and people can go directly to consultants who provide highly specialized services that may not be considered as primary health care. In the United Kingdom and other countries, what is called primary health care is more likely to be determined by the organizations or professionals providing services and not by the type of services provided. Also, some services necessary to meeting the basic health needs of the population, such as dentistry or social services, may be organized in separate organizational or financial structures, which could hinder the multidisciplinary and integrated development of comprehensive primary health care.

The situation becomes even more complex because the Declaration of Alma-Ata includes a concept of health policy that also deals with lifestyles and the environmental determinants of health. This implies that primary health care must be concerned with intersectoral issues.

Scope of the study
This study did not seek answers to these complex questions of definition but rather explored the following questions.

- Are countries shifting away from secondary and tertiary care towards primary care, defined as a widely accessible, locally organized system of service provision that meets the needs of the population in the health service structure in each country?
- Is the quality of primary health care changing, including stronger support for health promotion?
- Is the public participating more extensively in decision-making?
- Is there equitable access to the improvements being made?

Overview of core issues and main trends
Assessing whether health care in Europe is being reoriented towards primary health care requires examining countries or groups of countries with very different circumstances and at different starting points during the period of study.

The Nordic countries have long had a carefully planned interface between hospitals and primary health care to provide seamless service for maternity care or when elderly people are discharged from hospital into the care of community-based health and social services. This system of networking tries to ensure not only an easy flow of paperwork, including test results, but advice and guidance from hospital-based specialists to professionals in community-based care. It can work well, except that it cannot usually tolerate severe financial constraints, as the hospital sector is reluctant to transfer funds to primary health care so that high-quality services can be delivered in the community.

Elsewhere, more recent reforms and structural changes have aimed to create networks between primary and secondary care. The Mediterranean countries, especially Portugal and Spain and, to a lesser extent, Greece and Italy, have shifted towards primary health care and devolved responsibility for health and other matters to the regional and local levels. The role of general practitioners as gatekeepers to health care services has been strengthened, as has the role of multidisciplinary teams involving physicians, social workers and other health professionals, usually attached to the newly established primary health care centres.

In the United Kingdom, the health service reforms that introduced a quasi-market system and separated the roles of purchasers and providers of health care appear to have had a perhaps unintended but beneficial consequence. The reforms gave purchasers, or commissioners, which can include general practitioner fundholders as well as local health authorities, greater scope to assess the health care needs of their populations and more power and choice to purchase services from the primary health care sector wherever they believe these services to be best placed to provide effective solutions and value for money. One drawback, however, is the poor evidence base on which such choices can be exercised. Demonstrating short-term benefits is relatively easy for many types of hospital treatment, at least for individual patients. Nevertheless, the longer-term nature and population-based approach of many types of primary health care interventions, especially those related to health promotion and disease prevention, makes their value more difficult to assess. This problem was compounded in the United Kingdom by the need for purchasing managers, many of whom were on fixed-term renewable contracts, to show immediate results and short-term financial savings. The reforms are now being amended, so that general practitioners will no longer be fundholders. Instead there will be primary care groups, which will eventually function like very small health authorities commissioning services for catchment areas of about 100 000 people.

Some countries in central and eastern Europe, such as the Czech Republic, Hungary and Poland, have made far-reaching attempts at reorienting towards primary health care, which has become a main element explicitly underpinning current government moves to reform health care. In practice, the process has had limited success. Under the former systems, central funds financed the large-scale construction of hospitals and care was financed based on such variables as the number of beds and length of stay. This resulted in hospitals having many more beds than were actually needed, leading to a structural distortion away from primary health care. Poor motivation among physicians working outside the hospital sector, reluctance among newly qualified doctors to enter general practice and very strong resistance from medical lobbies has hampered the intended reorientation.

Nevertheless, innovative financial mechanisms designed to shift the balance in favour of primary health care services have been introduced on a pilot basis in some countries in the eastern part of the Region. Contracting of general practitioner services is being introduced, and some countries are aiming to use their limited funds more efficiently by allocating for primary health care based on demographic data and mortality indicators.

In the newly independent states, progress has also been hampered but for different reasons. Health services were built on a sectoral model, and there is a poor tradition of primary health care. Patients' lack of experience in receiving care in primary care settings, coupled with the poorly established function of gatekeeping, means that the primary care facilities that do exist are often underused and underdeveloped. This results in poor choice for patients, reinforcing the recourse to hospital care. As a result, governments, health professionals and the public have difficulty in imagining a health service based on primary health care. Nevertheless, the number of bodies specifically responsible for primary health care is increasing in some of the newly independent states, and there is very often multidisciplinary consultation with associations representing, for example, home care, general practitioners and paediatricians. Responsibility for primary health care is thus being decentralized to the community level, and the number of family physician centres and self-governing hospitals is increasing, albeit very slowly.

Primary health care and the link to other services
For primary health care to function properly it needs to provide a full range of basic services that are of high quality, adequately funded and staffed by appropriately trained professionals whose status is at least the same as that of their counterparts in secondary and tertiary care. Under such circumstances, populations would probably not only use primary health care services for maintaining health (health promotion and disease prevention, including screening) but also choose primary health care as a first stop when accessing secondary health services. Gatekeeping can therefore be a key issue that must be seen in and tailored to specific historical, structural, cultural and economic circumstances, with no single model being appropriate or relevant across the whole European Region. In almost half the Member States, people have direct access to specialists. In France and Germany, for example, the majority of the population would not accept the idea of gatekeeping by general practitioners. In other countries, certain groups of people have direct access to certain types of specialist, as in Croatia, Romania and Slovenia, where women have direct access to gynaecologists and obstetricians. In some countries that already have a tradition of gatekeeping by primary health care practitioners, such as Finland and Sweden, people increasingly tend to bypass their general practitioners and go directly to a high-technology specialist medical centre for care. Although this is part of people's free choice, it may be inappropriate and expensive and lead to inequity.

Which tools were used in reorienting towards primary health care?
As indicated above, ongoing health care reforms have generated considerable action in reorienting towards primary health care. In some cases this has been part of or closely linked to the development of a health for all policy, but in most cases it has been a parallel movement. Examining some of the tools used can help to determine how far the changes made were in accordance with the health for all philosophy.

A number of issues must be considered, however. First, the choice of policy instruments considered appropriate for a specific purpose in a country relates not only to the culture and tradition but to a specific time in the country's history. During the period covered by this study, the health care systems of the countries in the eastern part of the Region were going through tremendous changes largely related to their general shift towards a market economy. This skews the balance of the instruments they mentioned more frequently as promoting reorientation towards primary health care. Second, we have relied on two main sources of information: the replies to the questionnaire and work carried out at the Regional Office in preparation for a conference on health care reform *(8)*. As explained previously, lists of examples of the countries using a specific policy instrument should not be considered complete. Other countries using similar instruments may simply not have mentioned this.

Research and information

About three quarters of the countries reporting that they had increased research and improved information networks for reorienting health care towards primary health care are in the eastern part of the Region. Research was focused on aspects such as registering available services, assessing needs and demands for primary health care (in Albania and Armenia), reducing the number of hospital beds (in Bulgaria and Hungary), and assessing the level of existing resources being allocated to primary health care (in Poland and the Republic of Moldova). Countries reported that the European Union's Phare Programme and the World Bank were funding some of these projects.

These countries have only recently been introducing family physician or general practitioner systems as part of the reorientation to primary health care, and Estonia, Poland, Romania, Slovakia and Slovenia reported simultaneously improving the information network of such systems. A small number of countries in western Europe also reported improving their information systems: Ireland was computerizing information from general practitioners, Malta was introducing child health care records, and Spain was carrying out extensive research to examine the financing, provision and quality of primary care.

In the Netherlands, which already has a strong primary health care sector, a research centre has been set up specifically to support the development of primary health care. The reply to the questionnaire emphasized assessing medical technology and introducing programmed prevention (prevention consciously integrated into work practice) for general practitioners as new research areas.

The type of research seen in the Netherlands relates to the movement towards improving outcome and the "growing awareness that there are large gaps in knowledge of which treatments are effective and for whom" and to "the fact that even when research-based evidence is available, it is frequently neither well known nor acted on" *(8)*. Governments typically play a role in assessing technology and the quality of care; in Belgium, France, Germany, Israel and the Netherlands, the insurance organizations that pay for health care also carry out such research, and more recently, in the Russian Federation, regions such as St Petersburg and Samara have shown interest in such research.

The recent changes in Finland towards some increase in private health care has also apparently triggered research to assess how the activities of the public and private health care sectors could be coordinated.

Health education and building awareness
Sensitizing health professionals. A number of countries in the eastern part of the Region reported using health education and awareness-building techniques to reorient action towards primary health care. This related mainly to making the health services themselves aware that health promotion and disease prevention programmes need to be integrated into their work. Estonia, Georgia and Israel were developing broad-based health promotion programmes including health education. Some countries referred to using general practitioners for reaching out to vulnerable groups and people at risk for certain diseases. Countries in both east and west mentioned screening: Ireland, Poland, Turkmenistan and the United Kingdom. The system of contracts for general practitioners developed during the health care reforms in the United Kingdom specifically required that general practitioners advise on health promotion.

The European Network of Health Promoting Hospitals *(96)* has expanded considerably in Europe in recent years, and one of the aims of the hospitals in this Network is to build links to primary health care.

Using the mass media. Slovakia and Tajikistan reported using the mass media to reach out to the public and make them aware of the need for early assessment of health problems. Malta reported distributing information bulletins on the availability of primary health care services and services for immunization.

Consultation and negotiation
Consultation and negotiation appear to be quite frequently used in both the east and west of the Region to reorient health services towards primary health care. Those most frequently mentioned as being consulted or as participating in negotiations are the medical associations. Consultation related largely to the need for training general practitioners and changing their roles to ensure a smoother interface between hospital and community care, but there were also other examples. In the United Kingdom in particular, many examples of purchasing authorities commissioning health promotion and disease prevention services have been documented *(97)*.

Austria mentioned efforts to increase cooperation between the health and social sectors, which was facilitated by creating small health and social welfare districts and integrated health and welfare facilities. Spain mentioned very specific contracts developed following consensus group discussion, not only with the health professions but also with interested nongovernmental organizations. Ireland and the Nether-lands, among others, mentioned the need to negotiate over protocols to be developed on a continuing basis to ensure effective treatment in primary health care. In the Netherlands, the role of the Ministry of Health, Welfare and Sport was seen as being facilitative, supportive and corrective.

Linked to the attempts to improve research and information on the quality of primary health care, some countries have recognized the "importance of understanding how to change professional behaviour, in order that more effective and efficient treatments can be provided" *(8)*. There are already good examples of physicians sharing information on clinical activities, with the intention of changing behaviour in the direction of those who achieve the best practice, and the professional associations have played an important role in this *(98)*.

Interestingly, a number of countries in both the east and the west of the Region referred to the need for consultation to ensure better links between the primary health care sector and other levels of care, and Ireland mentioned the importance of consensus being reached between general practitioners and consultants.

Structural, administrative and management measures
Structural, administrative and management measures was the category of tools most frequently referred to by countries in both the east and west of the Region.

The total number of hospital beds has fallen significantly in recent years in almost all western European countries, mostly acute inpatient beds. At the same time, however, admission rates have increased and the length of stay has declined. This is caused by cost-containment policies and changing methods of treatment as well as changes in the roles of primary health care and social care *(8)*.

The countries in the eastern part of the Region have more hospital beds and higher admission rates than do countries in western Europe. The eastern countries reported trying to bring about three main changes:

- reducing the number of hospital beds: Albania, Hungary, Kazakhstan, Kyrgyzstan, Republic of Moldova, Turkmenistan and Uzbekistan;
- developing primary health care centres: Albania, Bulgaria, Czech Republic, Poland and Romania; and
- introducing a system of general practitioners or family physicians: Belarus, Bulgaria, Kazakhstan, Kyrgyzstan, Latvia, Republic of Moldova, Turkmenistan and Uzbekistan.

Lithuania and Turkmenistan linked the development of primary health care to the establishment of community health councils; for other countries, ensuring a free choice of physician was seen as an important move in the reorientation process.

Introducing such changes was not always smooth. Albania, Bulgaria and Estonia mentioned such problems as developing adequate services in rural areas and gaining acceptance for the concept of family physicians. Certain countries faced special problems such as reconstructing and revitalizing primary health care and emergency services destroyed during wars in their regions.

Some countries in western Europe mentioned the need to expand primary health care services geographically. Iceland, Malta, Portugal and Spain, for example, referred to the need to reduce the distances people need to travel to reach primary health care services. Austria established mobile primary health care services in 1991.

The overall emphasis in western European countries was linked to the content and quality of care. The United Kingdom viewed this in the mid-1990s as being linked to giving general practitioners the role of fundholders for their patients' care and developing contracts for care; as mentioned above, these developments are now being reversed. Belgium, Denmark and Slovenia have developed national policies for continuous quality of care development *(99)*.

Another frequent concern in western Europe was creating more effective links between general practitioners or family physicians and secondary care. Ireland was establishing pilot primary health care centres with close links to hospital services and was giving general practitioners access to investigative facilities in hospitals. Finland, France, the Netherlands, Portugal and Switzerland mentioned developing or strengthening similar close links between primary and secondary services. In France, primary health care is available either through the hospitals or in separate primary health care centres. Finland also reported on plans to ensure links between outpatient services and services dealing with housing and social welfare. The Netherlands reported on establishing alliances between primary and secondary sectors to treat terminally ill people and those with AIDS, but also mentioned that the participation of general practitioners in the secondary sector is facilitated by an integrated budget.

Attempts have also been made to improve service in community clinics and domiciliary care. In Israel, weekly home visits to older people with severe congestive heart failure appeared to reduce annual admission rates for hospital care by half *(100)*. Home nursing has been expanded in Denmark, Ireland and Spain (the Basque Country) and the United Kingdom. In parts of western Europe and for many people in the eastern part of the Region, the quality of housing presents an obstacle to the potential success of home nursing, especially when such housing is cold or damp.

Financial measures
Most of the countries that reported using financial measures to reorient health services towards primary health care are in the eastern part of the Region. Eight of the countries using financial measures mentioned the use of a specific formula to allocate resources to primary health care. Others referred to new financing mechanisms for family physicians, and Belarus was considering linking their remuneration to their performance. Poland attempted first to establish a framework for future development by clearing debts in care institutions and by investing support from the United States in equipping primary health care services. Both Georgia and the Republic of Moldova reported that the economic and fiscal crisis was inhibiting the switch from hospital-centred care towards primary health care.

This was echoed in Finland, where primary care services had borne a disproportionate share of the burden of fiscal cutbacks. Initiatives later introduced to support the development of primary health care included investing further funds in training for primary health care and shifting funds from institutional to open care. Ireland, the Netherlands and Spain emphasized getting value for money and trying to achieve greater accountability; funds had been made available for such activities as clinical audits, developing an integral model for estimating utilization and costs and, in Spain, developing contracts linking objectives and activities and monitoring the outcomes. Spain and the United Kingdom mentioned income-related incentives for physicians to carry out more disease prevention work. Reflecting the structural changes in some western European countries to create better links between the different levels of care, Israel was using financial incentives to encourage hospitals to support other levels of care.

Legislation and regulation

Legislative and regulatory tools were not so frequently mentioned as a means of reorienting towards primary health care, although a number of countries in the eastern part of the Region, such as the Russian Federation and Slovakia, mentioned recently passed comprehensive health care laws. Slovenia and Turkmenistan referred to specific regulations designed to determine the functions and obligations of the primary health care services and to provide guidance on the referral system and on how negotiations between partners should be carried out.

Western European countries mentioned laws and regulations infrequently, except to emphasize the legal provisions making primary health care services accessible to all. One area of concern was regulations clarifying the role of the national and local levels in delivering and assuring the quality of primary health care. In what has been considered a landmark in the development of legislation in Europe *(8)*, however, in 1993 Finland defined patients' rights by law. One of the more important aspects of this legislation is the role of the patients' omsbudsman, which includes advising patients on the practical implementation of the law and assisting them in writing complaints or applications for compensation. The Netherlands has taken the most comprehensive approach in legislation: treating the relationship between patient and physician as a "special contract" within civil contract law. This gives patients a direct claim on physicians and the ability to enforce their rights through the courts.

Human resource development

Almost all the countries in the eastern part of the Region said that they were using human resource development to orient their health care systems towards primary health care. Training general practitioners or family physicians was receiving the greatest attention, although eight countries also referred to changing the curricula for nursing education to prepare nurses for home nursing and community care. A WHO study *(101)* indicates that more attention is being given to the development of nursing than would appear from the replies to our questionnaire. According to this assessment there is renewed interest in nursing education, both in relation to reviewing curricula, especially for university education, and in relation to continuing education schemes. In the United Kingdom, a review of existing research demonstrated a direct correlation between the employment of nurses with higher levels of qualifications and better patient outcomes.

Slovenia mentioned the need for primary health care to focus more on women's health.

Disappointingly little attention seems to be given to the possibility of changing the proportions of different types of staff to develop health care along the lines suggested at Alma-Ata, or to reassessing the traditional roles of health professionals and the division of responsibilities between them.

The countries in the eastern part of the Region emphasized undergraduate and postgraduate education. Countries in western Europe focused more on measures for team-building, developing interdisciplinary action and improving performance on the job. Norway, for example, referred to increasing interaction between professional groups during basic and postgraduate training. Joint training for health and welfare professionals has already been initiated in Norway. Israel, Spain and the United Kingdom were providing guidelines for workers in primary health care on treating chronic diseases and on helping people to change their behaviour. The Netherlands reported developing hundreds of treatment protocols to improve performance and reduce the use of unnecessary tests and prescribing. Ireland mentioned measures to improve management capacity. Although the countries in the eastern part of the Region did not mention management training in their replies to the questionnaire, the work of the World Bank and the European Union's Phare Programme demonstrates that these countries are strongly emphasizing management training for improved primary health care.

Monitoring and evaluation

Reflecting the structural changes reported in the eastern part of the region, nine countries in central and eastern Europe reported monitoring changes in the number and use of hospital beds. Estonia and Poland were evaluating the quality and efficiency of primary health care services provided.

Ireland and Spain were evaluating the effectiveness of services in terms of costs and health outcome, and the United Kingdom also reported measuring variation in the utilization of services.

General conclusions

Can we follow the leaders?

The health for all approach has taken root in a small number of countries, even surviving changes in the governing parties. Can other countries follow their lead? As with many questions, the answer is both yes and no. Part of the success of the pioneers seems to be related to historical opportunities that cannot be replicated, but they also appear to have some common attributes.

The right people in the right place at the right time

In the countries and regions where health for all moved from policy formulation to action, the right politician was in place to initiate the process, and without this political commitment the policy process cannot go forward. In some cases the politicians of the time were enthusiastically and personally committed to health for all, and this had a widespread impact *(102)*. Perhaps even more importantly, there was a strong group of committed experts, who were often civil servants. The leaders of political parties change, but when skilled and committed civil servants stay in place they can keep the health for all approach on the agenda, developing a credible policy and strategy.

In examining the prospects for developing a successful health for all policy, countries need to be concerned not only with the ministry of health and its structure and staffing but with the general role and remit of the civil service, career structures, links between the national and subnational levels and provision for continued education and training. The civil service is only one of the many players in the process of developing health for all policy, but skilled and committed civil servants are required to manage the complex interaction that is essential between government departments and between the public and private sectors on a continuing basis and over an extended period of time.

Universal values

Where the health for all approach has stood the test of time despite political changes, the values and philosophy of the policy had been made explicit from the beginning. A kind of moral pressure was created such that most political parties had to come on board or to state openly that they would not favour ensuring that vulnerable people get a fair chance, which is not an easy political stance for most mainstream parties. Whether they all maintained these principles in implementing the policy is another story. The process of discussing the main ethical issues very openly, however, is useful in gaining broad support for what must be a long-term effort. In the shorter term (the average life of governments), a certain amount of stop and go and even backtracking may be unavoidable, but if consensus has been reached on the important values, then at the very least, any diverge will have to be explained.

A reasonably broad network

The policy documents that had been formulated by a small inside group (sometimes attached personally to the minister without also being linked to the normal bureaucracy of the ministry of health) or by outside experts died an early death. Where broader groups were involved in formulating the policy, although this did not usually include much lay participation, the mentality of professionals and experts seems to have been affected somewhat, which created ownership and kept the health for all approach on the agenda.

Bottom-up

Some countries had a strong grassroots movement for health for all, partly influenced by the WHO Healthy Cities project, the emerging WHO Regions for Health Network and similar movements inspired, for example, by Agenda 21. In some countries, the national government explicitly instructed local areas to develop their own policies; in others, local initiatives that predated national health for all efforts gained recognition later. Such grassroots developments created many more health for all supporters throughout countries. Their influence appears to have been quite decisive, not only in their local areas but through their participation in national discussions and discussions in professional associations and other organizations. This created a ripple effect that is difficult to stop.

Exchange of information

This ripple effect has been strong, and the roots are really taking hold in countries that have provided the means for local areas to exchange experience. This is clear in the United Kingdom; almost 30 issues of the newsletter *Target* have kept people informed of activities around the country. Notes are scribbled and information and addresses exchanged at national policy conferences and at the "health days" organized regularly in some countries in the eastern part of the Region. Several countries have also very successfully begun to exchange information with others, either to initiate a process of developing health for all policy or to legitimize and strengthen an ongoing process.

Guidance and feedback

Health for all is a complex and new process for many. There are excellent examples of guidelines, protocols and newsletters being used to support local areas in implementing health for all policies, in giving feedback on progress and in generating friendly competition as an incentive for action. The process of preparing such guidelines and protocols can involve different disciplines and broadens the circle of people who are involved in and understand the health for all approach.

An irreversible process

In countries in which the health for all process has been initiated and a solid base of support established, returning to a monosectoral, vertical approach to health policy development is virtually impossible.

Clear influence of the health for all approach

Even countries in which the development of a comprehensive health for all policy is not yet an accepted practice have attempted to formulate and implement policies for health in accordance with the health for all approach. About 90% of the countries replying to the questionnaire report using one or more policy instruments to tackle equity in health, to increase public participation in decision-making and to promote intersectoral action to influence lifestyles and reorient towards primary health care. Slightly fewer (about 80%) have initiated intersectoral action to improve environmental health, and cited concerns related to health care and orientation towards health outcome.

What about the latecomers?

If just over half the Member States have taken the health for all road or are now embarking on it, then just less than half have not. Does this mean that they are still drifting from day to day in an ad hoc, crisis management mode? Are they still focusing on inputs or organizational changes to health care with little relevance for health outcome? Do they still work in what has been shown to be an outmoded, ineffective, vertical manner adhering to narrow, disease-oriented policies? The present study does not answer these questions, which must be posed if we are to understand how to bring the latecomers on board.

Use of specific policy instruments

The kinds of policy instruments or measures countries have used vary depending on the area of concern. For some health for all principles, notably an orientation towards health outcome, intersectoral action for the environment and intersectoral action for health care, the range of policy instruments used has been more restricted than might have been expected. For example, the environmental health measures recorded relate most frequently to restricting the emission of pollutants or to occupational safety rather than to broader issues such as ensuring violence-free environments or easy access to public facilities.

For other health for all principles, especially equity in health, public participation, intersectoral action for lifestyles and reorientation towards primary health care, countries frequently use a wider range of tools: financial measures, legislation and regulation, structural, administrative and manage- ment measures and consultation. However, the broad picture tends to be working in rather traditional ways with rather traditional partners. This might be expected, since many people and organizations feel more comfortable working in familiar ways with partners they know.

For example, the financial instruments used in promoting equity are mainly measures to exempt vulnerable groups from co-payments for health care rather than broader financial measures to change income distribution. Measures related to lifestyles focus heavily on classroom-based health education. Human resource development and training and other more innovative measures may be used regionally and locally, as demonstrated by some of the case studies, but they are less commonly reported at the national level.

What hinders more lateral thinking? What are the main factors obstructing reaching out to new partners? These issues are urgent if we are to ensure more rapid progress in the future and to begin at least to restrict the growing inequities in health.

Although a few countries have attempted to link research and information to policy development, the use of this developmental tool also appears to be limited. On the whole, reference to research relates to specific projects rather than to an overall strategy, and an information strategy is seen mainly as a way of monitoring health status.

This pattern is perhaps not surprising given that the national government is responsible for legislation and regulation, fiscal measures and structural issues in most countries, whereas respon- sibility for human resource development and research may be delegated to professional bodies or academic institutions. However, addressing the complex issues related to the health for all approach by using the possible types of policy measures only in a restricted and rather conventional way raises some concerns and carries a number of risks for the future.

First, it suggests that the focus has failed to move sufficiently from health risk and health care treatment towards tackling the wider determinants of health such as the societal and related environmental conditions that are so crucial to tackling inequity in health. In this sense, medical rather than social models and concepts of health continue to prevail.

Second, the absence of strong leadership in training and research carries the risk of a patchy attempt to implement health for all now, and a lack of the necessary continuity and momentum to ensure adequate management capacity in the future.

Third, this study has revealed that the use of tools to monitor the process of policy development and to evaluate policy action is rather limited. Given that the implementation of public policy across

Europe has been subjected to stringent resource constraints and this trend is likely to continue, it is increasingly important to ensure that the limited resources available are being used as effectively and efficiently as possible. In a few countries, monitoring and evaluation of the effectiveness of interventions in the health care and social services is gaining momentum, with far-reaching impact on resource allocation and, to some extent, on individuals' health and social outcome. The rigour applied to measuring health outcome needs to be applied to the wider implementation of health policy and activities to assess the extent to which policy objectives are being met in the short, medium and long term. The evidence so far suggests that this is not happening widely. This has serious implications for the longer-term sustainability of the policy, and indicates the need for clearly focused research and information strategies developed and carried out by appropriately educated and trained staff.

Linking the various levels of policy development

Although it is appropriate that national or, in the case of federal states, regional health policies set overall goals and objectives, the huge variation in needs and resources at the local level requires that similar objectives be set at the local level, to ensure both that local circumstances are adequately dealt with and that local strategies are contributing to national or regional goals. There must be a smooth interface between policies and strategies at all levels. If this is missing, there are strong negative implications, especially for the health for all principles of equity in health, public participation and an orientation towards health outcome. Some of the case studies partly address this issue, but it was not a strong focus of this study.

Future studies should focus on the extent to which the vital role of the local level in policy implementation is recognized, and the essential links between the various levels of policy development are explicitly addressed.

References

1. COLOMER, C. ET AL. *Building healthy public policies with tourism and agriculture as partners: notes from the first phase of a WHO/EURO demonstration project in the Valencian Community.* Copenhagen, WHO Regional Office for Europe, 1996 (Regions for Health Network, Leading Edge Series, No. 2, document EUR/ICP/POLC 05 02 02(2)).
2. *Communication from the Commission to the Council, the European Parliament, the Economic and Social Committee and the Committee of the Regions on the development of public health policy in the European Community.* Brussels, European Commission, 15 April 1998 (COM/98/0230 final).
3. UNITED NATIONS DEVELOPMENT PROGRAMME. *Human development report 1997.* Oxford, Oxford University Press, 1997, p. 235.
4. NYKÄNEN, E. National programme on aging workers – dispelling the myths of age. *Socius*, 1: 4–5 (1998).

5. *Health in Europe – report on the third evaluation of progress towards health for all in the European Region of WHO (1996–1997)*. Copenhagen, WHO Regional Office for Europe, 1998 (WHO Regional Publications, European Series, No. 83).

6. *First cohesion report*. Brussels, European Commission, 1996 (document CM-97-96-928-C).

7. *Our healthier nation: a contract for health. A consultation document*. London, Stationery Office, 1998 (Cm 3852).

8. SALTMAN, R.B. & FIGUERAS, J. *European health care reform: analysis of current strategies*. Copenhagen, WHO Regional Office for Europe, 1997 (WHO Regional Publications, European Series, No. 72).

9. WILKINSON, R.G. *Unhealthy societies. The afflictions of inequality*. London, Routledge, 1996.

10. KUNST, A. *Cross-national comparisons of socioeconomic differences in mortality*. Thesis, Erasmus University, Rotterdam, 1997.

11. *Lithuanian health report – 1990's*. Kaunas, Medical Academy Press, 1994.

12. *Bulgaria's road to health for all*. Sofia, Ministry of Health, 1987.

13. *Promoting health in Hungary. Report of a group established by the Council of Ministers of the Hungarian People's Republic*. Budapest, Central Statistical Office, 1987.

14. MINISTRY OF HEALTH AND SOCIAL WELFARE. *Health for all by the year 2000. Polish strategy and targets*. Warsaw, Polish Medical Publishers, 1983.

15. *WHO's strategy for health for all by the year 2000 as reflected in the health policy of the German Democratic Republic*. Berlin, Ministry of Health of the German Democratic Republic, 1988.

16. *Consultation of countries with national health for all policy documents*: report on a WHO meeting, Sofia, 12–13 December, 1989. Copenhagen, WHO Regional Office for Europe, 1990 (document EUR/ICP/MPN 040).

17. *The health of the nation: a consultative document for health in England*. London, Stationery Office, 1991.

18. FLORIO, N. Working together for health: the federal and cantonal collaboration in Switzerland. *In*: *The process of health policy development: report of a working group on the development of subnational policies for health*. Copenhagen, WHO Regional Office for Europe, 1992, pp. 109–136 (document EUR/ICP/HSC 418).

19. *Better health, better Wales? Strategic framework*. Cardiff, Welsh Office, 1998.

20. SCOTTISH OFFICE DEPARTMENT OF HEALTH. *Working together for a healthier Scotland. A consultation paper*. Edinburgh, Stationery Office, 1998 (cm 3584).

21. *Well into 2000 – a positive agenda for health and wellbeing*. Belfast, Department of Health, 1998.

22. Ottawa Charter for Health Promotion. *Health promotion international*, **1**(4): iii–v (1986) and *Canadian journal of public health*, **77**(6): 425–430 (1986).

23. *Health for all policy in Finland*. Copenhagen, WHO Regional Office for Europe, 1991 (document EUR/FIN/HSC 410).

24. TSOUROS, A.D., ED. *World Health Organization Healthy Cities project: a project becomes a movement. Review of progress 1987 to 1990*. Copenhagen, FADL Publishers and Milan, SOGESS, 1991.

25. *Regions for Health Network annual report.* Copenhagen, WHO Regional Office for Europe, 1993–1998 (documents).
26. *Protocol and guidelines: countrywide integrated noncommunicable diseases intervention (CINDI) programme.* Copenhagen, WHO Regional Office for Europe, 1996 (document EUR/ICP/CIND 94 02/PB04).
27. WORLD BANK. *World development report 1993: investing in health.* Oxford, Oxford University Press, 1993.
28. *Health for all targets. The health policy for Europe.* Copenhagen, WHO Regional Office for Europe, 1993 (European Health for All Series, No. 4).
29. *Strategy of Tajikistan for future health by 2005.* Dushanbe, Ministry of Health, 1995.
30. *Health for the nation. Bulgarian health strategy.* Sofia, Ministry of Health, 1995.
31. *Lithuanian health programme.* Vilnius, Ministry of Health (in press).
32. *Health for all by the year 2000. The Finnish national strategy.* Helsinki, Ministry of Social Affairs and Health, 1987.
33. *Nota 2000* [Note 2000]. The Hague, Ministry of Health, Welfare and Culture, 1986.
34. *HEALTH21: the health for all policy framework for the WHO European Region.* Copenhagen, WHO Regional Office for Europe, 1999 (European Health for All Series, No. 6).
35. *Health for all by the year 2000. Revised strategy for cooperation.* Helsinki, Ministry of Social Affairs and Health, 1993.
36. *Health vision 2000.* Valletta, Ministry of Social Development, 1996.
37. *Shaping a healthier future. A strategy for effective healthcare in the 1990s.* Dublin, Department of Health, 1993.
38. Bättre hälsa för alla Östgötar – reviderat målprogram för landstingets folkhälsoarbete 1995–2000 [*Better health for all in Östergötland. Measurable outcome target programme for County Council health work, 1990–2000*]. Linköping, Östergötland County Council, 1990 (English summary available).
39. *Health plan for Catalonia, 1993–1995.* Barcelona, Department of Health and Social Security, 1993.
40. *National health policy of Turkey.* Ankara, Ministry of Health, 1993.
41. *Developing a policy for women's health. A discussion document.* Dublin, Department of Health, 1995.
42. JACOBSON, B. & YEN, L. Health action zones. *British medical journal,* **316**: 164 (1998).
43. *Healthy city plan of the City of Copenhagen, 1994–1997.* Copenhagen, Healthy City Project, Copenhagen Health Services, 1994.
44. *Health and wellbeing: into the next millennium.* Belfast, Department of Health, 1998.
45. *The world health report 1998. Life in the 21st century – a vision for all.* Geneva, World Health Organization, 1998.
46. *Research policies for health for all.* Copenhagen, WHO Regional Office for Europe, 1988 (European Health for All Series, No. 2).
47. *Priority research for health for all,* Copenhagen, WHO Regional Office for Europe, 1988 (European Health for All Series, No. 3).

48. RITSATAKIS, A. Opening address from WHO EURO. *In*: OLLILA, E. ET AL., ED. *Equity in health through public policy. Report on the expert meeting in Kellokoski, Finland, November 1996.* Helsinki, National Research and Development Centre for Welfare and Health, 1997, pp. 7–18.

49. *Level of living and inequality in the Nordic countries: a comparative analysis of the Nordic comprehensive surveys.* Stockholm, Nordic Council and Nordic Statistical Secretariat, 1984.

50. KUNST, A.E. ET AL., ED. *Socioeconomic inequalities in morbidity and mortality in Europe: a comparative study. Vol. 3. Country reports.* Rotterdam, Department of Public Health, Erasmus University, 1996.

51. *Variations in health: what can the Department of Health and the NHS do?* London, Department of Health, 1995.

52. *Independent Inquiry into Inequalities in Health.* London, Stationery Office, 1998.

53. FLYNN, P. & KNIGHT, D. *Inequalities in health in the North West.* Liverpool, NHS Executive, North West, 1998.

54. *Desigualdades sociales en salud en España: Informe de la Comision Cientifica de estudios de las Desigualdades Sociales en Salud en España.* Madrid, Ministry of Health and Consumer Affairs, 1996.

55. RASMUSSEN, N.K. Long-term health effects of unemployment – the case of Denmark. *In*: OLLILA, E. et al., ed. *Equity in health through public policy: report on the expert meeting in Kellokoski, Finland, November 1996.* Helsinki, STAKES, 1997, pp. 107–113.

56. GUNNING-SCHEPERS, L.J. ET AL., ED. *Socioeconomic inequalities in health: questions on trends and explanations.* The Hague, Ministry of Welfare, Health and Cultural Affairs, 1989.

57. MIELCK, A. & GIRALDES, M. DO R., ED. *Inequalities in health and health care. Review of selected publications from 18 western European countries.* New York, Waxmann Münster, 1993.

58. ROOM, G. ET AL. *Observatory on national policies to combat social exclusion. Second annual report.* Lille, European Economic Interest Group, 1992.

59. *Inequalities in health: report of a working group (the Black report).* London, Department of Health and Social Security, 1980.

60. WHITEHEAD, M. *The health divide.* London, Penguin Books, 1988.

61. Inequalities in health (editorial). *Lancet,* **2**(8193): 513 (1980).

62. MACKENBACH, J. Socioeconomic inequalities in health in the Netherlands: impact of a five-year research programme. *British medical journal,* **309**: 1487–1491 (1994).

63. *Equity in health and health care: a WHO/SIDA initiative.* Geneva, World Health Organization, 1996 (document WHO/ARA/96.1).

64. BENZEVAL, M. ET AL., ED. *Tackling inequalities in health: an agenda for action.* London, King's Fund, 1995.

65. LEVI, L. Managing stress in work settings at the national level in Sweden. *In: Preventing stress at work.* Geneva, International Labour Office, 1992, pp. 139–143 (Conditions of Work Digest, Vol. 11, No. 2).

66. *Policy appraisal and health – a guide from the Department of Health.* London, Department of Health, 1995.

67. *Lancashire's green audit 2: a sustainability report.* Preston, Lancashire County Council, 1997.

68. BERENSSON, K. Focusing on health in the political arena. *EUROHEALTH,* **4** (3): 34–36 (1998).

69. GEPKENS, A. & GUNNING-SCHEPERS, L.J. Interventions to reduce socioeconomic health differences. A review of the international literature. *European journal of public health*, **6**: 218–226 (1996).

70. DEKKER, E. & VAN DER WERFF, A., ED. *Policies for health in European countries with pluralistic systems*. Houten, Netherlands, Bohn Staflen Van Loghum, 1990.

71. KRASSOVSKY, C.S. Public health alcohol policy in the NIS: opportunities for a small nongovernmental organization. *In*: Harrington, P. & Ritsatakis, A., ed. *European Health Policy Conference: opportunities for the future. Vol. 5. Health challenges in central and eastern Europe and the newly independent states*. Copenhagen, WHO Regional Office for Europe, 1995, pp. 281–285 (document EUR/ICP/HFAP 94 01/CN01(V)).

72. *Human development under transition – country report for Turkmenistan*. New York, United Nations Development Programme, 1996.

73. MACNAGHTEN, P. ET AL. *Public perceptions and sustainability in Lancashire: indicators, institutions, participation*. Preston, Lancashire County Council, 1995.

74. *Priorities in health care. Ethics, economy, implementation. Final report from the Swedish Parliamentary Priorities Commission*. Stockholm, Ministry of Health and Social Affairs, 1995 (Swedish Government Official Reports 1995:5).

75. *Choices in health care. A report by the Government Committee on Choices in Health Care*. Rijswijk, Ministry of Welfare, Health and Cultural Affairs, 1991.

76. *Briefing on priority setting*, No. 4, 1998. Birmingham, Health Services Management Centre, School of Public Policy, University of Birmingham, 1998.

77. HANSSON, L.R. & VANG, J. *Health facilitators: an investment in local health work*. Copenhagen, WHO Regional Office for Europe, 1997 (Regions for Health Network, Leading Edge Series, No. 3, document EUR/ICP/POLC 05 02 02(3)).

78. *Healthy and sound. Framework for health policy in the Netherlands 1995–1998*. Rijswijk, Ministry of Health, Welfare and Sport, 1996.

79. PEDERSON, A.P. ET AL. *Coordinating healthy public policy. An analytic literature review and bibliography*. Ottawa, Ministry of National Health and Welfare, 1988.

80. *Environment for sustainable development – an action plan for Sweden*. Stockholm, Ministry of Health and Social Affairs, 1996.

81. TAKET, A.R., ED. Making partners – intersectoral action for health. *In*: *Proceedings and outcome of a joint working group on intersectoral action for health, Utrecht, 30 November–2 December 1988*. The Hague, Ministry of Welfare, Health and Cultural Affairs, 1990.

82. Scenarios and other methods to support long-term health planning. *In*: *Proceedings and outcome of a Steering Committee on Future Health Scenarios – WHO Workshop, the Netherlands, 1986*. Rijswijk, Steering Committee on Future Health Scenarios, 1986.

83. RITSATAKIS, A. Parliamentarians for health. *In*: Harrington, P. & Ritsatakis, A., ed. *European Health Policy Conference: opportunities for the future. Vol. 3. Implementing policies for health at country, regional and city levels*. Copenhagen, WHO Regional Office for Europe, 1995, pp. 227–235 (document EUR/ICP/HFAP 94 01/CN01(III)).

84. *Environment and health: report on the Second European Conference, Helsinki, Finland, 20–22 June 1994.* Copenhagen, WHO Regional Office for Europe, 1995 (document EUR/ICP/CEH 212(FIN)).

85. *Corporate health, corporate action – action pack.* Cardiff, Health Promotion Wales, 1995.

86. CSÁKÓ, M. *Towards a safe and healthy working environment in CCEE. A trade union view. In:* Harrington, P. & Ritsatakis, A., ed. *European Health Policy Conference: opportunities for the future. Vol. 5. Health challenges in central and eastern Europe and the newly independent states.* Copenhagen, WHO Regional Office for Europe, 1995, pp. 168–196 (document EUR/ICP/HFAP 94 01/CN01(V)).

87. MILIO N. Food and nutrition policy. *In: Health for all policy in Finland.* Copenhagen, WHO Regional Office for Europe, 1991, pp. 153–177 (document EUR/FIN/HSC 410).

88. *North Rhine–Westphalians together for better health.* Bielefeld, Ministry of Work, Health and Social Services, North Rhine–Westphalia, 1992.

89. *Environment for sustainable development – an action plan for Sweden.* Stockholm, Ministry of Health and Social Affairs, 1996 (Swedish Official Reports Series 1996:124).

90. *Press release 98/329 Tuesday 11 August 1998*, London, Department of Health, 1998.

91. *Tackling inequalities in health: an agenda for action.* London, King's Fund, 1995.

92. *Working together for better health.* London, Department of Health, 1993.

93. WARNER, M. *Implementing health care reforms through substitution.* Cardiff, Welsh Institute for Health and Social Care, 1996.

94. RUWAARD, D. ET AL., ED. *Public health status and forecasts. The health status of the Dutch population over the period 1995–2010.* The Hague, National Institute of Public Health and Environmental Protection, 1994.

95. *Alma-Ata 1978: primary health care.* Geneva, World Health Organization, 1978 ("Health for All" Series, No. 1).

96. PELIKAN, J.M. ET AL., ED. *Pathways to a health promoting hospital. Experiences from the European Pilot hospital project 1993–1997.* Gamburg, Germany, Health Promotion Publications, 1998 (Health Promoting Hospital Series, No. 2).

97. KILLORAN, A. *Putting health into contracts. The role of purchasing authorities in commissioning health promotion and disease prevention services.* London, Health Education Authority, 1992.

98. ANKONÉ, A. & SPREEUWENBERG, C. Artsen werken samen van Ierland tot Kyrgyzstan [Physicians collaborate from Ireland to Kyrgyzstan]. *Medisch contact,* **48**(6): 165–167 (1993).

99. BLOMHOJ, G. et al. *Continuous quality development: a proposed national policy.* Copenhagen, WHO Regional Office for Europe, 1993 (document EUR/ICP/CLR 059).

100. KORNOWSKI, R. ET AL. Intensive home-care surveillance prevents hospitalization and improves morbidity rates among elderly patients with severe congestive heart failure. *American heart journal,* **129**: 762–766 (1995).

101. SALVAGE, J. & HEIJNEN, S., ED. *Nursing in Europe: a resource for better health.* Copenhagen, WHO Regional Office for Europe, 1997 (WHO Regional Publications, European Series, No. 74).

102. Politicians look at the lessons from their experience (full report of Plenary E). *In:* Harrington, P. & Ritsatakis, A., ed. *European Health Policy Conference: opportunities for the future. Vol. 1. Overviews and outcomes.* Copenhagen, WHO Regional Office for Europe, 1995, pp. 75–82 (document EUR/ICP/HFAP 94 01/CN01(I)).

4

Learning from the past, looking to the future

Anna Ritsatakis

Understanding the past

The context of health for all development

The health for all approach, with its clear ethical basis and advocacy of working across sectors, is not unique to the health field. It reflects years of similar thinking and experience at the international level over a wide range of fields. For example, the need for a more unified approach to managing change and development was recognized as far back as the late 1960s and early 1970s *(1)*, by organizations such as the International Labour Organization with its "basic-needs" approach *(2)*, the United Nations Research Institute for Social Development with its unified approach to development *(3)* and the Organisation for Economic Co-operation and Development, which attempted to develop a set of social indicators in order to measure the quality of life *(4)*. The International Development Strategy proclaimed by the United Nations General Assembly on 24 October 1970 (see Box 4.1) expresses the essence of such a unified, multisectoral approach, which could well act as a preamble to a health for all policy today *(5)*.

Box 4.1. International Development Strategy, United Nations General Assembly, 1974

The ultimate objective of development must be to bring about sustained improvement in the well-being of the individual and bestow benefits on all. It undue privileges, extremes of wealth and social injustices persist, then development fails in its essential purpose. This calls for a global development strategy based on joint and concentrated action by developing and developed countries in all spheres of economic and social life: in industry and agriculture, in trade and finance, in employment and education, in health and housing, in science and technology.

Long-term commitment
The WHO intersectoral approach to promoting equity in health has regularly been formally reaffirmed over the past 20 years. This formal process started with a World Health Assembly resolution in 1977. It was followed by the approval by the WHO Regional Committee for Europe of the European strategy for health for all in 1980 and of the 38 regional targets for health for all in 1984 *(6)*. An updated version of the strategy was adopted by the Regional Committee in 1991 *(7)*. The recommendations from a European ministerial-level health policy conference in 1994 *(8)* urged countries to base their national policies for health on this revised policy. Two years later, the charter adopted during a second ministerial level conference held in Ljubljana to discuss health care reforms *(9)* called for countries to carry out such reforms within the framework of comprehensive health policies, with clearly defined objectives and targets for health. Following extensive consultation the Health Assembly, in May 1998, endorsed a renewed global health for all policy *(10)*, despite the recognized complexities and difficulties of taking intersectoral action for health. In September of the same year the Regional Committee reaffirmed its commitment to this approach by approving HEALTH21, the health for all policy framework for Europe for the twenty-first century *(11)*.

Recognition by other international organizations
Recognition of the health for all approach to developing policies for health has not been restricted to WHO or to the health sector. It has been reflected in the work of many international organizations, but notably in that of UNICEF, UNDP, the World Bank and the Council of Europe. Much of the more recent work of the European Union, although not always referring explicitly to health for all, reflects similar thinking. This can clearly be seen, for example, in the recent Communication from the Commission on the development of public health policy in the European Community *(12)*.

Both a political and an evidence-based approach
Evidence compiled over many years, and broad discussion in scientific and political circles on the causes and effects of social and economic trends, have underpinned a long-term commitment in a number of sectors to an integrated approach to development. One of the earliest social reports, produced in 1933 by President Hoover's Committee on Social Trends *(13)*, tried to "interrelate the disjointed factors and elements in the social life of America, in the attempt to view the situation as a whole rather than a cluster of the parts". From the early 1960s, well known development economists such as Gunnar Myrdal *(14)* were providing the evidence to show the complexity of the impact of social and economic policies, indicating that what were termed their "backwash" effects could be much greater than their intended direct effects. This was reflected in a greatly expanded interest in social reporting and the development of social indicators during the 1960s and 1970s, in order to meet a "scarcity of precise and reliable data on existing social conditions and problems, and of instruments to measure the real impact of social policies and programmes" *(15)*.

World events sharpen the focus on poverty and inequities
In more recent years, following the fall of the Berlin wall in 1989, the United Nations and particularly the WHO European Region experienced a sudden increase in the number of Member States, many of which

had a very low per capita income. The rapid changes that accompany transition to market economies in these countries are exacerbating an already deteriorating situation, and a new openness of attitude has brought to the forefront a host of hitherto veiled social and economic problems. In parts of western Europe, persistent unemployment and pockets of severe deprivation in some regions are graphic reminders that wealth created in a free-market economy does not necessarily filter down, and can lead to greater division between rich and poor. From other parts of the world also, television and the news media have brought the plight of hundreds of thousands of people dying of hunger into living rooms across Europe. The 1990s provided a sharp focus to the issue of poverty and, it has been argued, may have created a public saturation or weariness with issues of deprivation.

The international organizations have also refocused their attention on these issues. Pressure from many sides caused the World Bank to reassess the impact of its policies on the most vulnerable, and this was reflected in its 1993 report on investing in health *(16)*. The first *World health report* published in 1995 *(17)* stated that poverty was a major cause of ill health and mortality. UNDP has advocated its human development index, which combines indicators related to life expectancy, education and income as a more appropriate indicator than per capita income for ranking countries' development. In its *Human development report* for 1997 *(18)*, UNDP strongly reiterated that poverty is not only a question of lack of income but encompassed a shorter life, lack of education, lack of material means and social exclusion, and that the way to deal with this was to take action to enhance people's capacities in all these areas. This was backed by an increasing body of research indicating that, particularly when countries have reached a certain level of economic development, it is no longer differences in absolute material standards that affect health in society but relative poverty, social position and issues such as control over one's work environment *(19)*.

The World Summit for Social Development, which took place in Copenhagen in 1995, was called to examine what were considered to be manifestations of a deep-seated social crisis faced by almost all societies: poverty, high unemployment and social disintegration. A WHO position paper prepared for the Summit *(20)* suggested that, rather than treating the symptoms of these conditions, an attempt should be made to eradicate the structural causes of inequity, by focusing on empowerment and equal access to all that society has to offer, including health.

Within the European Community

This period also witnessed the shifting of considerable funds across western Europe as the European Union redoubled its efforts to combat poverty. In 1985 the launch of the Single Market was swiftly followed by a consensus that steps were needed to raise the quality of social protection. The ensuing European Social Fund (ESF) is the European Union's most important financial instrument for promoting employment and developing human resources. As an integral part of the Union's policy of economic and social cohesion, the ESF contributes to bridging the gaps between the wealthier and less advanced regions of the Union. Between 1994 and 1999 it is expected to have transferred a total of ECU 47 000 million from the Union's budget in order to co-finance actions undertaken by the Member States.

Although not designed specifically for this purpose, the main priorities of the ESF also affect the determinants of health, since they are to:

- combat long-term unemployment and exclusion from the labour market;
- develop the professional skills and qualifications of potential job seekers;
- help young unemployed people to enter the labour market;
- promote equal opportunities between men and women in the labour market;
- foster the creation of new jobs;
- pre-empt unemployment by adapting workers to industrial change; and
- improve educational and training systems.

The European Union's Social Charter, adopted by 11 member states in 1989, contained 47 initiatives, including 29 that required Council approval. Nearly two thirds of these have been adopted.

In November 1993, the Commission published a consultative paper on the future of European social policy. It was clear that European citizens needed to feel that the Union and social Europe was of greater relevance to them than in the past. The key messages emanating from the consultative process were that there was a distinctive European social model based on democracy and individual rights, free collective bargaining, a market economy, the need for equality of opportunity for all and the importance of social welfare and solidarity.

In July 1994, the Commission published its proposals for future directions in a White Paper on European social policy. It argued for a new mix between social and economic policy, insisting that competitiveness and social progress could flourish together. It said that Europe needed above all an adaptable, educated and motivated workforce, something that only social policy could create. The main themes of the White Paper were employment, how to develop the legislative base, and the vital need for a society in which all were active and all could contribute (21).

There have also been significant developments in European Union legislation that relate to the achievement of greater equity in some of the determinants of health. Over the last 30 years, the Union's social policy legislation has dealt with aspects of the free movement of labour, equal treatment for men and women, health and safety standards at the workplace, worker information and consultation, and the terms and conditions of employment.

Health policy response from countries

Much of the scientific evidence indicating a need to shift from a narrow focus on health care to a broader focus on community health had been available for many years. As mentioned above, discussion on the need to take an integrated approach to economic and social development, including health development, has come from many quarters. The health policy response from countries, however, has been extremely varied.

Formulating policies for health

As seen in Chapter 3, since the early 1980s more than half of the Member States in the WHO European Region have at some point at least undertaken the process of formulating what they claimed to be comprehensive policies for health. Of these early policy documents, some provided realistic frameworks for action whereas some seemed to be little more than printed "wish-lists", while others had hardly been formulated before they became politically redundant.

Following a dip in interest around the time of the immediate changes in the CCEE, when privatization and so-called health care reforms were the vogue, in the last five years there has been considerable renewed concern with the development of overall health policy. Since 1992, 18 of the 51 countries in the Region have either formulated policies based on health for all or are actively engaged in the process. In Finland, the Netherlands and the United Kingdom, this policy formulation was part of a normal revision process of previously valid policy documents. A further nine countries have already indicated to WHO that they are keen to discuss possible support for developing a health for all policy. It is expected that even greater interest will be kindled in those countries that have not yet embarked on the health for all approach, following the publication of HEALTH21 *(11)*.

Many ways to do it

These written policy documents represent a wide variety of approaches. They range from policies that largely retain a traditional health care focus to those that perhaps over-ambitiously try to cover the full span of the original 38 European health for all targets. Some have set numerous quantified targets, while others have felt it was politically (or in some cases scientifically) safer to rely on qualitative policy statements, indicating the intended direction for action rather than putting a quantified value on complex issues of concern.

The main focus of the documents also varies. Some concentrate more or less heavily on dealing with specific diseases, while others are concerned with tackling the problems of certain population groups or with settings for action. Most use a mix of these approaches. In many cases, these general policy documents are accompanied by, or exist parallel to, issue-specific policies such as those on food and nutrition, controlling substance abuse or environmental protection.

What is common to practically all these documents is that they pay at least lip-service to the need for an intersectoral approach to health, and in some cases present the need for working with partners in other sectors with some enthusiasm (though perhaps still with little recognition of the possible objectives of prospective partners). Almost without exception, these policy documents refer to the need to achieve greater equity in health.

Under different circumstances

Health for all policies have reached the political agenda in very varied country situations, at different times, and in different economic climates over the past 20 years or so. There has been a similar experience in other WHO regions, even in countries with a low level of economic development, some of which have taken innovative approaches to integrating health and development. This indicates that when the political will is present, the health for all approach is a flexible tool that can be adapted to suit different political and administrative systems and different sets of economic and social circumstances.

Finland was the first country in the WHO European Region to try this approach. It was, however, a rather special case. Finland is a relatively small, homogeneous country; it was blessed with prosperity and stability at the time when the process was initiated; it has a strong commitment to a health for all approach; it had sound information, research and experts already in place; it had high-quality health care and skilled and motivated civil servants; and it had a population used to the benign guiding role of the state, a search for consensus being the usual way of working. Even when Finland was hard hit by economic recession in the early 1990s, this approach, though hard-pressed, was not abandoned.

Although WHO's health for all approach is sufficiently flexible to be adapted to conditions anywhere, the type of system and culture in which it is taken up and the social and economic climate prevailing when a country implements it will obviously influence the policy options that are feasible and the chances of making rapid progress. But this way of trying to approach health challenges from different aspects, of attempting to understand the challenges from the perspective of many partners and sectors, or applying "joined up thinking" to health policy development (as this was described at a recent conference of local authority leaders in England (22)) is one that can be used to tackle socioeconomic inequalities in health at any time and in any place. The strength of the approach is in its flexibility, but this means that it should not be applied like a "cookie cutter". Wherever and at whatever level the approach is used, it is important that the wider policy environment and its implications for health policy development are also taken into account.

Different entry points

Many countries have formulated intersectoral policies that are issue-specific but health-related, such as environmental policies under the Agenda 21 initiative (23) or food and nutrition policies. For example, following the International Conference on Nutrition in 1992 (24) and the endorsement of the World Declaration and Plan of Action for Nutrition by the World Health Assembly in 1993 (resolution WHA46.7), a survey carried out in the European Region (25) showed that of the 35 responding Member States, 27 had initiated, were currently planning or had already implemented activities on nutrition policy. Respondents felt, however, that there was insufficient awareness and understanding of nutrition problems among policy-makers and planners.

Some countries have developed separate policies for health promotion or for health services. Ideally, issue-specific policies such as those for food and nutrition or for health care, would come under the umbrella of a wider policy setting objectives for health, as a means of expanding on its general directions. In other countries, such issue-specific policies have been utilized as an entry point to the later development of a more comprehensive policy for health. The latter way of working can create problems, however, as indicated by a recent review of the implementation of *The health of the nation* in England *(26)*, where it is stated that for many health care practitioners, as well as those from other agencies, the health strategy came too late because by then the policy agenda had largely been determined by changes in health care delivery arrangements.

It would be interesting to compare the impact of issue-specific policies developed as stand-alone policies, against those that are part of more comprehensive efforts to improve health.

Obstacles and facilitators to progress

Persistent problems – insufficient capacity to manage change
Many of the problems faced by the then 32 European Member States at the end of the 1980s still plague most of the present 51 countries in the Region. Foremost among these problems has been that of achieving intersectoral action for health. Collaboration with certain sectors such as social welfare has been traditional, and this is frequently mentioned by countries. Other sectors and players fortunately take the initiative themselves for interventions that have an impact on reducing inequities in health, such as the efforts of the environment or transport sectors to reduce pollution or to limit road accidents. As yet, however, there appears to be little evidence of countries even monitoring who these potential self-motivated partners for health might be.

On the whole, the health sector still appears to act largely alone, and tends to be dominated by medical models. Even when attempts have been made to carry out more community-based programmes for health promotion, it is not unusual for this to be carried out almost as a sideline, parallel to actions in the traditional health care sector where it is "business as usual".

Another seemingly intractable problem is that of securing effective links between short- and long-term actions. Politicians tend to be interested in the short-term issues, which can be addressed within their term of office; management incentives also focus on tackling the short-term issues, without necessarily linking these to longer-term strategic aims.

Encouraging signs for the future
There are, however, some positive signs that indicate a greater potential for managing change in the future.

More transparent values and criteria.   It is clear that tough choices have to be made. In recent years, there appears to have been a greater willingness to openly discuss the ethical values that will guide these choices. There is also some indication of a stronger attempt to set priorities, and some good examples of trying to do this on the basis of transparent criteria, such as in countries like the Netherlands, Sweden and the United Kingdom, and regions such as Catalonia.

Additional backing for the ethical arguments.   Evidence from recent research has shown that, in addition to the ethical argument for investing in equity in health, this also makes good economic sense. A fairer society seems to have multiple benefits including better health and, as suggested by data from 16 countries, bigger increases in labour productivity *(27)*.

Strengthening participation in decision-making.   Strong pressure for decentralization and pluralism in partnerships, which is becoming more usual with the delegation of power to lower levels, together with spreading privatization, strongly organized interest groups and the appearance of new players on the scene, have led to some innovative attempts to improve channels of participation in decision-making, including the use of modern technology such as the Internet.

Making a virtue of necessity.   When not used as an excuse to cut health promotion activities, continuing cost constraints have sometimes proved a powerful incentive for more imaginative thinking regarding alternative uses of resources, particularly at the local level.

Gains experienced in taking the health for all road

The value of going through the process
Whatever the facilitators or obstacles, it appears that even the attempt to take a health for all approach can bring some added value. In other words, even when the formulation of the policy leaves much to be desired, its implementation proves difficult, or progress in achieving the targets set has been disappointing, simply the experience of going through the process can be useful for a number of reasons:

- it has led to an improvement in information for health policy development, particularly of information reflecting possible inequities;
- mechanisms for wider participation have been tried and, once the opportunity to participate has been given, it is difficult to retract;
- cross-sectoral attempts at collaboration have been tried and, even when these have not been widespread, successful new partnerships have provided an example for others;
- even when policies have not been strongly implemented, discussions with prospective partners have opened a window of opportunity to new ways of working; and
- in some cases, a reasonable policy framework has provided guidelines for broad political consensus, so that even incremental steps can be kept in the right direction.

Building consensus
When the underlying principles have been presented as being of broad concern for society, and where cross-party political understanding and support has been sought from the beginning and systematically maintained, this seems to have kept the health for all approach on the agenda for an extended period. The presentation of health as a human right, and of equity as being a fair chance for

all, may have contributed to its more general acceptance and to the development of cross-party consensus in some countries, which is essential for a long-term policy. Available research results indicate that greater equity in health is in everyone's interest. Tackling inequalities in health is, however, a long-term process, and frequently needs strong efforts to repackage and revitalize the process in order to keep the momentum going.

The discussion has not yet been sufficiently broadened. Much of it still takes place within the health sector and between health experts. There are some good examples whereby countries, regions or cities have organized public discussion on health-related issues, although it is doubtful whether a survey of the general public would reveal much awareness of the health policy as opposed to health education issues. There are still only rare examples of the health sector exploring with other sectors possible common problems and health opportunities.

A clear map of the way forward

Where clearly written documentation has existed on countries' goals and objectives, the priorities between them and the strategies to achieve them, it appears that interested individuals and groups have been able to use it as a means of keeping even small incremental steps on track.

For the CCEE and NIS, it is not yet clear whether the formulation of national policy frameworks have had any noticeable influence on negotiations with the large investment organizations or donor countries. As national policy-making and management skills improve, and as local people gain stronger ownership of such processes, they should be in a position to exert greater pressure and have a better chance of determining their own future, even when powerful institutions or specific donors still come with their own agendas.

Regular and reliable reporting

There are good examples whereby public health reporting seems to be influencing the decision-making process. In some countries, reporting to parliament or local authorities has had a considerable impact on the health policy discussion. Recent attempts in a number of countries to monitor and report on inequities in health in particular seem to have prompted reconsideration of the issues when local politicians were able to compare their local constituencies with those of their neighbours.

Interpretation, presentation and working with the media

A sound evidence base is not sufficient to ensure action. There are, however, some good examples whereby skilful interpretation and presentation of the information has ensured that the evidence has had an impact outside academic circles and has contributed to initiating or sustaining the health for all process. Obviously this is an area where much more could be done. Watching television, listening to the radio and reading newspapers and magazines are still the most usual forms of recreation for the great majority of people; so far only a few countries seem to be developing this as a means of focusing the health policy discussion, rather than merely as a channel for health education.

Working on all levels

The countries where the process of health for all development seems to continue to go forward, however haltingly, are those where there has been simultaneous progress on national, regional and city levels. This may be explained partly by the fact that working on different levels has created a critical mass of people who understand the need for and advocate an intersectoral approach. It also seems to have facilitated the development of alternative approaches to similar problems in different parts of certain countries, creating possibilities for learning and improvement.

Where necessary changes lagged behind

The case studies and country profiles in this study indicate serious attempts to go beyond rhetoric to action. Where, however, change in countries was essential to make the health for all approach work, some aspects of policy development lagged far behind expectations.

Capacity for making partnerships

On the whole, there are still few people with the training and skills to open a fruitful intersectoral dialogue. The business world affords a wealth of material on getting to know potential partners, taking into account that they may have different organizational cultures and ways of working *(28)* and the importance of understanding that they may have different perceptions of the same issues *(29)*. Many of the tools used for this purpose outside the health sector could be usefully explored.

Increasing participation

Broad participation in decision-making is still not the norm. Some innovative attempts are being made, however, and new information technology such as the Internet is already being used as one means of doing this. This type of development raises the question of ensuring that the information available is of high quality and that a wider gap is not created between those who have access to it and those who do not.

Finding effective structures, processes and incentives

There is no clear consensus on the most effective way to change behaviour and to develop partnerships for health across sectors. The matrix we used as a tool for analysis in this study included a complex set of eight possible groups of policy measures. In contrast, Winsemius *(28)*, for example, has grouped these into three basic categories: legislation/regulation (using the whip); offering incentives (using the carrot); and consensus-building and cooperation brought about by communication, mediation, advocacy and education.

The health for all policy suggests that countries should establish specific structures for the promotion of intersectorality at government level, but only a handful of them report setting up and operating specific intersectoral bodies (variously named health committees, councils and working groups) at national level. There appears to have been more experience in doing this at regional and local levels, and in some countries interesting joint health and development mechanisms are emerging at the local level.

Drawing upon a comparative study of policy coordination capacities in 12 European Union member states, Metcalfe *(30)* suggested a simple nine-point scale along which administrations could be placed according to their degree of development in policy coordination. At the lowest level of coordination, departments work independently, simply informing others of their decisions; at the next level, they engage in consultation and in actively searching for agreement; at the third level they arbitrate policy differences; and at the most advanced end of the scale they are involved in establishing a government policy coordination strategy that draws on clearly established central priorities. Mechanisms to antici-pate, detect and resolve policy conflicts early in the process, to help identify inconsistencies and to reduce incoherence are essential if a higher level of coordination is to be achieved *(31)*.

Surprisingly little is as yet known about the full range of structures, processes and incentives employed by countries to promote intersectoral action for health. WHO's European Centre for Health Policy in Brussels is at present trying to map out some of the mechanisms being used and to address questions such as whether countries find the setting up of new intersectoral bodies effective and feasible for screening the possible impact on health of policies in other sectors; and whether they should be given the responsibility for ensuring that, when necessary, such policies are revised to mitigate deleterious impacts and enhance beneficial impacts. Alternatively, what would be the effect of adapting the way in which existing structures operate, and of strengthening and encouraging them to work with new partners by providing training and financial and other incentives? Would it be more appropriate to both establish an overall guiding body to act as a "health watchdog", provide the vision and monitor progress, and at the same time to adapt existing structures and mechanisms in order to promote intersectoral action for health in development? Discussion of these and the many other possible options does not yet appear to have begun.

Despite 20 years of effort to introduce a health for all approach, the necessary shift in thinking has not yet happened on a wide enough scale. Even in many of those countries where an attempt is being made to move from narrowly focused policies for health care to broader policies for health, there is little evidence of discussion on the possible impact of emerging social, cultural and economic changes. In 1996, the World Bank *(32)* stressed the importance of considering the effects of the policy environment, asking whether differences in transition policies and outcomes reflect different reform strategies or whether they primarily reflect country-specific factors such as history, the level of development or, just as important, the impact of political change taking place at the same time. By examining the strengths and weaknesses, the opportunities and threats to health gain, or what is known as SWOT analysis, policy-makers form some idea of the measure of control they may have over seemingly indeterminate happenings in the broader policy environment. They will gain some indication of what is unique about the particular country or local environment in which they are operating, what are its assets, which of the obstacles to promoting equity in health can be influenced, and what must be accepted as given, at least in the short term.

On the whole, the health sector still appears to be rather introspective, sticking to traditional ways of working; there are comparatively few examples of its readiness to pick up simple tools being developed in other sectors. For example, an analysis of the population in a country by the type of socioeconomic category used by those carrying out market surveys in the private sector, might give a better understanding of potential needs, constraints and opportunities than the traditional categories of sex and five-year age groups used for years by national statistical services. Techniques developed in the world of advertising could no doubt improve communication skills for health policy development.

Looking to the future

As a concept, the WHO definition of health as "a state of complete physical, mental and social well-being and not merely the absence of disease or infirmity" *(33)* has stood the test of time remarkably well, although it has not proved easy to measure across countries and over time. Consequently, the scientific community has found it easier to measure changes in mortality rates, since death is more precisely defined and the public probably also finds death and disease easier to grasp than "complete physical, mental and social well-being".

Patterns of disease

There have been shifts in the burden of disease. In view of the fact that people are now living longer, growing importance is being given to the concept of healthy life expectancy. The burden of morbidity among the very old (particularly dementia and Alzheimer's disease) will have a tremendous impact on carers and health and social services. The increasingly skewed dependency ratio (in terms not only of age ratios but of the numbers of years people are not working due to longer education and retirement), and the imbalance between social security contributions and benefits, have major implications for sustainability. Governments must face increasingly difficult ethical choices regarding the rationing of resources.

Improvements in health status are unevenly distributed across the European Region. Some countries, mainly the CCEE and NIS, are witnessing a re-emergence of some of the old public health issues. Communicable diseases such as diphtheria and poliomyelitis are increasing, partly as a result of poor socioeconomic conditions and the lack of vaccines. New lifestyles and behavioural patterns are also bringing their own problems in the CCEE and NIS, such as a rise in sexually transmitted diseases, including AIDS, and increased levels of cardiovascular disease. In some of the CCEE and NIS, basic services such as clean water and waste disposal are still an issue. Rates of infant and maternal mortality also tend to be much higher in the NIS and some CCEE.

Although the main causes of death remain quite stable, conditions in the modern world, particularly in the workplace, are influencing the patterns of disease, with increasing levels of stress and poor mental health playing an important role. Across the Region, we are witnessing uncertainty in employment, changing patterns of industrial production, changing roles of men and women and increasing disease, such as that resulting from repetitive physical work. The extensive welfare systems in place in most of western Europe since the middle of the century are becoming increasingly difficult to support. Policy-makers have been wrestling for some time with the task of cutting back on welfare state expenditure, but this has been largely unsuccessful as the number of claimants, such as the elderly and the unemployed, continue to rise.

People living in the CCEE and NIS are experiencing a different type of stress linked to the trauma of transition. Increased levels of stress are evident in people's recourse to high-risk behaviour as shown by levels of smoking, alcohol consumption and traffic accidents.

Obviously we must be concerned with the level and distribution of disease, but if we are to achieve a shift in the way we think and act in policy terms, then we must go further. In creating its development index, UNDP has shifted the focus from the traditional measure of development in terms of per capita GNP to examining the *capacity* of populations for development in terms of their income, their education and their health. Unless we think in terms of an individual's and a community's capacity for health, then we will not make the essential shift in thinking to focus on the complex web of determinants of, risks to and opportunities for health development.

In looking to the future, therefore, we need to remind ourselves of the determinants of health and of some of the main issues with which we must be concerned. Various models can be used to show the interconnections between health risks or between the various levels of policy intervention *(34)*. Rather than using one of these well known models, Fig. 4.1 depicts their components in a rather different way. On the one hand it shows the complexity of and the interactions between the main categories of determinants and risks that affect health, and on the other it disaggregates these components to highlight concerns that will need greater emphasis in the future.

General socioeconomic and political conditions

Peace, war and conflict

Unfortunately, one of the basic prerequisites for health – peace – is not secure in parts of the European Region. Armed conflicts continue almost on a daily basis in a number of the CCEE and NIS. The situation in the Balkans is still volatile but, if further instability and violence can be avoided, new options for collaboration could emerge. Although improved in recent years, the situation in Northern Ireland is still not without conflict, and separist groups in France and Spain continue to operate. More recently, the Kurds, although venting their frustration more against buildings than people, have shown that they can bring the effects of conflict right across Europe.

The social cost of war must also be assessed, in terms of destruction of the health services infrastructure and loss of health professionals, and the long-term impact on those disabled by war or affected by its violence, such as victims of rape and those who have lost close family members. Countries must pay particular attention to some groups such as refugees and migrants, whose health is at risk from poor living conditions and who often fall outside the social safety net. War has implications for the stability of social networks, many of which are disrupted, and for the escalation in civil violence and suicide.

Fig. 4.1. The determinants of and risks to health

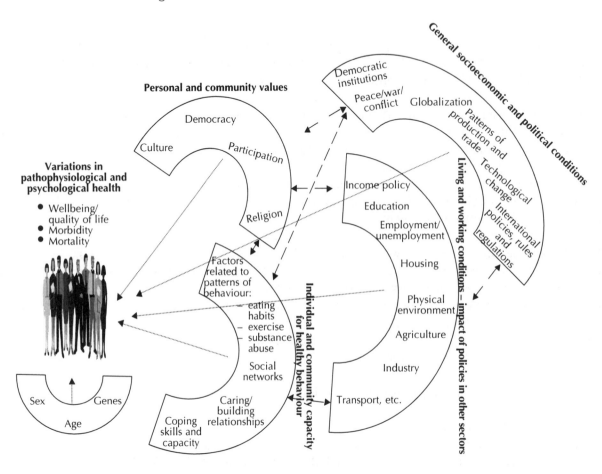

War and conflict bring extreme feelings of loss of control. Other socioeconomic and political trends, however, also affect the capacity of national, regional and local authorities to influence the factors that affect health within the areas of their own jurisdiction, while individual citizens feel a growing sense of alienation. As stated in the WHO global health for all policy *(10)*, "National and local decisions are affected as never before by global forces and policies". A number of the vastly complex issues involved are mentioned briefly in the following sections to indicate the conditions under which we shall be developing policies for health in the future.

Globalization – a new political reality
Europe, like the rest of the world, is caught up in increasing levels of globalization as the dramatic growth in trade, travel, migration and communications continues, transnational companies spread their area of

operation even wider, and actors and events in one part of the world affect the livelihoods and lifestyles of people everywhere.

Potentially, the process of globalization could lead to increased economic wealth, or to a further weakening of some disadvantaged areas. There are considerable differences in how countries and groups within countries stand to benefit. Globalization represents the possibility of a concentration of power without accountability, as an array of new multisectoral actors transcend the nation state to take possession of a new international arena. Many of these agencies are operating without controls, one example being the impact of international currency speculation on national economic policies, which can be to the detriment of health and welfare expenditure.

Ensuring that the potential of globalization can be tapped so that the impact on humanity is positive rather than negative represents a major political challenge. This was reflected in the choice of "Responsible globality?" as the theme for the thirtieth annual meeting of the World Economic Forum in Davos *(35)*. Sir Geoffrey Chandler *(36)*, for example, feels that transnational companies were wholly unprepared for the changes that they face. Their supply chains may involve working conditions where starvation wages, sexual or racial discrimination or child labour are the norm, and in some cases they face serious problems of physical security for their plants and people. On the other hand, the heightened scrutiny of corporate behaviour and companies' self-interest in a good reputation, as well as their need for a stable investment environment, has created in some companies greater concern for issues of social cohesion.

Globalization and changing patterns of production and trade

Access to all kinds of products, including information, has greatly expanded but it can be difficult to control the *quality* of some of these products and information. On the positive side, the increased potential for sharing knowledge could conceivably prevent or mitigate the impact of disease outbreaks or environmental health threats, or hasten the spread of good practice in health care. On the other hand, the effects of new lifestyles, tastes in food and leisure activities may bring mixed blessings for health. Easy access to information on technological advances in health care will certainly create demands that cannot be met, and access to pharmaceuticals and other products without the control and supervision of experts could have serious implications for health.

The forces of globalization have been felt in the labour market. Although, in theory, globalization allows the free movement of labour, in reality it is capital that flows to where labour is cheapest. The protective power of labour market legislation can be diminished as workers are increasingly detached from their companies, and people lacking a high level of education and skills are being devalued in an increasingly competitive economy. These issues pertain very closely to social exclusion, social cohesion and employment, which are among the prime determinants of health. Although some enterprises may be trying to take a more socially responsible approach to their own company policies, it is not clear where responsibility for the collective impact of these global trends now lies, and how their possible impact on health can be put on the global and national agendas.

Globalization poses other challenges, such as the abolition of so-called barriers to trade. In some cases these acted as a safeguard against threats to the environment and public health; on the other hand the development of regional trading blocks has serious implications for less developed countries. As capital, goods and ideas cross borders in response to supply and demand, however, there is a faster growth in productivity, trade volumes and national income; without growth it could be more difficult to tackle some of the serious issues of inequity with which we are faced. Taking an optimistic view, the World Bank *(32)* contends that such "integration helps lock countries onto the path toward more-open trade, while membership in international institutions spurs domestic institution building".

Supranational bases of power

In addition to the increased internationalization of knowledge systems, changed patterns of communication, technology, production and consumption, and the promotion of internationalism as a cultural value – all of which accompany globalization – greater world regionalization is bringing about shifts in power, for example in the growing European Union, the Association of South East Asian Nations (ASEAN) and the North American Free Trade Agreement (NAFTA). When the health for all policy was launched, no-one would have predicted the break-up of the USSR and Yugoslavia, and the converging of what had seemed like opposing east–west camps.

Although the European Union countries retain much of their national independence, they act together on many issues, some of which have a strong impact on health. There are now 15 member states, with another 6–7 negotiating entry. Within a few years' time, about half of the WHO Member States in the European Region will probably be members of the European Union. It will be vital for health policy purposes to analyse how the policies of a rapidly expanding Union will impact on health, both within the Union and in other countries, and what will be the health impact of socioeconomic policies implemented by these rather small, new European Union countries as they make their entrance to world markets.

Rapid and full integration into the global economy in recent years seems to have taken precedence as the main goal of economic development, and balanced budgets and cutbacks have dominated the political scene. Thus the 1990s have seen an erosion of some of the structures for health care, education and social security that were established following the Second World War. The push for some of the European Union countries to meet the criteria for monetary union is also causing cutbacks in spending on health and other public services. It is difficult to see how far these trends will continue in the future, or whether the general public will call for protection of its hard-won gains.

Other regroupings of countries have taken place on the international level as the CCEE have become members of many "clubs", each with its own culture, way of working and rules of behaviour. For example, the Council of Europe, with its strong focus on human rights and long tradition of working with local authorities, can be expected to influence issues of equity and participation in decision-making. OECD, with its tradition of peer review of economic and other policies and its well established mechanisms for in-depth discussions of policy issues at the highest levels, can be expected to influence a wide range of issues related to health development. A small number of the CCEE have already joined the World Trade Organization with its multilaterally agreed trade rules on goods and services. These groupings and regroupings will have an impact on how the member countries will deal with health policy issues in the future and how they will see their own role in shaping changes internationally.

International policies, rules and regulations

Supranational organizations have an increasingly strong influence on national social and economic policies, so that issues of redistribution, regulation and social empowerment may be raised to regional and even global levels. It has been argued that globalization and international policies have set welfare states in competition with each other and generate the "danger of social dumping, deregulation and a race to the welfare bottom" *(37)* and that there is a need for a more socially responsible globalization.

Democratic institutions and changing international and subnational configurations

While changing configurations of countries are shifting the power base at the international level, new groupings of subnational units both within countries and across national borders are also creating fresh challenges for democratic institutions.

In both the east and the west of Europe, decentralization is an increasing trend, with more decision-making power and responsibilities being given to lower levels in countries. One of the challenges of the future, particularly for the CCEE and NIS, is that this move has not always been accompanied by equivalent funds or clarification of roles and responsibilities.

Greater decentralization brings the possibility of increased participation in decision-making, if the essential information and structures are in place, but can also be very time consuming (to which the Swiss, with their long tradition of searching for consensus, would testify). It can pose difficulties in coordinating the actions of increasing numbers of partners, when a countrywide effort is needed. There is also a danger of greater inequities if more advantaged regions and districts move faster to pick up new opportunities. Small, well organized groups may articulate felt local needs, but they can sometimes effectively obstruct actions that may be necessary for a wider societal good.

Whatever the pros and cons, the parallel move to concentrate power at the supranational level and to decentralize at the local level seems to continue. In the United Kingdom, for example, Scotland and Wales are moving rapidly ahead to establish new representative bodies. The Italian Parliament recently devolved further rights to the regions. Poland and Sweden are regrouping subnational units into stronger regions. In the Russian Federation, as the federal level struggles to cope with a legacy of heavy legal and administrative problems, some of the federal units (republics, regions, territories and districts) seem to be filling the gap and taking their own initiative. It was reported, for example, that during the economic crisis in 1998, despite restrictive federal laws, some regions quickly put limits on the prices of food, gas and electricity and banned or limited food exports in order to protect their own populations *(38)*.

Even the concept of regions has itself become much more blurred *(39)*. The Council of Europe and the European Union have long worked with regions characterized as such, not necessarily because they are a subunit of a country but because they share similar geographical or physical characteristics, or because they have a particular main area of interest such as tourism. Moves towards both integration and decentralization have contributed to changing what is recognized as a "region", with important implications for decision-making, responsibility and accountability for health policy. Cross-border regions are proliferating. The German town of Herzogenrath and the town of Kerkrade in the Netherlands, for example, are integrating services such as the fire service as they gradually become the binational community of Eurode. The European Union is funding at least 17 cross-border regions in such places as the French–Italian Riviera, Copenhagen in Denmark and Malmö across the sea in Sweden, and even spilling beyond its borders in, for example, neighbouring regions of Albania, Bulgaria and Greece.

The number of networks of regions has been growing in recent years. Frequently, regions see themselves as "regions in Europe" just as much (and in some cases where there has been a struggle for greater political autonomy perhaps more) than they see themselves simply as a subdivision of a national entity.

There have long been strong reasons for border regions to work closely together to tackle problems of environmental pollution or to stop the spread of communicable diseases. The classification of regions in European Union countries according to their level of disadvantage and eligibility for priority funding also gives clear common interests that cut across national boundaries.

Technological developments

Much more attention will need to be paid by health policy-makers to the technological developments taking place throughout the world. Despite the fact that technology has been harnessed to cut out much of the physical strain of lifting heavy weights, for example, repetitive stress injuries are growing. Linked to the expanding information society are the increasing numbers of sufferers who spend long hours on the keyboard in front of a computer screen. A rough estimate of the total number of keyboards in daily use across Europe, and of the hours that today's infants might expect to spend at a keyboard and screen during their lifetime, might give an indication of trouble in store for the future.

Technological advances in health care

In 1998, an article referred to "the development of new technologies and ever larger amounts of information" as the first driver of change *(40)*. The article refers to some of the new technological developments that could become part of normal medical practice over the next 20 years (see Box 4.2).

The rate of technological advance in medical treatment offers tremendous opportunities but also threats. On the one hand, there have been tremendous improvements in the knowledge of diseases and how technology can assist their prevention and treatment. On the other, increasing demands for high-tech care may push up the health care budget and also raise considerations of equity. Some of the new drugs for treating HIV infection and AIDS, for example, are expensive and not everyone has equal access to them.

Box 4.2. Predictions on health technology

Year	Predicted development
2000	Artificial blood
	Full patient records on smart cards
2005	Personal wearable health monitors
	Determination of entire human DNA sequence
2010	Artificial heart
	Artificial sense
2012	Robots extensively used for routine hospital tasks
	Genetic links to all diseases identified
2015	Individual's genome part of medical record
	Artificial lungs
2016	Artificial brain cells
	Artificial liver
2020	Extension of human life span to 100 years

Technology can be expensive because of the initial cost of the equipment or because skilled staff are needed to use it. Technology assessment includes the evaluation of technical performance, clinical efficacy, safety, economic efficiency, organizational impact, social consequences and ethical implications *(41)*.

Genetics is another area of interest that offers high hopes of medical advances. Molecular genetics has greatly increased the understanding of diseases, such as cystic fibrosis, in which there is a single gene defect *(42)*. The human genome project should make the search for "disease" genes much quicker. Genetic technology also poses ethical challenges, the high hopes offered by early diagnosis being tempered by issues such as discrimination on the basis of genetic make-up.

There is also some concern that a preoccupation with technology should not erode public health research. This has been one of the debates raised in relation to the European Union's Fifth Framework Programme, with some pressure groups within the European Parliament advocating that the Programme adopt technological research as its main area for support. Public health groups maintain, however, that the health of populations depends less on technological "fixes" than on social determinants and individual choices, and that essentially a balance must be struck between the two *(43)*.

Information technology
The third millennium is already being heralded as the information age. In relation to health care, patients will have access to the same information as their doctors, and possibly even glean more information than

their doctors about rare conditions. But who, if anyone, will be validating this information? Although individuals will be able to access more information, it will be increasingly hard to know the reliability of that information and may mean that individuals in the end choose to go to trusted organizations that can provide them with validated information. Some are predicting a central role for the "informed consumer" in the future, whereby health care providers will be seen to progress from managing disease to promoting health and self-care on the basis of lifetime plans built on intimate and detailed knowledge of customers *(44)*.

Need for good governance

This brief indication of some of the main areas of concern in looking at general socioeconomic and political conditions leads to one conclusion in particular: the need for good governance. "Financial crises are really human crises. Politicians can no longer ignore the manifest urgency of building economic development in parallel with an environment of social and human justice" *(45)*.

There is an even stronger need than in the past to facilitate open discussion at all levels and to link international, national, regional and local attempts to develop health. The essential mechanisms and process are not yet in place, or are not yet working effectively at all levels or in all countries.

The European Union, with which about half the WHO Member States in the European Region are in some way linked, is beleaguered by a crisis of confidence that led the Parliament to create a committee of independent experts to report on alleged mismanagement, corruption and nepotism. The Court of Auditors found that some 5% of the US $93 billion annual budget had been carelessly or fraudulently spent, usually by member governments *(46)*. At the same time, however, the Union is forging ahead with the ambitious monetary union, and there is still the intention to enlarge the Union and to introduce the major structural reforms required by enlargement. This has been described by one writer as being a situation in which there is "no ringmaster, no efficient executive authority and no real democratic accountability. The most urgent decisions will be left, as always, to horse trading" *(47)*.

Even as there are problems at the supranational level, the national level is apparently weakening as power is ceded to the Union. At the same time, from below, the regions in countries are reassessing their own role in Europe. The Committee of the Regions appears to be playing an increasingly active though perhaps not yet clearly defined and recognized role. Individual regions and federations of local authorities obviously consider it to be worthwhile setting up their own links, and there are at present at least 160 regions with offices of representatives based in Brussels. The whole issue of ensuring a democratic dialogue and good governance in the expanding and changing European Union is creating a great deal of discussion.

Decentralization, privatization and a greater pluralism of partners have led to momentous changes in the role and responsibilities of the state. Correspondingly, the changing policy environment has opened new opportunities for other partners to influence the policy process. What is clear is that national policies must increasingly be drawn up in line with external, global or other supranational factors, while remaining in harmony with regional and local centres of power.

Living and working conditions – impact of policies in other sectors

In addition to taking into account the general socioeconomic and political conditions, Fig. 4.1 indicates that in developing policies for health we must be particularly concerned with the impact on health of policies in other sectors. As in the previous section, some of the issues that need much greater attention from health policy-makers in the future are indicated.

Breaking the cycle of poverty

This continues to be one of the greatest challenges to promoting and protecting health in the European Region. Poverty exacerbates the spread of disease but, equally importantly, the impact of ill health has the capacity to intensify poverty or push groups and societies below the poverty line. Research has created a better understanding of the contribution that good health makes to economic activity, and of the importance of enabling individuals to lead a socially and economic productive life. Poverty is linked not only to low income but to malnutrition, ill health, poor education, bad housing, chronic unemployment or underemployment, poor access to many legal, social and information services, and the inability to assert legal or political rights. Older people and children, and vulnerable minorities such as migrants and refugees, are most at risk.

The challenge is to break the cycle of poverty and safeguard the economic and social rights of future generations. Despite substantial efforts to create jobs in some countries poverty persists, partly due to unemployment, partly due to low-paying jobs and partly due to increasing financial difficulties faced by those on retirement pensions. Such inequities have been institutionalized in the distribution of land, capital, infrastructure and markets, as well as in the provision of services. It will take some radically new approaches if this situation is to be changed in the near future.

Problems are particularly serious for countries experiencing slow economic growth. In Europe, the most serious problems have been felt in the CCEE and some of the NIS. The World Bank's *World development report 1996 (32)* groups countries according to how quickly they have moved towards liberalization. Group 1 (Croatia, the Czech Republic, Hungary, Poland, Slovakia, Slovenia and the former Yugoslav Republic of Macedonia) is the fastest moving. Albania, Bulgaria, Estonia, Latvia, Lithuania and Romania form group 2, followed by Armenia, Georgia, Kazakhstan, Kyrgyzstan, the Republic of Moldova and the Russian Federation in group 3. The slowest is group 4, comprising Azerbaijan, Belarus, Tajikistan, Turkmenistan, Ukraine and Uzbekistan. Some countries' economies have been affected by war or economic blockades. The *World development report* suggests that what may be important is not so much the path countries choose to take towards liberalization of their economies – the "big bang" or the gradual approach – but the fact that change is decisive and consistent.

In the country profiles, information is given on the share of national income enjoyed by the richest and poorest population groups in countries. In the CCEE we are witnessing almost a "Latin-americanization" of the situation: in Brazil, for example, the richest 20% of the population earn more than 30 times that of the poorest, whereas in Switzerland and the United Kingdom this is about 10-fold. Such differences represent a real threat to social cohesiveness and solidarity. Social disintegration related to poverty and unemployment, and illustrated by an increase in harmful behaviour patterns such as the use of alcohol and drugs, violence and suicide, signals a failure of development.

Relating income policy and health

Countries rarely assess income policy in terms of its impact on health, despite the fact that evidence shows a very strong correlation between income and health. Health improves from the low- to medium- to high-income groups, until very high levels of income are reached at which point the correlation disappears on some of the measures used *(48)*. It also appears that a fall in the prevalence of relative poverty is related to a more rapid improvement in life expectancy *(49)*, but income policy tends to be assessed mainly in terms of its impact on the public budget or competitiveness, not in relation to its potential impact on health.

For a low-income family, an officially recommended healthy diet, for example, may cost 30% more than they can typically afford to spend *(50)*. A warm coat or the travel costs to go for health care may also be out of their reach. Relative prices strongly affect the way in which low-income families dispose of their income. In some countries, the adjustment from industry towards services has meant huge shifts in relative prices. In the Russian Federation the price of paid services relative to that of goods in the average consumer basket rose five-fold between 1990 and 1994 *(32)*.

It would be extremely difficult to tease out the health impact of income policies, but closely monitoring and reporting on the health of the lowest income groups would at least begin to shed new light on income policy and health.

Unemployment is a major cause of poverty, ill health and dysfunction

Youth unemployment in particular is a stark indicator of the failure of development, yet it is still unacceptably high and shows little sign of falling. This is particularly severe in certain local areas. In the European Union countries in 1995, for example, in the 10 worst affected regions, the average unemployment rate was 26.4% – nearly 7 times the average rate (just under 4%) in the 10 least affected regions. The *First cohesion report (51)* states that "even though a process of convergence between the member states is apparent, economic and social cohesion *within* most member states seems to have experienced a setback during the 1990s in the form of widening disparities in income and unemployment". In 1993, average GDP per head in the 10 richest regions was 3.3 times higher than in the 10 poorest regions. The average disparity in incomes per head in the European Union is twice that of comparable regions in the United States.

Economic growth alone does not always bring jobs. In most economies, for example, smaller companies generate job growth, not the larger firms. Particularly in local areas there may be a mismatch between job opportunities and the skills of local workers. In many countries women account for a disproportionate share in the unemployed. Particularly in central and eastern Europe, women seem to be affected by labour market discrimination, as evidenced by layoffs of women before men and open discrimination in job advertisements *(32)*. In certain areas, particularly where there has been a decline in heavy industry and a rise in the service sector, it is the men who have suffered disproportionally from unemployment, as their wives find work more easily and the men see their traditional roles reversed. The stress, isolation and low income of the unemployed, and particularly long-term and youth unemployment, represent a serious threat to health, yet it does not appear that this situation will be improved for a number of years to come.

Health at the workplace

Having a job does not ensure better health. There are also rising levels of stress caused by uncertainty in employment and the fear of unemployment. On the other hand, we have referred to the stress-related threat to health from overemployment in some groups. The uncontrolled working conditions in the so-called "black economy" also give rise to concern. The hours of unofficial activity in the economy in a sample of NIS, based on electricity consumption, was estimated in 1994 to be some 37% of the total *(32)*.

Other prerequisites for health

Globally, the countries that experience the least inequities, despite their level of economic growth, are those whose governments have invested in health, public spending on classrooms and textbooks, safe drinking-water and sanitation, nutrition and immunization programmes, and family planning.

Europe is extremely fortunate in the advances made in providing education and training for its population. The length of formal education has increased throughout the Region, and there is little indication that the trend towards expanding further education will change. Many countries are trying to provide the flexibility and choices that lifelong education allows for working-age and older people. Together with the improved skills this implies, comes the need for society to support young people for a longer period of time and also to give adults the possibility of leaving the workforce for extended periods of additional education or retraining. This, together with the increasing numbers of elderly people needing care and the persistently large numbers of unemployed people, puts a considerable burden of dependency on those who are working. The need for lifelong learning, for supporting those without a job, and caring for those in need of care is not disputed in societies governed by solidarity. The limited capacity to meet such needs will require some serious rethinking on how such essential services and care can be best provided.

The continued expansion of formal and informal education will create a better informed and demanding public. The information sector has made such tremendous technological advances in recent years that a whole new information and learning environment has been created. The information and ideas to fuel aspirations and to question the choices made by policy-makers are becoming ever more readily available to broader groups of people and to younger age groups. Kindergarten children now play on computers that were the domain of university students not too long ago. Access to information and know-how allows questioning of the "experts", changing the traditional pupil/teacher and patient/doctor relationships for those who have access to the information. Those without such access will find themselves at a disadvantage, and it should be remembered that in parts of the European Region, such as remote parts of the Russian Federation, some people do not have telephones or television, which are considered necessities in western Europe. On the other hand, goods and people are moving faster and further, bringing multi-ethnic cultures and foods, new ideas and new ways of behaving to societies that were much more homogenous just a few years ago. The challenge for the future is to improve the distribution of information and choice without creating unsustainable demands or relinquishing some of the habits of the past that were good for health. In most countries, the potential role of the health sector in such a societal discussion has yet to be explored.

For most of Europe, overall improvements in housing have been impressive, and life-threatening factors such as those related to communicable diseases have been largely removed. There are still, however, huge gains to be made in terms of reducing health hazards as reflected in accidents in the home, particularly for children and older people.

Large numbers of people in some parts of the Region have been made homeless through war and it will take years to repair this damage. In many CCEE, the cost of housing as a proportion of family income is rising, with a consequent reduction in income available for other purposes. Across Europe, as people congregate in urban areas, the needs of young children to play and experiment, of people who need quiet to rest or study, and of those who indulge in noisy forms of recreation come into conflict, creating considerable psychosocial health hazards.

Physical environment
Degradation of the environment is not only a European but a global issue. This was one of the clear messages of the 1987 Brundtland Report and nothing has happened since then to change its validity: one fifth of consumers use four fifths of the earth's resources *(52)*. Though consumption patterns may highlight deficiencies in societies' behaviour, they also indicate that the state of science and technology has not yet reached the level whereby it is easy to balance sustainability with the level of economic activity necessary to ensure what has come to be perceived in the west as an adequate quality of life, with its reliance on the use of cars and high-technology domestic appliances. Technological developments may affect these trends – more and cheaper microchips, for example, allow increasingly efficient use of energy – but there is obviously an opportunity for the health sector to present more convincingly the impact of the degradation of the environment on human health. This could contribute more forcefully to the discussion on a need for patterns of production that emphasize quality more than quantity, and for patterns of consumption that satisfy requirements of global responsibility to meet basic needs and contribute to a better quality of life, while minimizing the use of natural resources and toxic materials and the emission of wastes and pollutants.

In the CCEE and NIS, the expansion of traditional heavy industries, often using coal as the main source of energy, has had disastrous effects on the environment. Despite valiant efforts, this heavy legacy will take many years to deal with. The environmental liabilities created by haphazard disposal of wastes are mostly unknown, but could be large *(32)*. Some environmental damage, such as the destruction of the Aral Sea and pollution of the Black Sea, are extremely serious and pose long-term problems. In the NIS, contamination from nuclear waste is of particular concern, as are unsafe nuclear reactors. Bosnia and Herzegovina faces the problem of the safe destruction of tons of pharmaceuticals sent by some donor countries when their expiry date was due.

The agricultural sector still accounts for a considerable proportion of employment in parts of the Region. It also has a responsibility to conserve freshwater resources, protect the environment, preserve food safety and contribute to good nutrition *(11)*. About 30% of energy consumption in industrialized countries is attributable to the agriculture and food sector, and 90% of this is used for the transport, packaging and preparation of food. The pending accession to the European Union of countries with a comparatively large agricultural sector, the expected reform of the Common Agriculture Policy, public concern with the development of genetically modified agricultural products, and developments in the World Trade Organization all provide strong reasons for the health sector to take a strong stand on implications for nutrition and health.

During the preparatory discussions for the Third Ministerial Conference on Environment and Health, held in London in June 1999, there was a strongly felt need to tackle the effects of transport on the environment and health. Currently road accidents in the European Region result each year in 120 000 deaths and 2.5 million injuries, and one third of those who die are under 25 years of age. Increased reliance on private motorized transport is a major contributor to exposure to air pollution and noise. Major car manufacturers are attempting to develop more environmentally friendly cars, but the highways needed for even such green transport can cut across communities, limiting opportunities for social interaction. Fear of accidents is reported by parents as the main reason for taking children to school by car, a practice that limits the development of their independence and reduces the chances of their becoming habitual walkers or cyclists. On the other hand, those who do not have a car are frequently isolated from places of entertainment and cheap shopping outlets.

This is not an issue for the transport and health sectors alone. It relates to wider issues of land use and community development, to how far locally produced agricultural and other products, for example, are locally consumed and whether the transport of some goods could be avoided. It will take a much more comprehensive approach to health and development for such issues to be dealt with in the future.

Individual and community capacity for healthy behaviour
As the summary table of the results of our enquiry indicates (see Fig. 3.3), even where countries are implementing measures to promote health the balance is tilted towards health education measures. They seem to assume that if people simply know what is good for their health they can and will do it. Fig. 4.1 attempts to indicate that the capacity of individuals and communities to act in a way that is beneficial to health is very much determined by the overall socioeconomic climate, the conditions in which they live

and work, and their personal and community values. It is also governed by the support they receive from social networks and their capacity to develop and maintain relationships and to cope with the life events that affect their health.

Caring relationships and coping with stress

Both the structure and the distribution of populations are changing more quickly than in the past, affecting social networks and the capacity to cope. For example, the continuing urbanization and rural depopulization in some countries can go hand in hand with an erosion of traditional cultures, changes in family structure and breakdown in civic structure. In particular, the plight of older people in rural areas that is causing concern in some countries could become acute if present trends continue. On the other hand, cities can "provide excitement and variation and opportunities for extending experiences, breaking out of traditional moulds or meeting new people. They are also centres of learning, invention and innovation that benefit from cultural diversity" *(53)*.

In countries such as the Russian Federation, few can expect to live to enjoy their retirement, but for much of Europe the greying of the population is undoubtedly one of the triumphs of public health and the general improvement in the level of living. On the whole, the elderly today are more healthy than their peers of previous generations. With life expectancy nearing 80 years in some countries, many people will still have 20 or 30 years or more to live after their formal retirement from paid employment. It is doubtful whether society has changed sufficiently to take advantage of this increased potential, or to meet the needs of the greater numbers who reach the fourth age and are in need of extra care and support. Many societies are still geared to a situation wherein most people did not reach the age of 70, and there is ample evidence that our perception of aging debilitates and creates premature dependency *(54)*.

Changing patterns of social support

The form and structure of the basic human unit, the family or household, is also changing. It is more usual for people to marry more than once, with the various combinations of stepchildren, half siblings and "double" parents and grandparents that this brings. One-parent families are also more usual, with the lack of social support that this can entail. Women who have been the traditional carers of the young and old in the family are more likely to hold a job outside the home and be unavailable for this traditional role, or try to do it anyway on top of their other responsibilities, to the detriment of their own health. In the Nordic countries, for example *(55)*, the changing female role has entailed a shift for elderly parents from a relationship in which they were dependent on their children to one in which families complement publicly provided services, and this has apparently been welcomed. Even in countries where a move from such traditional family support is seen with less enthusiasm, the two-way support between grandparents and grandchildren and between children and parents may be less feasible in increasingly urban societies, particularly given that fewer people now stay all their lives in the place where they were born. In the European Union, the subsidiarity principle is likely to rule out the granting of any powers to the Commission with regard to the care of older people *(56)*; nevertheless, the resulting increase in exchange of information on examples of good practice may result in pressure for change from an increasingly vocal older population.

Eating, exercise and substance abuse
What one eats and drinks, whether one smokes or takes drugs, how much exercise one takes and whether one enjoys safe and satisfactory sexual behaviour are among the main risk factors for the main causes of death and disease. These are often termed the lifestyle issues. This gives the impression that the "lifestyle" followed is freely chosen, whereas a rapidly expanding body of research shows that this is frequently not the case. This is what Fig. 4.1 attempts to reflect by separating out the general socioeconomic conditions under which people live and the impact on their lives of policies in other sectors.

Eating habits are strongly influenced by experience in early childhood, so that some people start with an advantage. They are also strongly influenced by the level of disposable income; low-income parents report wanting to buy more fruit and vegetables for their children, or cutting down themselves on food to make sure other family members have enough *(57)*. One of the most frequent reasons for older people eating inadequate meals is ill-fitting dentures *(58)*.

Long working hours and the double burden of employment and caring for families reduce the time and inclination for exercise, as does the lack of safe places for walking and cycling.

Totally unprecedented social and economic changes in eastern Europe have placed tremendous stress on those populations. In countries such as Hungary, for example, statistics indicate increasing levels of smoking and drinking and higher rates of suicide and crime. "Society's answer … was to strengthen its traditional stress management strategy, resulting in greater withdrawal and self-inflicted harm" *(59)*.

New policies for health that facilitate community action and strengthen social networks will be needed to bring about the necessary changes in lifestyles.

Personal and community values
Values, culture, religion and spiritual wellbeing are not factors that have hitherto been given a high profile in countries in relation to health policy development. They do have a strong impact, however, on the capacity to cope and on the scope for action for health gain by individuals and communities.

Culture and religion
Among the most prominent aspects of culture and religion that impinge on health are those related to eating habits and to the expected role of men and women. These can affect directly such basic risk factors as nutritional status and reproductive health and indirectly such determinants of health as income and employment. Signatories to the 1994 Declaration on the Promotion of Patients' Rights in Europe resolved that "Everyone has the right to have his or her moral and cultural values and religious and philosophical convictions respected" *(60)*.

Multi-ethnic societies

Many countries in the Region have a long experience of being multi-ethnic societies. For others, recent movements of migrants and refugees have brought them face to face with the challenge of ensuring health for all without a shared culture or traditions or, in some cases, even a common language. "Women who follow working spouses to a foreign country may be among the most marginalized, particularly if the home culture discourages them from mixing with strangers" *(61)*.

Democracy and participation

It is not only democratic institutions that are important but also attitudes and traditions in relation to democratic behaviour and participation. In the Scandinavian countries, for example, people on the whole expect the right to participate in decision-making and tend to exercise that right. In a review of health policy development in Finland for example *(62)*, Finns were described as "joiners" and, as part of their tradition, it was felt that voluntary organizations would quickly move to meet new needs rather than waiting for the state to act.

This is not always the case in other parts of Europe. The legacy of the previous system in the CCEE has left its own particular problems – in some countries there are few people who have experience of the processes for running a democratic dialogue. In addition, unlike the post-war democracies of Finland, the Federal Republic of Germany and Italy or the southern European countries that emerged from military dictatorships in the 1970s (Greece, Portugal and Spain), the CCEE have to deal not only with political and constitutional challenges but a transfer of the ownership of production and the development of the market. There is no precedent for them to follow, and some feel that it is all too much.

Summarizing the challenges for the future

The pace of change seems to have gathered momentum in recent years. We cannot know the face of Europe five or ten years hence. From the brief discussion above, however, it appears that certain health challenges will still be important as we enter the 21st century. These are summarized in Box 4.3.

Is the health for all approach still valid?

In any policy-making process, the policy options would be theoretically endless in the absence of values and principles to define a workable policy framework. In most of the countries in the WHO European Region, aspirations are high but financial resources – and in some cases human resources – are either stable or decreasing. Some countries or some groups do not enjoy what are now considered to be acceptable standards of the prerequisites for health. Tough choices will have to be made as to how best to use and share available resources. The need for clear values and principles to provide an ethical framework for health policy development stands out particularly starkly, therefore, as we face the 21st century.

The WHO health for all policy provides clear principles that have been refined over the years. Fig. 4.2 shows how the health for all principles are interrelated, with equity acting as the fundamental and linking principle.

Box 4.3. Challenges for health policy development

Continued domination of the main causes of death
Assuming no new illnesses arise, the pattern of disease will be broadly as we know it now, requiring action in many sectors to tackle the underlying causes of morbidity and mortality.

Unequal chances
Large numbers of people will continue to be excluded owing to their lack of employment, income, education or health, unless measures are taken to enhance their capacities to cope and provide them with the necessary skills and opportunities to use their full potential. A sense of solidarity will need to be maintained.

Increasing demands and limited resources
The demand for goods and services will surpass sustainable production processes. There will consequently be a need to make critical choices and set priorities in order to use available resources more effectively. This will require a transparent and broad participatory approach to decision-making.

Conflicts of interests and a pluralism of partners
Certain actors, such as some multinational corporations, those with access to the means of mass communication or even small vociferous lobbying groups, may wield more power than is desirable in a healthy civic society. The state will need to play a strong role in orchestrating an open discussion, enforcing standards and protecting the vulnerable.

Societies in a state of flux
Societies in which some of the institutions and relationships that had hitherto seemed rather stable will be constantly shifting: relationships between national and local authorities, public services and amenities, employers, employees and workmates, and family members. The need will be for readiness for change rather than a readiness to fill a predefined role.

Information explosion
Seemingly boundless information will be available for some, improving their chance for informed participation, but leaving at a disadvantage those who cannot access this wealth of knowledge. There will be a strong need to access and utilize available information and to employ democratic systems to deter its misuse.

Technological and scientific advances
We shall no doubt be surprised by unexpected technological and scientific breakthroughs, which may have a positive or negative impact on health and the health services. The health sector will need to be vigilant in uncovering and dealing with the opportunities and threats to health.

New skills and ways of working
Intersectoral action, building and maintaining new partnerships for health and development, requires new skills and approaches. There is an urgent need for training and capacity-building for achieving consensus and managing change.

Fig. 4.2. The five interlocking principles of health for all

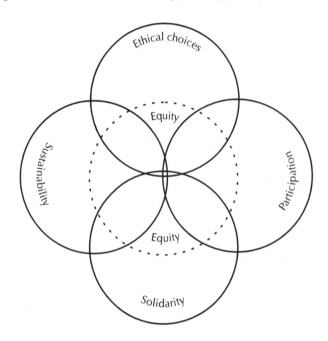

A definition of equity in health is given in Chapter 1. What it means in practical terms is ensuring a fair chance for all. The concept of fairness and justice is the thread drawing together the other four principles. As UNDP work has clearly shown, the gaps are to be closed by empowering the disadvantaged, by ensuring that they have access to and are supported to take advantage of the prerequisites for health (income, education, employment, housing, food, social support, health care, etc.).

Acceptance of the equity principle implies acceptance of the principle of solidarity. Solidarity assumes society's will to survive, and the expressed wish of all the people to assist the survival of some people. This is an ethical and human rights issue. It assumes that society is willing to shift resources to improve the lot of the disadvantaged, to empower them by specific actions to enhance their own capacity to reach their full potential, and at the same time to ensure that they are not hampered by conditions beyond their control.

The principle of sustainability is partly an extension of the equity principle, since it states that humanity should ensure that it "meets the needs of the present without compromising the ability of future generations to meet their own needs" (63).

The reiteration of the principle of participation, which is also defined in Chapter 1, is an issue of human rights, democratization and a well functioning civic society. The increasingly difficult ethical issues that will have to be faced demand an even stronger focus on achieving broad participation in decision-making. A health policy of the health for all type, which requires action in so many areas and on so many levels, can only be implemented with the involvement of those affected by it.

Since the other principles are in themselves issues of ethics, why include ethical choices separately? There are two main reasons:

- the intransigence of the problems related to the first three principles, and the apparent ease with which they are sometimes ignored when other more materialistic values come to the fore; and
- recent advances in science and technology that relate not only to issues of equity but are challenging even the concepts of death, parenthood and the very notion of what makes us human.

Highlighting ethical choices as a principle for health for all also allows room for considering the necessary balance between solidarity and individual rights, including the need to "respect … individual choice, personal autonomy and the avoidance of harm" *(10)* in guiding matters that influence health, including developments in science and technology and their application.

Strategic approach
As we look to the future, the basic strategic approach of health for all, described in a 1986 WHO report on intersectoral action for health *(64)*, remains intact. This states that the capacity of individuals to deal with health hazards such as smoking or obesity is less, and the obstacles to success are greater, when they also have to cope with problems such as poverty, poor education or unemployment. People in vulnerable groups are frequently faced with a combination of these obstacles, thus compounding their difficulties. Society must take action to deal with these issues, so that the individual will have a better chance to take effective action in the areas over which he or she has control. In the light of more recent research, community action would also need to deal with issues related to the strengthening of social networks and social cohesion.

Same dance, new steps
The steps of the past will not be sufficient to meet the challenges of the future. If Europe is to reduce the health gaps, their root causes must be dealt with in terms of ensuring that individuals have the personal capacities to improve and protect their own health and that of the communities in which they live; that they are not hindered by cultural, economic or structural obstacles; that a wide range of actors are made aware of the implications of their actions for health and that they feel responsible for this; and that there is a strong system of surveillance and reporting to ensure that all people and groups are enabled to participate in the process of health gain.

Many of the changes that need to be made take time and perseverance. "Muddling through" is not going to be a feasible option in this rapidly changing and closely interconnected world. The demands and pressures can be expected to be so great, and the means of expressing such demands increasingly available to large sections of the population, that there will be a need for a more transparent process of using available resources and know-how more effectively, and for a strong stand to protect and promote the rights of the vulnerable.

From the general conclusions in Chapter 3, there are some broad strategic implications.

- Countries will have to make an even stronger shift towards intersectoral action for health so that health is seen as an integral part of overall socioeconomic development.
- Much of the action must take place earlier, tackling the underlying determinants of health.
- It is no longer sufficient to try to put health on the agenda of other sectors; there must also be an attempt from the health sector to contribute to the achievement of objectives in other sectors, by looking for common or converging objectives.
- This means making new alliances and building new skills, including those required for presenting a more convincing health argument; creating awareness of health issues; reaching consensus and dealing with conflicts; assessing the health impact of social and economic policies; evaluating strategies and interventions; monitoring progress; and adapting to change.

This should result in investing for health where the greatest gains in public health and equity in health can be achieved. Although this is by no means an easy task, the case studies and country profiles in this study show that there are good practices in some countries that could provide examples for wider implementation. To paraphrase the 7-S management system, countries could make a shift in their thinking and approach through a "10-S system" for health for all (Box 4.4) *(65)*.

According to Kriegel & Brandt *(66)* "change is *un*comfortable, *un*predictable, and often seems *un*safe. It's fraught with *un*certainty and always looks harder than it is. 75% of American business leaders are not well prepared to manage change". We might ask what hope is there for the health sector, but what is certain is that time must be made for such a shift.

In many countries the present environment of downsizing and cost constraints, and the consequent stress and overwork for many, puts time at a premium. Good communication takes time, building trust takes time, understanding someone's feelings or point of view takes time. This is an essential element in building new partnerships. Many decision-makers have little time to listen and respond, or opportunity to clarify, restate and summarize. Many people have little time to think beyond dealing with the next crisis or getting through the next day. The health sector in particular and decision-makers in general have a heavy responsibility in providing the information and mechanisms to ensure that the ethical issues and critical decisions facing the health sector and its partners get the time they need.

WHO's functions in policy analysis and support to countries

Working with international partners
The equity principle has been strengthened in WHO's own policies for health for all at global and regional levels. A recent European Union communication on the development of public health policy highlights

Box 4.4. Thinking it through – the 10-S system for health in development

- **Socially acceptable** – advocate and facilitate consensus on the health for all values

- **Sensitive** – respond appropriately to differing needs, for example on gender issues and the needs of vulnerable groups, providing evidence to inform this discussion and ensuring that the voice of these groups is heard

- **Sustainable and feasible** – promote environmentally friendly solutions, tested to suit new patterns of living, working and caring for family members

- **Seamless** – press the case for an integrated approach to health and development, assessing the health impact of global, national and local policies, looking for both threats to and opportunities for health across sectors and boundaries

- **Smarter** – adapt quickly to technological advances, through flexibility in the face of rapid change while maintaining consistency of purpose

- **Simple not simplistic** – avoid expert terminology, speak the language of both those with the problems and those with the solutions, finding strategies and policy measures that are in line with felt needs

- **Scientific** – provide sound evidence, utilizing quantified and qualitative data and the best available experience to match problems and opportunities to the resources and solutions most likely to succeed

- **Selective** – in the complex health for all process, choose priorities on the basis of clear criteria and a democratic process, setting out a clear timetable, designation of responsibilities and means of arbitrating conflicts of interest

- **Skilful** – master the new competencies (consulting, negotiating and advocating for health) needed to sustain a health for all approach over time, and to work with new partners at the international, national, regional and local levels and with communities, groups and individuals; put in place mechanisms that facilitate the development of such partnerships and counteract possible financial, structural and cultural obstacles

- **Steadfast** – argue for equity, ethics, solidarity, participation and sustainability even in the teeth of opposition, and stick by those principles even in hard times

the need to address inequities in health and to assess the impact on health of policies in other sectors. International organizations such as the Council of Europe, the World Bank, UNICEF and UNDP are shifting the focus of their work to deal with the determinants of inequities in health. The widening health gaps both between and within countries are causing growing political concern, and some concern even in certain business circles. Finally, academics are renewing their interest in the scale and distribution and determinants of inequities in health. Although much more needs to be known, particularly about selecting the most effective interventions for the achievement of health gain, already there is sufficient knowledge to justify policy action.

The time appears to be ripe for WHO to play a more energetic role in the international arena, in advocating the health for all values of equity and solidarity in health, participation in making ethical choices and achieving sustainability in development. This entails raising awareness of the concepts and the implications for society if such values are not adhered to. It means being more active in efforts to improve research and information, and facilitating an international discussion on the validity and transferability of the results and of their implications for policy purposes.

Together with other international partners, a contribution could be made by:

- assessing the impact of socioeconomic policies (at international, national and local levels) and specific programmes and projects on equity in health;
- evaluating the effectiveness of interventions to promote equity in health;
- building stronger links to socioeconomic decision-making bodies such as:
  - IGOs, the European Union, the World Bank and the World Trade Organization
  - parliaments (international, national and regional) and city councils
  - ministries of finance
  - associations of entrepreneurs and trade unions
  - consumers (including focus on women as purse-holders of family income);
- improving the use of mass media and new information technology;
- encouraging the use of changes in health of low-income groups as an indicator of overall development; and
- supporting countries to make the policy shift that is essential for closing the gaps, including policy support linked to the preparation of candidate countries for entrance to the European Union.

Implications for the Regional Office and follow-up to the present study
This study was designed as a first step in a continuing analysis of policy development in Europe. It was also seen as a learning exercise, and a means of highlighting issues to be examined further in the future.

Clearly, it will also be necessary to evaluate the way in which the present study was carried out and to suggest improvements for similar activities in the future. It is already clear, however, that a number of issues need to be explored in more detail. The newly established European Centre for Health Policy, which is jointly funded by a number of European Member States and has the main part of its staff based in its Brussels office, will be able to play an active role in this work.

Information exchange

An important central role for WHO is to disseminate information, knowledge and experience as a "clearing house" on health policy development for the European Region's 51 Member States.

The present study was facilitated by initiating an *information base* on the process of policy development. This is one of the most important outputs of the whole effort, and already provides a valuable starting point for future work. The database will be developed further and much of the information will be available on a *web site*.

Case studies of the type included in this study are also a valuable source of information for policy-makers, whether they are embarking on a process of health policy development or reassessing their own efforts in the light of the experience of others. Why and how policies are developed is frequently information that lies only in the heads of those who were responsible for the process, and case studies are an effective way of preserving such information and presenting it for discussion and analysis. It is hoped that a regular health policy forum can be created to facilitate in-depth discussion of such country or regional case studies.

Regular *comparative studies* of health policy development and processes would also provide information in a format accessible to policy-makers.

Developing expertise and methods for health policy analysis

The role of the Regional Office in supporting health policy development must be underpinned by rigorous and credible expertise in health policy analysis at an international level. This is a comparatively new field, and the methodology for carrying out such policy analysis needs to be further developed. OECD has shown that regular analysis of economic, environmental and education policies can be extremely valuable for the countries under review, for the international experts who carry out the review process, and for the international community when the results are disseminated and discussed. The Regional Office is in a unique position to develop a similar service for health policy analysis. The planned health policy forum could provide a venue for the in-depth discussion of such reviews. Systematic work of this nature at the international level would contribute to the development of a strong network of experts with broad international experience.

Networking the networks

Europe is well endowed with strong research institutions and experts with very varied experience, many of whom are linked through networks and associations. With its experience and health mandate, the Regional Office is in a valuable position to act as a hub, linking up networks, institutions and people with interests in health policy development, analysis and assessment. The Office has two additional strengths in this respect: it covers 51 countries; and its long-term commitment ensures continuity to networks that are otherwise extremely sensitive to the availability of funding for their survival.

Direct policy support to countries

There is immense scope and demand for continuing support to countries in health policy development. This could include systematic reviews of national experiences, and advising on possible processes for health policy formulation, implementation, monitoring and evaluation. This would include sharing information on issues touched upon in this study such as:

- setting up effective structures and mechanisms for achieving consensus on the values and principles that underpin policies for health and development, and for the definition of objectives and priorities;
- examining the advantages and problems encountered in setting targets for health and the criteria, methodology and processes for target-setting;
- developing a democratic dialogue for health; for some countries this would entail a new way of working to create a realistic policy "vision", clarifying non-negotiable positions or values, possible trade-offs between sets of values, determination of criteria for priority-setting, and balancing conflicting and converging interests;
- reaching out for possible new alliances through consultation and negotiation in order to look for common and converging objectives (in non-health sectors and with new partners); reaching consensus on what to do about conflicting interests; setting standards by defining non-negotiable positions (and sticking to them); and supporting and enhancing the negotiation skills of weaker groups; and
- learning more about existing structures, strategies, mechanisms and incentives for intersectoral action, how these can be more effective in different policy environments, and how decision-makers in increasingly pluralistic societies can be engaged in such action over the longer term.

Broadening the range of policy tools considered

This might include providing examples of good practice in integrating health in national, regional and local development efforts, evaluating the effectiveness of policy interventions, and presenting possible policy options.

Mechanisms for monitoring and evaluation of policy outcomes

The work carried out for this study has shown this to be a relatively neglected area, as is that of setting up structures to monitor and evaluate progress in policy implementation, enhancing the necessary skills, sharing results, and revising policy on the basis of results.

Improving skills and capacities for health for all policy development

This has been one of the most neglected areas since the launch of the health for all policy in Europe. Much more needs to be learnt about the appropriate support mechanisms for education and training, by identifying places where effective support mechanisms are in place and why they seem to be effective.

Maintaining continuity and momentum
This has proven difficult for countries, particularly in times of political or social uncertainty or during periods of economic crisis. Areas of interest that might be explored would include the possible roles of parliamentary health committees, expert institutions and NGOs.

Opening a health dialogue with other sectors
It is high time to start a dialogue for health and development with other sectors on an international level. There is a need to discuss with key stakeholders in other sectors possible common or converging objectives, conflicting interests and how they might be dealt with, and whether certain principles and strategies for future collaboration could be agreed.

With health as its sole mandate, WHO is in a particularly favourable position to play a wider role in working with many other international organizations, both public and private, to bring such issues to public attention. The European Union also can be expected to turn much greater attention to this issue in relation to its own policies, as stated in Article 152 of the Treaty of Amsterdam.

Health impact assessment
Closely linked to the above is the need for the development of health impact assessment, using methods that are rigorous and credible but simple enough to be carried out on a regular basis, and processes that encourage and facilitate democratic participation. The United Kingdom for example, is developing a methodology for rapid health impact assessment of urban regeneration programmes *(67)*. The Minister of Health, Welfare and Sport in the Netherlands commissioned a report on this issue in order to "make a significant contribution to reinforcing the interests of public health in intra-departmental and inter-departmental policy deliberations and thus to the establishment of healthy cabinet policy" *(68)*. The Federation of Swedish County Councils is developing three types of health impact assessment, with varying levels of sophistication, depending on the issue to be assessed *(69)*. These and other examples will be reviewed by WHO's European Centre for Health Policy in an attempt to broaden the discussion and, through a process of consensus-building, testing and evaluation in the field, to provide some general guidelines for countries and regions in Europe.

Development of learning and information packs
Much of the available information related to the issues addressed in this section is at present not in an easily accessible and usable form for groups such as key decision-makers, educators or the general public. There is a need to build on information created in the academic field through the involvement of lay people and democratic processes, and to present this in innovative ways, including support and where necessary training on how to use it.

Development of models to coordinate health and health services policies
In only a few cases are health care reforms, health care policies and other public policies found within overall policies for health. The study had shown that in many countries, even when there is experience of

broad health policy development, this frequently runs parallel to and separate from developments in health care.

Evaluation of the settings approach
Many countries have started to use a settings approach, the most common settings being the family, school and work environment and, more recently, universities, kindergartens, night clubs and prisons. An exploration of these various examples could throw light on which settings or mix of settings appear most effective for which target groups, and how similar work might be encouraged in other settings.

In all these areas of concern, the emphasis must be on evaluating and sharing experiences so that countries can benefit by building on the successes and learning from the failures of their peers. In many cases general principles and guidelines can be developed for countries to adapt to their own needs. WHO networks such as the Regions for Health Network or Healthy Cities could be involved as testing grounds. Equally important will be the growing portfolio of examples and experiences that can be shared, and the informal networks through which policy-makers across Europe can consult and advise each other.

References

1. WOOD-RITSATAKIS, A. *Unified social planning in the Greek context*. Athens, Centre for Planning and Economic Research, 1986 (Studies 23).
2. LISK, F. Conventional development strategies and basic-needs fulfilment. *International labour review,* **115**: 175–191 (1977).
3. *Preliminary report of a unified approach to development and planning*. Geneva, United Nations Research Institute for Social Development, 1972 (document 72/C.66).
4. *Measuring social wellbeing*. Paris, Organisation for Economic Co-operation and Development, 1976.
5. *International Development Strategy. Action programme of the General Assembly for the Second United Nations Development Decade*. New York, United Nations, 1970.
6. *Targets for health for all. Targets in support of the European regional strategy for health for all*. Copenhagen, WHO Regional Office for Europe, 1985 (European Health for All Series, No. 1).
7. *Health for all targets. The health policy for Europe*. Copenhagen, WHO Regional Office for Europe, 1993 (European Health for All Series, No. 4).
8. *European Health Policy Conference: opportunities for the future. Report on a WHO Conference*. Copenhagen, WHO Regional Office for Europe, 1996 (document EUR/ICP/HFAP 94 01/CN01).
9. *The Ljubljana Charter on Reforming Health Care*. Copenhagen, WHO Regional Office for Europe, 1996 (document EUR/ICP/CARE 9401/CN01).
10. *Health for all in the twenty-first century*. Geneva, World Health Organization, 1998 (document A51/5).
11. *HEALTH21: the health for all policy framework for the WHO European Region*. Copenhagen, WHO Regional Office for Europe, 1999 (European Health for All Series, No. 6).

12. *Communication from the Commission to the Council, the European Parliament, the Economic and Social Committee and the Committee of the Regions on the development of public health policy in the European Community.* Brussels, Commission of the European Communities, 1998 (document COM(98)230 final).

13. Horn, R.V. Social indicators: meaning, methods and applications. *International journal of social economics,* **7**: 421–460 (1980).

14. Myrdal, G. *Asian drama – an inquiry into the poverty of nations.* London, Allen Lane Penguin Press, 1963.

15. *Social reports: their contribution to integrated development planning. Vol.1. Report of seminar, Saint-Pierre, Italy, April 1976.* New York, United Nations, 1976.

16. World Bank. *World development report 1993: investing in health.* New York, Oxford University press, 1993.

17. *World health report 1995. Bridging the gaps.* Geneva, World Health Organization, 1995.

18. United Nations Development Programme. *Human development report 1997.* New York, Oxford University Press, 1997.

19. Wilkinson, R. G. *Unhealthy societies: the afflictions of inequality.* New York, Routledge, 1996.

20. *Health in social development. WHO position paper, World Summit for Social Development, Copenhagen, March 1995.* Geneva, World Health Organization, 1995 (document WHO/DGH/95.1).

21. European Union. *Employment and social policy.* (http://europa.eu.int/pol/socio/info_en.htm) (accessed 25 October 1999).

22. Stringfellow, R. Partners in health. *TARGET,* No. 28, p. 22 (1998).

23. *Report of the United Nations Conference on Environment and Development, Rio de Janeiro, 3–14 June 1992.* New York, United Nations, 1992 (document A/Conf. 151/26 (Vol. 1)).

24. *International Conference on Nutrition. Final report of the Conference, Rome, December 1992.* Geneva, World Health Organization, 1992 (document).

25. *A comparative analysis of the situation regarding nutrition policies in WHO European Member States.* Copenhagen, WHO Regional Office for Europe, 1998 (document EUR/ICP/LVNG 01 02 01(A)).

26. Nuffield Institute for Health, University of Leeds; Welsh Institute for Health and Social Care, University of Glamorgan; & London School of Hygiene and Tropical Medicine. *The health of the nation – a policy assessed. Two reports commissioned for the department of health from the Universities of Leeds and Glamorgan and the London School of Hygiene and Tropical Medicine.* London, Stationery Office, 1998.

27. Glyn, A. & Miliband, D., ed. *Paying for inequality: the costs of social injustice.* London, Rivers Oram Press, 1994.

28. Winsemius, P. Intersectoral negotiation. *In:* Taket, A.R., ed. *Making partners: intersectoral action for health. Proceedings and outcome of a joint working group on intersectoral action for health, Utrecht, Netherlands, 30 November – 2 December 1988.* The Hague, Ministry of Welfare, Health and Cultural Affairs, 1990.

29. Fisher, R. & Ury, W. *Getting to yes: negotiating agreement without giving in.* London, Arrow Books, 1986.

30. METCALFE, L. International policy coordination and public management reform. *International review of administrative sciences*, **60**: 271–290 (1996).
31. *Building policy coherence: tools and tensions.* Paris, Organisation for Economic Co-operation and Development, 1996 (Public Management Occasional Paper No. 12).
32. WORLD BANK. *World development report 1996: from plan to market.* New York, Oxford University press, 1996.
33. *Constitution of the World Health Organization.* Geneva, World Health Organization, 1985.
34. ACHESON, D. *Independent inquiry into inequalities in health.* London, Stationery Office, 1998.
35. Economics and social cohesion. *Time*, 15 February 1999, p. 46.
36. CHANDLER, G. The new corporate challenge. *Time*, 1 February 1999, p. 64.
37. DEACON, B. *Towards a socially responsible globalization: international actors and discourses.* Helsinki, STAKES, 1998 (GASPP Occasional Papers, No. 1/1999).
38. ZARAKHOVICH, Y. A clash of Kremlins. *Time*, 14 December 1998, p. 19.
39. *The process of health policy development. Report of a working group on the development of subnational policies for health.* Copenhagen, WHO Regional Office for Europe, 1992 (document EUR/ICP/HSC 418).
40. SMITH, R. Imagining futures for the NHS. *British medical journal*, **317**: 3–4 (1998).
41. ABEL-SMITH B. ET AL. *Choices in health policy: an agenda for the European Union.* Aldershot, Dartmouth, 1995.
42. SAVILL, J. Science, medicine, and the future: Molecular genetic approaches to understanding disease. *British medical journal*, **314**: 126 (1997).
43. SARACCI, R. ET AL. Europe's health research: getting the right balance. *British medical journal*, **316**: 795 (1998).
44. SMITH, R. The future of healthcare systems. *British medical journal*, **314**: 1495 (1997).
45. KIM DAE JUNG & WOLFENSOHN, J. D. Economic growth requires good governance. *International Herald Tribune*, 26 February 1999.
46. GRAFF, J. L. Big buildup to a Euro letdown. *Time*, 25 January 1999, p. 19.
47. DAVIES, N. Wandering borders. *Time*, Winter 1998–1999, p. 32.
48. BLAXTER, M. *Health and lifestyles.* London, Tavistock/Routledge, 1990.
49. WILKINSON, R. Income distribution and life expectancy. *British medical journal,* **304**: 165–168 (1991).
50. COLE-HAMILTON, I. & LANG, T. *Tightening belts: a report on the impact of poverty on food.* London, London Food Commission, 1986.
51. *First cohesion report.* Brussels, European Commission, 1996.
52. *Caring for the future. Report of the Independent Commission on Population and Quality of Life.* New York, Oxford University Press, 1996.
53. *City planning for health and sustainable development.* Copenhagen, WHO Regional Office for Europe, 1997 (European Sustainable Development and Health Series, No. 2; document EUR/ICP/POLC 06 03 05(B)).
54. CHUPRA, D. *Ageless body, timeless mind. A practical alternative to growing old.* New York, Harmony Books, 1993.

55. WAERNESS, K. The "welfare mix" of social care for the elderly: a Nordic perspective. *In:* Harrington, P. & Ritsatakis, A., ed. *European Health Policy Conference: opportunities for the future. Vol. II. Intersectoral action for health.* Copenhagen, WHO Regional Office for Europe, 1995 (document EUR/ICP/HFAP 94 01/CN01(II)).

56. WALKER, A. The social care of older people in the European Union – deconstructing dependency in old age. *In:* Harrington, P. & Ritsatakis, A., ed. *European Health Policy Conference: opportunities for the future. Vol. II. Intersectoral action for health.* Copenhagen, WHO Regional Office for Europe, 1995 (document EUR/ICP/HFAP 94 01/CN01(II)).

57. WHITEHEAD, M. Counting the human costs: opportunities for and barriers to promoting health. *In: Economic change, social welfare and health in Europe.* Copenhagen, WHO Regional Office for Europe, 1994 (WHO Regional Publications, European Series, No. 54), p. 69.

58. *The art of aging – a contribution to the technical discussions on healthy aging.* Copenhagen, WHO Regional Office for Europe, 1990 (document).

59. MAKARA, P. The effect of social changes on the population's way of life and health: a Hungarian case study. *In: Economic change, social welfare and health in Europe.* Copenhagen, WHO Regional Office for Europe, 1994 (WHO Regional Publications, European Series, No. 54), p. 93.

60. WORLD HEALTH ORGANIZATION. *Promotion of the rights of patients in Europe.* The Hague, Kluwer Academic Publishers, 1995.

61. BRANDRUP-LUKANOW, A. The forgotten women of western Europe. *Entre nous,* No. 38, 1998, p. 3.

62. *Health for all policy in Finland – WHO health policy review.* Copenhagen, WHO Regional Office for Europe, 1991 (document EUR/FIN/HSC 410).

63. WORLD COMMISSION ON ENVIRONMENT AND DEVELOPMENT. *Our common future.* Oxford, Oxford University Press, 1987.

64. *Intersectoral action for health. The role of intersectoral cooperation in national strategies for Health for All. Background document for the Technical Discussions, Thirty-ninth World Health Assembly, May 1986.* Geneva, World Health Organization, 1986 (document A39/Technical Discussions/1).

65. SILBERGER, S. *The 10-day MBA: a step-by step guide to mastering the skills taught in top business schools.* New York, Piaticus, 1993.

66. KRIEGEL, R. & BRANDT, D. *Sacred cows make the best burgers. Developing change-ready people and organizations.* New York, Warner Books, 1996.

67. SCOTT-SAMUEL, A. ET AL. *The Merseyside guidelines for health impact assessment.* Liverpool, Merseyside Health Impact Assessment Steering Group, University of Liverpool, 1998.

68. PUTTERS, K. *Health impact screening: rational models in their administrative context.* Rijswijk, Ministry of Health, Welfare and Sport, 1997.

69. *Focusing on health. How can the health impact of policy decisions be assessed?* Stockholm, Federation of Swedish County Councils, 1998.

Annex

Country profiles

Albania

Demography, policy environment and health care system

Albania is located in the Balkan peninsula, neighbouring the Federal Republic of Yugoslavia to the north, the former Yugoslav Republic of Macedonia to the east, the Adriatic and Ionian Seas to the west and Greece to the south. Since general elections in March 1991, Albania has been governed by a package of constitutional provisions that declared the Republic of Albania as a sovereign and democratic state. Albania is divided into 36 districts and 315 communes.

In 1995 the population was 3.2 million. The average population density is 110 per km^2 (1994); 37% of the population live in urban areas (1993); 6% of the population is aged ≥ 65 years and 34% aged 0–14 years (1994); and the dependency ratio is 60% (1993).

In 1995 the mean income per person was US $700. The inflation rate is 22.6% (1994) and the unemployment rate 13% (1995).

The infant mortality rate was 32.9 per 1000 live births in 1995; the average life expectancy at birth in 1994 was 72.1 years.

Private practice and private insurance have been legalized and the Health Insurance Institute was launched in 1995. Most pharmacies and dentists have been privatized, and health service financing and delivery are being reorganized substantially.

Approach towards achieving health for all

A major process of economic reform was instituted in 1992, and from 1993 there were signs of economic recovery led by the agricultural sector. The main objective of health care reform is to develop an outcome-oriented system based on health insurance. Health care reform is part of the overall process of social and economic reform. Plans to develop an overall health policy are being undertaken in two stages, beginning with the development of a health care policy and building to a more comprehensive policy covering lifestyles and environmental issues. In 1997, the Government planned to assess the capacity of the existing infrastructure and institutions to develop and implement health promotion policies.

Two information documents, on situation analysis and on policy options and implementation issues, have been formulated in support of the effort to improve health services. The second phase of the policy development process is on hold because the political situation is unstable.

Focus on health outcomes and reorientation towards primary health care

Traditionally, a high proportion of health care in Albania has been provided in primary health care, and preventive services have been widely accessible. There were, however, a number of shortcomings, including: low motivation of physicians, lack of a family physician approach and failure to respect the gatekeeping function; insufficient freedom of choice for patients; inadequate public health and community orientation; and lack of intersectoral coordination. Early in 1997, primary health care services were disrupted further and are now the most poorly serviced area of the health care sector. Much of the equipment used in primary health care has been stolen, and primary health centres have sometimes been occupied by squatters, especially those in remote areas.

To address these issues, a document on primary health care policy was elaborated in a participatory process involving the staff of the Ministry of Health and Environmental Protection, the Medical Faculty of the University of Tirana and the Institute of Public Health, with the assistance of the EU Phare Programme. The main objectives of this consensus document include: renovation of primary health care centres and a rapid needs assessment in primary health care; training the people who will train general practitioners and nurses; initiatives on infant and maternal mortality, nutrition and perinatal mortality; and reducing the number of hospital beds. As a result, a number of rural hospitals have already been closed.

The Institute of Statistics collects demographic, mortality, social and lifestyle data and economic indicators in Albania using a centralized system. The system makes data collection relatively easy, but there is poor feedback to the local level and information is not linked to management and monitoring processes. Modern information technology and national information experts are severely lacking because of the country's previous long isolation. Steps are now being taken to upgrade the information system and encourage it to be used better for orienting health care decisions.

Promotion of equity, public participation and intersectoral action

Equity
In contrast to the situation in a number of the countries of central and eastern Europe, life expectancy has continued to improve in Albania, mainly because of better nutrition and past investment in education of girls and women. Immunization rates are high and infant mortality has fallen dramatically since the 1960s, although it is still well above the European regional health for all target. Equity of access to health care services is expected to be improved, mainly through the renewed primary health care centres. Other targets that should improve equity are:

- to increase the coverage of preventive services by 20% (from 60% to 80%) for rural areas and by 5% (from 95% to 100%) for urban areas by 2005;
- to reduce infant mortality to 25 per 1000 live births and maternal mortality to 0.25 per 1000 live births;

- to increase the percentage of households with access to safe water by about 20% (from 65% to 85%) for rural areas and by 3% (from 97% to 100%) for urban areas; and
- to reduce malnutrition and undernutrition to less than 10% of children under 5 years of age by 2000.

Education is another determinant of health. The mean number of years of schooling in Albania compares well with international standards. During the present transition, however, enrolment in secondary school has declined; a lack of resources to repair schools, pay teachers' salaries and develop new curricula has meant that standards of education are falling. Remittances from emigrants, mainly to Greece and Italy, have become an important source of income. Approximately one quarter of the work force has found work in other countries, and most are sending back money to their families. This money and money earned through other business ventures abroad may approach a sum representing 25% of GDP, but there is also concern that many villages in eastern and southern Albania have few working-age men and women.

The official rates of unemployment are high, but hidden unemployment figures are of more concern, especially in some cities with unofficial unemployment rates of 80%. The Government is under pressure to reduce the costs of the social safety net while continuing to meet the needs of the most vulnerable groups. Elderly people have fared especially poorly from attempts to keep the budget deficit under control; the factor saving many from even worse socioeconomic conditions is that many elderly people live with their children.

Rapid change has brought paradoxical situations of incongruous living conditions, with some families, for example, enjoying a colour television but no running water. There are signs that the changing family structure and new roles for women are leading to conflicts within the family and to rising levels of family violence.

Public participation
Albania is implementing democratic institutions and moving towards a market-based economic system, and an active civic society that supports individual freedom within limits is developing. One of the most important recent laws has been the Bill of Human Rights, which guarantees human rights and fundamental freedoms. The number of privately and legally recognized associations and voluntary organizations has increased. Special support has been given to nongovernmental organizations related to youth and women's affairs, which are some of the most active; they deal with, for example, creating jobs for women; family planning; collecting and analysing data related to divorce; and family violence. Surveys currently indicate that people are more oriented towards nongovernmental organizations than towards political parties, but membership is still very limited and tends to be more in urban areas. The mass media have been a powerful means of disseminating information and involving people in policy issues including those related to health.

Intersectoral action
Housing is in short supply and often in severe disrepair; about 4% of the population are homeless. Privatization of about 230 000 state-owned dwellings and construction of new flats has somewhat

improved the situation, but further initiatives are needed. Water supplies are often inadequate and infrequent, which creates particular stress for women, who traditionally collect water if the home does not have running water or water is only available for a few hours each day. Poor sanitation and waste disposal are also a problem. Nevertheless, the capacity to generate hydroelectric power means that 98% of Albanians have electricity in their homes.

Other environmental challenges include deforestation, soil erosion, air and water pollution and loss of biodiversity. As of 1994, the industry perceived to be causing the most pollution was the oil and gas industry. The virtual lack of treatment of municipal waste poses a serious problem. Dumping of untreated sewage constitutes a major health challenge, polluting groundwater needed for drinking-water or beaches intended for recreation and tourism. Environmental legislation in line with European standards is gradually being put in place. Nevertheless, other challenges such as unemployment that are considered more pressing are taking precedence over environmental problems. Albania lacks a functional system for monitoring air pollution, although one is being planned. One result of the failure to control pollution has been the rise in the prevalence of occupational diseases. More research is being undertaken on the nature and causes of occupational health risks, and legislation is in process to protect workers in the work environment.

Transport and communication are especially poor because investment has been limited. Only 5% of total investment was devoted to these sectors; the next lowest level of investment in any other formerly socialist country in central or eastern Europe was 15%. The number of telephones has increased seven times since 1989, which has implications for everything from business dealings to medical emergencies. Until the communist regime collapsed, Albania had no privately owned cars. Car ownership rose from 2.1 vehicles per 100 inhabitants in 1990 to 12.7 per 100 in 1993, which has led to a dramatic increase in the number of road accidents.

Environmental education and increased public awareness have played a key role both in the workplace and in the general living environment in changing people's behaviour. New nongovernmental organizations have been crucial to this process, organizing scientific activities such as symposia and conferences and producing the first environmental newsletter with the assistance of the Ministry of Education and the Committee for the Protection of the Environment.

The law on privatization of agricultural property provided for the dissolution of cooperatives and equal distribution of land to village members. Today, a unique egalitarian rural economy exists, although those in close proximity to rural markets enjoy more than twice the income of those in remote areas. After the transition, farmers were producing mainly for their own consumption; by 1995, many were producing for urban markets. Nevertheless, only one or two people can be supported on the smallholdings, with the result that many young people have had to migrate to the city, leading to high levels of urban unemployment.

Andorra

Demography, policy environment and health care system

Andorra lies in one of the high lands in the central Pyrenees, between France and Spain. The territory, 468 km^2, ranges in altitude from 838 to 2942 metres above sea level. It has a border with France of 56.6 km to the north and east at an average altitude of 2500 m. To the east, south and west the border with Spain is 63.7 km at an average altitude of 2200 m. Andorra has been a sovereign constitutional principality since 1993. There are seven parishes with an elected local government (*Comú*) with substantial powers. The General Council of the Valleys (Parliament) has 28 members.

In 1996 the population was 64 000. The average population density is 138 per km^2 (1996); 96% of the population live in urban areas (1996); 11% of the population is aged ≥ 65 years and 15% aged 0–14 years (1996); and the dependency ratio is 42%.

In 1995 the mean income per person was US $18 100.

The infant mortality rate was 2.9 per 1000 live births in 1996; the average life expectancy at birth in 1996 was 80.1 years for males and 83.5 years for females.

In 1994 total health expenditure was 5% of estimated GDP.

The health care system is based on social security, which covers about 85% of the population, and health care services are provided and financed by both private and public actors. The Government formulates policies for health, influencing the social security system, health care professionals and institutions and the public. By law all residents are entitled to health services, at government expense if they are unable to pay.

Approach towards achieving health for all

The General Health Act passed in 1989 considers the determinants of health and focuses on health. A health plan for 1990–1991 was based on the needs determined by more than 70 local experts and other participants and formulated 18 strategic targets based on the framework of the WHO European strategy for health for all. Current work includes evaluation and preparing a new plan. National health surveys (1991 and 1997) and other specific surveys on satisfaction by both consumers and professionals are used to plan services.

Focus on health outcomes and reorientation towards primary health care

The Department of Health has contracted the development of guidelines for five clinical conditions with the college of general practitioners. Common software is being adopted and used to manage patient records by a group of selected general practitioners, including the use of minimum basic common data. The package of services delivered by community health centres, especially home services, is being extended.

Promotion of equity, public participation and intersectoral action

Equity
Public funding ensures access to services for all residents who are not covered by social security and are unable to pay. Special arrangements apply to groups such as handicapped people, people with HIV infection or AIDS, and people serving prison sentences.

Public participation
The public has substantial choice and freedom within the system of health care services. Participation through specific channels (such as patient or consumer associations) is still unusual.

Intersectoral action
The Department of Health works with other sectors and groups such as:

- the Department of Education concerning health and nutrition in schools and the training of nurses;
- the Department of the Environment concerning air and water quality and noise pollution;
- the Department of Finance in obtaining and using adequate funds;
- the Home Department regarding safety in some public places and health in prisons;
- the Department of Foreign Affairs concerning international relations in health;
- the Department of Public Works regarding building and maintaining health facilities;
- the Department of Agriculture concerning health and hygiene in abattoirs;
- the Department of Industry regarding radiological safety control;
- the Department of Trade concerning healthy settings (hotels, restaurants, etc.); and
- the seven local governments regarding the quality of water supplies and health centres in their parishes.

Armenia

Demography, policy environment and health care system

Armenia is bordered by Georgia to the north, Azerbaijan to the east, Turkey to the west and Iran to the South. Armenia gained full independence in December 1991. The parliament is a National Assembly with 190 members, and the country is divided into 11 administrative districts.

In 1996 the population was 3.8 million. The average population density is 127 per km^2 (1996); 67% of the population live in urban areas (1996); 8% of the population is aged ≥ 65 years and 27% aged 0–14 years (1996); and the dependency ratio is 58%.

In 1994 the mean income per person was US $680. The inflation rate is 2000% (1995) and the unemployment rate 27% (1993).

The infant mortality rate was 15.5 per 1000 live births in 1996; the average life expectancy at birth in 1996 was 72.9 years.

Total health expenditure in 1991 accounted for 5% of GDP.

Armenia was previously one of more economically stable regions of the former USSR. The transition to a market economy had a destabilizing effect. A severe earthquake in 1988 left over 25 000 people dead and 500 000 homeless; this coupled with an influx of over 300 000 refugees from Azerbaijan has exacerbated the problem of migrants and refugees.

Approach towards achieving health for all

Armenia does not yet have an overall policy for health for all, but embarking on a process of radical social and economic development has emphasized broad-reaching policies for health care.

Focus on health outcomes and reorientation towards primary health care

One of the top priorities since independence has been the restructuring of the health care system. The National Programme on Reform Development in the Health System for 1996 includes:

- improving management of the health care system through decentralization;
- reforming the financing of the health care system and introducing health insurance;

- reforming the system of evaluation;
- regulating the privatization process in health care and in other sectors;
- improving the system of education for the health care workforce; and
- licensing procedures.

The possibility of introducing privatized health care has been discussed, and fees for services such as private rooms and private consultations with physicians have been incorporated in the new bill for health care reform. There are plans to strengthen primary health care and to introduce a general practice system, which will mean retraining physicians as general practitioners. The World Bank is supporting moves towards primary health care and public health initiatives as an integral part of overall development.

Recent laws include one on medical aid and services to the population (1996), and one on epidemiological safety of the population (1992). Both bills were disseminated for consultation, revised based on the comments received and approved by the National Assembly. They provide a legislative basis for people's right to health and government responsibility for providing health services. Specific programmes have been initiated in primary health care, licensing of medical institutions and health care providers, tuberculosis control and control of sexually transmitted diseases. A national action plan for nursing has also been developed.

Focus on health outcomes and reorientation towards primary health care

Health outcome orientation is still a relatively new concept for Armenia, and routinely collected health statistics and other health information are not yet sufficiently used for policy-making purposes. An Information Committee has therefore been set up and a monitoring system established in the Ministry of Health. The development of standards, licensing procedures and guidelines for health professionals are also being emphasized.

Promotion of equity, public participation and intersectoral action

Equity
The laws on health services and epidemiological safety provide for equal access to available health care according to need, and the right to safe living and working conditions. Additional measures to promote equity in health include:

- a research programme to determine the access to health care among groups with low socioeconomic status;
- health education programmes aimed at vulnerable groups, including programmes to encourage breastfeeding and education programmes on sexual health and tobacco consumption;
- subsidies for high-risk groups in maternal and child health, sexually transmitted diseases and cancer;
- measures to sensitize health professionals working with children and elderly people to the needs of those in lower socioeconomic groups;

- monitoring the impact of ongoing reforms and programmes for the general population and for certain target groups, including the development of a set of health indicators to monitor progress; and
- plans to establish a basic benefits package and to develop protocols for treatment of conditions covered under the basic package.

Public participation

Armenia declared its independence after large public demonstrations and strikes. The high level of public participation in these events may account for the relatively stable situation in recent years. Efforts to further democracy include the establishment of a multi-party state, the creation of a working parliament, establishment of trade unions, promotion of nongovernmental organizations and the passing of two laws on human rights. The law on medical aid and services ensures patients' right to participate in health care decisions; the law was published in the main newspapers as a draft and in final form, so that people would be informed of that right. Surveys to determine the views of health care providers and patients are being developed.

Intersectoral action

Lack of resources has caused the existing welfare system to collapse. The country has been immersed in a long-term energy crisis, and living standards have fallen dramatically. Nevertheless, the Ministry of Health works together with a number of other ministries, mainly on lifestyles, the environment and occupational health. There are severe environmental problems: 60% of the land is eroded and mining is responsible for large tracts of polluted land. Water resources are scarce, and industrial pollution is still a problem in urban areas. Research is being carried out on the development of a national environmental health action plan. A board consisting of representatives from the Ministries of Health and of the Environment has been established to evaluate the results of this research.

Together with the Ministry of Education, a number of campaigns have been organized to reduce the rates of sexually transmitted diseases and AIDS and to reduce tobacco and alcohol consumption. Duties are charged on imported tobacco and alcohol, and pilot studies are being conducted on smoking habits and behaviour.

Austria

Demography, policy environment and health care system

Austria is situated in southern central Europe, bordered by the Czech Republic and Germany to the north, Hungary and Slovakia to the east, Italy and Slovenia to the south and Liechtenstein and Switzerland to the west. Austria is a federation of nine federal states (*Länder*) on the basis of a parliamentary democracy. The head of the Austrian State is the federal president elected directly by popular vote. The Government is headed by the federal Chancellor. The main legislative bodies of the Republic are the *Nationalrat* (National Council) and the *Bundesrat* (Federal Council), the two houses of the Austrian Parliament. Each of the nine federal states is administered by its own government.

In 1995 the population was 8 million. The average population density is 96 per km^2 (1995); 56% of the population live in urban areas (1994); 15% of the population is aged $\geq$ 65 years and 18% aged 0–14 years (1994); and the dependency ratio is 48% (1994).

In 1994 the mean income per person was US \$24 950. The inflation rate is 2.2% (1995) and the unemployment rate 4.6% (1995).

The infant mortality rate was 5.4 per 1000 live births in 1995. The average life expectancy at birth is 73.7 years for men (1994) and 80.2 years for women (1996).

In 1995 total health care expenditure accounted for 9.6% of GDP.

The securing of health is a public task in Austria. Various ministries of the federation, federal states and municipalities, as well as the social security institutions as self-administrated public corporations, assume important responsibilities in public health. This legal fragmentation leads to a highly complex structure that creates considerable challenges in coming to consensus, especially in financing. The health care system is primarily financed by social insurance, which covers 59% of health expenditure; the regional public authorities pay about 18% and the private funding share is about 23%.

Approach towards achieving health for all

The federal Government is responsible for legislation, formulating health policy and general directives, technical supervision of health services and training and supervising the health insurance system, which is managed autonomously. The federal state authorities, assisted by health advisory councils, are responsible for carrying out directives and implementing laws and policies. Health officers at the federal state and district levels supervise the carrying out of national and federal state measures in the districts and the municipalities.

Focus on health outcomes and reorientation towards primary health care

Recent and planned reforms mainly relate to changes in hospital structure (especially financing), the development of integrated systems of outpatient medical care, nursing, social services and support, broader health promotion activities and preventive services, and the development of strategies for quality assurance and of quality standards at federal level for both infrastructure and treatment. A new model of hospital financing has already been introduced that provides the nine federal states with individual budgets and autonomy in the financial management of their hospitals. The service-oriented hospital financing system reimburses hospitals according to the diagnosis made rather than number of days of care. The remuneration of all providers in the health care sector is to be made transparent and consistent with the services rendered.

Access to primary health care facilities is guaranteed for the entire population, since everyone is protected by health insurance. Since 1991, the establishment of mobile services has been further extended and the financial security of those who need care assured. Further, preparatory steps have been taken towards coordinating and integrating the various health and social facilities by creating small health and social welfare districts. Virtually 100% of the population can reach primary health care facilities within one hour.

Promotion of equity, public participation and intersectoral action

Some of the characteristics already inherent in the Austrian health care system have helped to facilitate implementation of the principles of health for all.

Equity
More than 99% of the Austrian population are covered by a compulsory social security system and therefore have access to the facilities of the health care system. Considerable progress has been made towards enhancing equal opportunities through reforms to national insurance legislation. In 1991, psychotherapy was recognized as a service reimbursed by health insurance, and financing of preventive medicine and health promotion have become mandatory for the social insurance funds. In 1993, a preventive nursing scheme was introduced with the aim of granting people who need permanent care a statutory claim to nursing benefits. The amount of these payments depends on the degree of the handicap or the extent of the nursing needs.

Public participation
As with most pluralistic health care systems, the decision-making power is not predominantly concentrated in the hands of one person, group or institution. Policy decisions are generally the result of negotiation among various interest groups.

Decentralization of the health care system ensures health care adapted to the population's needs. Decentralized structures and administration in several sectors also means that decision-making within the health care system is widely dispersed. The individual social insurance funds, for instance, administer themselves and are coordinated by a central institution, the Main Association of the Austrian Social Insurance Institutions. The individual subgroups or carriers are formed by the federal states, professional groups or individual enterprises. Nongovernmental institutions are involved in the work of health authorities. Self-help groups also participate in providing health care.

Intersectoral action

In 1992, a Health Promotion Unit was created at the Ministry of Health, and the Austrian Healthy Cities Network was established. In 1993, Austria joined the European Network of Health Promoting Schools, and a WHO Collaborating Centre for Health Promoting Hospitals was established. University institutes contribute through health promotion research and interdisciplinary training in health promotion for health personnel and other professions.

There is no centralized decision-making or implementation of health promotion activities, basically because of the federal structure of Austria. The Minister of Health has launched a few nationwide programmes in AIDS, drugs and smoking. The Health Promotion Unit has become a focal point for the development of health promotion in specific settings (such as schools, workplaces and hospitals) and the Foundation Healthy Austria coordinates specific programmes (for example, on nutrition or physical activity).

The elaboration of fundamental principles for an environmental health information system has been the most important step in ensuring environmental health in Austria. The objective of the system is to compile at the smallest possible scale data on health status, provision of health care and socioeconomic and environmental conditions and to use this material as the basis for planning and political decision-making.

Important recent legislation includes the Tobacco Act (1995), the Act on Genetic Engineering (1996), the Act on New Hospital Financing System (1996), the Medical Devices Act (1996) and the Narcotic Substances Act (1997). A new Health and Nursing Care Act is pending.

Bodies at various levels (national, state, district and municipality) participate in health activities and closely cooperate in this field. Numerous nongovernmental organizations also play a part in providing health care, carrying out their activities in virtually all areas of the health care services.

Azerbaijan

Demography, policy environment and health care system

Azerbaijan is located on the western coast of the Caspian Sea, between the Islamic Republic of Iran and the Russian Federation, and has been an independent republic since August 1991. The political system is based on parliamentary democracy and strong presidential rule. There are 65 administrative districts (*rayons*). In addition to the districts, three cities have separate administrations: Baku, Ganja and Sumgayit.

Unfortunately, Azerbaijan continues to be in a state of undeclared war. Many people have been killed, and the disruption of former trade routes has contributed to a severe shortage of essential goods and supplies. There are acute shortages of vaccines, pharmaceuticals and medical equipment, and a large proportion are being provided through humanitarian assistance.

In 1994 the population was 7.4 million. The average population density is 84 per km^2 (1993); 55% of the population live in urban areas (1993); 5% of the population is aged $\geq$ 65 years and 33% aged 0–14 years (1993); and the dependency ratio is 61% (1993).

In 1995 the mean income per person was US $498. The inflation rate is 1780% (1994) and the unemployment rate 1% (1993).

The infant mortality rate is 26.9 per 1000 live births (1994) and the life expectancy at birth 67.9 years (1994).

In 1993 health care expenditure comprised 2.8% of GDP.

The health care system has deteriorated in Azerbaijan in the post-Soviet period because of the war and a lack of funding due to economic collapse. The organization of services has not changed significantly and still follows the traditional Soviet model. There is no private health insurance in Azerbaijan.

Approach towards achieving health for all

Azerbaijan has not yet developed an overall policy for health. A number of programmes are in operation that have been drawn up according to the principles of health for all.

Focus on health outcomes and reorientation towards primary health care

As in other former Soviet systems, there is no tradition of integrated primary health care. The current approach is medically oriented, based on the traditional model of sanitary-epidemiological services that prevailed in the former Soviet Union. The sanitary-epidemiological services are responsible for environmental health services and immunization coverage. Measures such as screening, family planning and health promotion have not yet been introduced.

One of the main priorities is to prevent communicable diseases such as diphtheria, tuberculosis and poliomyelitis. As a basis for future action, in 1994 the Ministry of Health together with UNICEF initiated a survey on health care demand, attitudes towards paid health care and health care expenditure in the Kuba district. The survey revealed that many current practices (particularly the excess capacity in hospitals) were not cost-effective or sustainable. There was also a high degree of inequity as most services require fees, putting the most vulnerable groups at risk. The Kuba project is an attempt to reform the health care system while retaining the best elements of the previous Soviet system, such as wide coverage of the population. If this is successful, it will be expanded to other regions of Azerbaijan. The project aims to promote:

- a shift from inpatient to outpatient care and merging of specialized services with the central hospital system;
- sharing of costs between the state and municipalities; and
- community involvement through the establishment of health councils consisting of influential individuals in the town, health committees in every health centre catchment area (this includes several villages) and district health advisory boards.

In 1995, the Ministry of Health established a steering committee at ministerial level to address issues of policy development, and an implementation committee at district level. The implementation committee has prepared plans to reorganize the district health care system. In 1996, the Minister for Health issued a decree stating plans for reform of the health care system. The main priorities include control of communicable diseases (tuberculosis and diphtheria control and poliomyelitis eradication). The Government will soon explore the options for reform in detail.

Promotion of equity, public participation and intersectoral action

Since plans are only at an initial stage of development, action is still being considered.

Equity
The vulnerable population will be exempted from a system of introducing fees for drugs.

Public participation
In Azerbaijan, there is not yet any tradition of community involvement in public services.

Intersectoral action

There are plans to develop a national policy for health reforms with the participation of various ministries (health, finance and social protection) under the auspices of the Prime Minister.

Belarus

Demography, policy environment and health care system

Belarus is bordered by Poland to the west, Latvia and Lithuania to the north, the Russian Federation to the east and Ukraine to the south. Belarus is an independent state. Parliament consists of two chambers: the Chamber of Representatives with 110 seats and the Council of the Republic with 64 seats. The country is divided into 6 regions (*oblasts*), 118 districts (*rayons*) and 1452 communities (towns, villages and settlements).

In 1995 the population was 10.3 million. The average population density is 50 per km^2 (1995); 69% of the population live in urban areas (1995); and 13% of the population is aged $\geq$ 65 years and 22% aged 0–14 years.

In 1995 the unemployment rate was 3%.

The infant mortality rate was 13.3 per 1000 live births in 1995. The average life expectancy at birth is 68.6 years (1995).

The central and regional governments have the leading role in planning and administering the health sector; the public sector provides facilities for health services. Private services are almost nonexistent.

Approach towards achieving health for all

A concept was prepared on the development of the health care system in Belarus. The short and long-term priorities were defined as:

- addressing the consequences of the Chernobyl accident, with special emphasis on thyroid cancer;
- maternal and child health, including a family planning component with the special aim of reducing infant mortality and strengthening training in neonatology;
- control of communicable diseases (target diseases of the Expanded Programme on Immunization, control of diarrhoeal diseases, tuberculosis and sexually transmitted diseases);
- drug policy development;
- reforms in the health care system (family physicians, privatization and training in public health, including training of nurses); and
- a countrywide integrated noncommunicable diseases intervention (CINDI) project, including an oral health component.

Other areas of concern were cardiovascular diseases, AIDS, diabetes and substance abuse.

Poor socioeconomic conditions have led to a marked deterioration in health status, with life expectancy, especially among men, declining to seriously low levels. The situation of communicable diseases, including tuberculosis and diphtheria, is also worrying, as are the consequences of the Chernobyl incident: about 22% of the population was directly exposed to radioactive contamination. The incidence of thyroid cancer per 10 000 population was 6.0 in 1995 and 6.3 in 1996.

Focus on health outcomes and reorientation towards primary health care

Belarus has a comparatively large number of medical institutions (both inpatient and outpatient), hospital beds and medical staff. Primary health care is given at polyclinics (both for adults and for children), at rural physicians' outpatient clinics and in hospitals. The system of general practitioners is being developed through postgraduate training in primary health care.

It is planned to try and eliminate some of the excessive specialization in health care and to introduce a system whereby physicians' salaries are linked to performance. Diversifying the services provided by the polyclinics, developing home nursing and primary health care training for nurses, and introducing a family physician system are some of the initiatives planned to facilitate the reorientation towards primary health care. A shift to a health care system based on health insurance is also being explored, as is increased decentralization.

The WHO CINDI programme aims to ensure that appropriate data on noncommunicable diseases are collected and used for policy purposes.

Promotion of equity, public participation and intersectoral action

Equity
The Law on Health Care, enacted by Parliament in 1993, proclaims the rights of all citizens to adequate medical care. According to the Law, funding of health care should comprise no less than 10% of GDP, but poor socioeconomic conditions prevent this. The economic crisis has resulted in sharply declining living standards. More than two thirds of the population live below the poverty line. In contrast to some countries in central and eastern Europe where pensioners fare poorly economically, pensions are indexed in Belarus. Families with dependants, people with low income and unemployed people are therefore the most vulnerable groups. Social assistance beneficiaries receive only minimal payments (in 1995 only 10% of the average income).

State support for socially vulnerable groups somewhat mitigates the effects of falling real incomes. Expenditure on health care as a proportion of GDP has remained high, although it has fallen in real terms with the decline in the GDP. Some of the subsidies previously available under the Soviet system, such as those for housing, electrical power and transport, are gradually being phased out. The salaries of public employees have been reduced, causing a brain drain, with the most promising professionals seeking employment outside the health, education and science sectors.

Public participation

Prior to the end of the Soviet Union, Belarus was one of the most economically and socially well-off republics. Rapid industrial and agricultural growth therefore required suitably qualified people to work in these sectors, and Belarus therefore developed a highly efficient educational sector. This scientific and intellectual capacity has been an important factor in establishing a participatory process.

A sound regional policy is important for health and sustainable development. A law on local administration and self-rule delegates to local administrations the responsibility for development in their respective areas, including health and environmental management. Nevertheless, responsibility needs to be decentralized along with the reform of the central government. Steps to involve the wider public include the formation of organizations of cooperatives and entrepreneurs, along with free and independent trade unions, foundations, associations and mass media.

Intersectoral action

Industrial activity has caused extensive damage to the natural environment. Large cities are becoming sources of continuous pollution, which is a serious challenge to people's health. About one quarter of the national territory is contaminated by radioactive fallout from the 1986 Chernobyl accident. In addition, intensive development of the chemical and petrochemical industries is producing vast quantities of hazardous waste. Environmental research is conducted by the scientific research institutes of the Ministry of Health, institutes for training of physicians, centres of hygiene and epidemiology, and health care institutions.

Substance abuse has been increasing, although the rapid rise in the price of alcoholic beverages from 1995 has curbed drinking somewhat. Other projects aimed at promoting healthier lifestyles have been introduced under the WHO countrywide integrated noncommunicable diseases intervention (CINDI) programme in the areas of nutrition, breastfeeding, smoke-free cities and physical activity. In 1996, an anti-smoking competition "Quit and Win" was held in Minsk, and the Ministry of Health and the Committee on Science and Technologies passed legislation for work to begin on the formation of a state scientific technical programme on preventing noncommunicable diseases.

Belgium

Demography, policy environment and health care system

Belgium is bordered by the Netherlands to the north, the North Sea to the north-west, France to the west and south, and Germany and Luxembourg to the east. In May 1993, Belgium became a federal state, composed of communities and regions. There are three regions based on language: Flemish, French and German. Since 1995, the federal Parliament has consisted of a Chamber of Representatives with 150 members.

In 1994 the population was 10.1 million. The average population density is 325 per km^2 (1993); 97% of the population live in urban areas (1994); 15% of the population is aged ≥ 65 years and 27% aged 0–14 years (1994); and the dependency ratio is 50% (1993).

In 1996 the mean income per person was US $26 100. The inflation rate is 2% (1996) and the unemployment rate 14% (1996).

The infant mortality rate is 8.5 per 1000 live births (1995) and the average life expectancy at birth 77 years (1992).

In 1995 the total health expenditure was 8% of estimated GDP.

The Belgian health care system is financed mainly by social insurance with a mix of public and private providers.

Approach towards achieving health for all

Given the federal nature of the country, health for all is not enshrined in an overall health policy in Belgium, but its principles are applied in practice. Public health policies take as their starting point WHO's definition that health is not only the absence of disease and infirmity, but a state of complete physical and mental wellbeing.

Focus on health outcomes and reorientation towards primary health care

At the national level, the Ministry of Social Affairs, Public Health and Environment is responsible for sickness insurance, hospitals, legislation, personnel training, health-related standards and international relations.

Responsibility for certain issues lies at the community and regional levels: for example, the provision of health care to the population, the management of social services, care of elderly people, health education and home care, as well as the aspects of environmental health not dealt with by central government.

The provinces and municipalities also have certain powers, notably in regard to sanitation and certain local services.

Priorities in the French Community include AIDS, drug abuse, elderly people, mental illness, immigrants and the disadvantaged.

The Flemish Community has developed a comprehensive health promotion and prevention strategy based on the following premises: coordination of local and regional initiatives; increasing intersectoral collaboration; ensuring adequate resources for specific preventive actions; and surveillance of trends in data related to public health. The latter is considered especially important to ascertain the health status of the population, as well as the quality of the health care system and of the care delivered and what future needs might be.

Promotion of equity, public participation and intersectoral action

Equity
Geographical access to health care poses little or no problem in Belgium. The country is highly urbanized and services are widely available. Almost the entire population is covered by an insurance system operated by the National Institute of Sickness and Disability Insurance. National welfare organizations may take responsibility for meeting the needs of certain groups such as elderly and disabled people. Less is known about equity in health status.

Public participation
The size of the private sector, the community-based arrangements, the influence of professional groups and the dominant role of the sickness insurance system all mean that the Belgian health system is a complex entity, making public participation in heath planning and programming difficult. Nevertheless, a policy of regionalization and community-based government facilitates decentralized decision-making. The distribution of power at the federal level, between health and other sectors and between the national government and the communities and regions, means that health policies are determined through a process of consultation and negotiation with all actors, including patients.

It is mainly at the local level that the population is involved in running the health system, although there are democratic mechanisms to ensure representation at the community and national levels. Numerous councils (in particular parents' and patients' councils) allow various groups to express their views and participate in health care decisions. Professional groups and other nongovernmental organizations are also involved.

Belgium is currently drafting a Patients' Rights Charter in accordance with the Council of Europe recommendations. These rights include:

* access to health care facilities;
* the right to know the name of the health care provider;
* respect for human dignity;
* the right to refuse medical treatment;
* the right to be informed exactly of one's state of health;
* the right to be informed fully of the risks involved in any given treatment or diagnosis; and
* the right to be informed of the overall costs and the personal contribution to the medical treatment costs.

Intersectoral action

At the local level, the use of a settings approach, emphasizing the contribution of such environments as homes, schools, workplaces and cities, promotes intersectoral action. These are some of the newer initiatives, but not all intersectoral policies are new. For example, for many years there have been joint planning programmes between health and social services on care for elderly people. Problems related to smoking, alcoholism, nutrition and the social reintegration of disabled and elderly people are high on the list of priorities.

Various financial and legislative measures that aim to promote environmental health have been initiated:

* substantial reductions in train fares (ranging from 20% to 60% to encourage people to use public transport instead of their private cars) during the summer months;
* tighter enforcement of speed limits, as speeding tends to increase levels of harmful gases in the atmosphere; and
* banning of all tobacco advertisements except on sales outlets from May 1997.

Bosnia and Herzegovina

Demography, policy environment and health care system

Bosnia and Herzegovina is located in the middle of the Balkan peninsula bordering Croatia in the north, west and south and the Federal Republic of Yugoslavia in the east and south. In 1992 Bosnia and Herzegovina was recognized as an independent country. Bosnia and Herzegovina has two entities, the Federation of Bosnia and Herzegovina (of which Sarajevo is the capital) and the Republic of Srpska (of which Pale is the capital). Sarajevo is the capital of the state of Bosnia and Herzegovina. Administration of health issues is delegated to the entity level, and the Federation of Bosnia and Herzegovina and the Republic of Srpska thus have separate ministries of health.

In 1996 the population was 3.7 million. The average population density is 89 per km^2 (1993); 62% of the population live in urban areas (1991); and 7% of the population is aged $\geq$ 65 years and 27% aged 0–14 years (1991).

In 1996 the mean income per person was US $890 (Federation of Bosnia and Herzegovina). The unemployment rate is 13.5% (Federation of Bosnia and Herzegovina, 1996).

The infant mortality rate is 13.6 per 1000 live births (Federation of Bosnia and Herzegovina, 1996) and the average life expectancy at birth 73 years for males (1995).

By the end of the 1980s Bosnia and Herzegovina had a well developed health system. In 1990 the total health expenditure was about 6.5% of estimated GDP and about US $245 per person. A four-year war, however, had serious repercussions for health status and led to widespread destruction of health and social services. Funds for health care were insufficient and the percentage of GDP spent on health care declined to 1.25%.

Bulgaria

Demography, policy environment and health care system

Bulgaria is bordered by Romania to the north, the Black Sea to the east, Greece and Turkey to the south and, to the west, the former Yugoslav Republic of Macedonia and the Federal Republic of Yugoslavia. The Bulgarian Parliament consists of a National Assembly with 240 members. A new constitution was adopted in July 1991, defining citizens' rights, including the right to health care, and providing fundamental changes in the role and function of government institutions. The country is divided into 9 regions composed of 278 districts.

In 1993 the population was 8.4 million. The average population density is 76 per km^2; 70% of the population live in urban areas (1994); 15% of the population is aged $\geq$ 65 years and 18% aged 0–14 years (1994); and the dependency ratio is 50%. Aging, particularly of the rural population, is of major concern.

In 1994 the mean income per person was US $1250; inflation hit a record high of 310% in 1996. The unemployment rate is 12% (1994); the lowest 10% of the population have a 3.3% share of income or consumption while the highest 10% have a 25% share (1994).

In 1994 the infant mortality rate was 15.5 per 1000 live births and average life expectancy at birth 71.1 years.

In 1994 the total health expenditure was 5% of estimated GDP.

All public medical services are free of charge, and private medical services were made legal in January 1991.

Approach towards achieving health for all

Efforts have been directed towards avoiding financial collapse and interruption in the delivery of health care activities, and towards formulating an overall health policy with clear priorities. The Bulgarian health strategy was drawn up in 1995, and a national plan of action for implementing of the strategy is currently being developed.

A modern telecommunications system for emergency health care is being developed with resources from the EU and the World Bank.

Legislation has been drafted for the establishment and organization of a health insurance fund. Further work is needed regarding changes in the tax system and public evaluation of health risk.

Focus on health outcomes and reorientation towards primary health care

A separate strategy aimed at reorienting services towards primary health care has been developed. Major changes are planned in outpatient and hospital care, which have been traditionally oriented towards treatment rather than prevention, in order to reduce the level of inappropriate specialized treatment.

Research is still being conducted on the reorganization and management of the health care system and possible new approaches to primary health care. To facilitate a shift to primary health care:

- a training programme for general practitioners is to be carried out in collaboration with the Bulgarian Medical Association, and there is to be free choice of general practitioners and paediatricians;
- preventive services will be introduced in schools, health services provided in the workplace and primary health care services expanded in rural areas;
- certain resources will be transferred from hospitals to nursing homes, hospices and day care; and
- services will be free of charge in polyclinics, consulting rooms and rural health centres.

Promotion of equity, public participation and intersectoral action

Equity
The social determinants of risk behaviour (such as tobacco smoking, alcohol consumption and sexual behaviour) in adolescence are being surveyed. Researchers are also examining the demographic and psychosocial characteristics of individuals who avoid screening programmes or have an unusually high or low level of contact with health services. Particular attention is being given to monitoring the situation of children living in difficult circumstances. In practical terms an intersectoral approach has been adopted to deal with inequity; the Ministry of Health has worked together with the Ministry of Social Affairs to organize direct food aid to vulnerable groups such as elderly and unemployed people, pregnant women, newborn babies and infants. The Ministry of Health is also working with the Ministry of Education, Science and Technologies and the Ministry of Labour and Social Affairs to regulate organizations and bodies that deal specifically with children in accordance with the United Nations Convention on the Rights of the Child.

Financial measures to promote equity include:

- partial reimbursement of the costs of medicines for certain population groups;
- financial allowances for children of preschool age, to ensure adequate nutrition; and
- provision of aid by municipalities to low-income elderly people requiring permanent medication or a special diet.

These programmes have not yet had the desired effect owing to a combination of unrealistic goals, inadequate financing and poor coordination.

Courses in medical ethics and health management are also being initiated for health personnel.

Public participation
In contrast to the previous policy document from 1987, *Bulgaria's road to health for all*, which was not disseminated for consultation or discussed in Parliament, the 1995 strategy *Health for the nation* was put out for consultation to a wide range of partners including state institutions, political bodies, the mass media and nongovernmental organizations. Surveys to determine the public awareness of health risks and perceptions of health services are planned.

Practical measures to promote public participation include:

- the use of settings such as schools, working environments and families to engage people in health issues (a number of schools are members of the European Network of Health Promoting Schools);
- consultation with community councils to democratize decision-making by actively involving workers and the wider community in the development of local health service plans; the family is being promoted as a new source of support;
- establishment of public coalitions for health involving representation from health services, schools, nongovernmental organizations, trade unions and local administrations in all regions; and
- promulgation of laws on patients' rights.

Intersectoral action
Research is being conducted on the relationship between disease, lifestyles and ecological and biological factors. Efforts to promote healthier lifestyles include:

- facilitating smoking cessation groups and using the mass media to spread the message to stop smoking;
- educating children on the dangers of tobacco and alcohol consumption, using a tone that informs rather than moralizes;
- providing information and training on the safe preparation of food, stressing the importance of food labelling; and
- using settings to promote an intersectoral approach and targeting certain groups such as woman and young people in relation to promoting healthy lifestyles and reproductive health.

The national plan of action reflects a wide intersectoral approach, and the Ministry of Social Affairs, Agriculture and Food Industry, the Ministry of the Environment, the Ministry of Education and Technology and others were involved in developing the plan, as were nongovernmental organizations (a project on palliative care is being developed in cooperation with charities and nongovernmental organizations) and insurance bodies (the National Insurance Institute).

Structures to strengthen intersectoral cooperation at the national level are being developed, including:

- an interdepartmental commission to combat drug abuse and trafficking;
- an interdepartmental commission on environment protection; and
- interdepartmental working groups for healthy schools and healthy hospitals.

Regional health centres have also been established. They include consultation bodies consisting of representatives from local municipalities, professional organizations, trade unions and health professions. The regional health centres have been assigned specific responsibilities but, due to financial problems and pressure from professional organizations and trade unions not to take certain decisions, they have not yet proved to be effective.

Croatia

Demography, policy environment and health care system

Croatia is bordered by Hungary and Slovenia to the north and by Bosnia and Herzegovina and by the Federal Republic of Yugoslavia to the east. A new constitution and a multi-party system were adopted in December 1990. The Croatian Parliament (*Sabor*) consists of 127 members. The country is divided into 21 counties (*zupanija*), 121 towns and 414 municipalities, all administered by elected councils.

In 1994 the population was 4.7 million. The average population density is 84 per km^2 (1993); 54% of the population live in urban areas (1993); and 12% of the population is aged $\geq$ 65 years and 20% aged 0–14 years (1994).

In 1996 the mean income per person was US $4300, the inflation rate 3.9% and the unemployment rate 12%.

In 1995 the infant mortality rate was 8.9 per 1000 live births and life expectancy at birth 73 years.

In 1994 health care expenditure comprised 7.5% of GDP.

Following the recent war, Croatia must rebuild its health and social systems, construct new water supply and wastewater drainage systems, and deal with refugees and those suffering from post-traumatic stress disorder.

Approach towards achieving health for all

In 1996 Croatia formulated an overall policy for health, entitled the Republic of Croatia policy and strategy for health for all by the year 2005. An implementation plan is being prepared for discussion in Parliament.

Focus on health outcomes and reorientation towards primary health care

The strategy focuses on the following key areas:

*   revitalization of primary health care and emergency, perinatal and intensive care services;
*   development of management information systems;
*   rehabilitation of war victims;

- health promotion and disease prevention; and
- environment and health.

The big push in restructuring health services is towards primary health care, with efforts being made to train physicians in general practice and family medicine.

Quantified targets have been set as a means of monitoring progress in areas ranging from perinatal mortality to adequate housing. Resources are also to be allocated for health systems research and for developing measures of effectiveness.

Promotion of equity, public participation and intersectoral action

Equity
According to the constitution, everyone living in Croatia is entitled to basic health care. In 1993 an insurance-based system was adopted, which, together with the many health facilities destroyed during the war, partly explains the proportionally higher expenditure (as a percentage of GDP) on health care than in other countries in central and eastern Europe that are still making this transition. Under the new system, financial responsibility was shifted from local authorities to the National Health Insurance Fund. This is a form of regulated market competition, and the state continues its lead role in supervising the delivery of health care to certain vulnerable groups, pregnant women, children up to 15 years, elderly people and the disabled. Special measures have been taken to support disadvantaged groups. Victims of war are especially vulnerable. Information is being collected on the extent of inequity.

Public participation
Measures to promote participation include informing the public, in order to foster understanding and cooperation in health-related matters; and the use of international standards such as the European Charter on Patient's Rights.

Intersectoral action
The Ministry of Health took the lead role in preparing the new overall health policy and in assuring legal provisions for its implementation. Further cooperation planned with other sectors and groups to implement the strategy includes:

- engaging the education sector and mass media in disseminating information and promoting healthy lifestyles;
- creating healthy work environments in cooperation with workers, employers and trade unions;
- using such settings as cities, schools and hospitals to promote health;
- occupational rehabilitation for those disabled by war: teams of professionals work together with victims both in rehabilitation centres and in their own homes, and funding is arranged from health insurance funds, pension funds and disability insurance funds;

- in collaboration with the food industry, introducing a programme of food enrichment and measures to reduce levels of salt and saturated fats in foods;
- legislation on cigarette advertising, smoke-free environments and a special tax for preventing disease;
- monitoring and evaluation of environmental health risks;
- establishment of the National Council on Environment and Health to strengthen interdepartmental cooperation on environmental and health issues;
- consolidation of various types of food legislation with that of the EU, FAO and WHO, including labelling of food products in accordance with EU regulations;
- food contaminant surveillance to assess health risks;
- establishment of a national centre for occupational health and register of occupational diseases, and analysis of jobs with special working conditions arising from new technologies;
- economic assistance to reconstruct housing and other facilities destroyed by war;
- surveys on causes of home accidents;
- participation of the health and environmental sectors in decisions about urban planning;
- in cooperation with the Association of Croatian War Veterans, development of a proposal for a project on multisectoral interventions in the treatment and prevention of post-traumatic stress disorder.

Czech Republic

Demography, policy environment and health care system

The Czech Republic is bordered by Germany to the west, Poland to the north, Slovakia to the east and Austria to the south. The 1993 constitution provides for a bicameral parliament, although an upper house (the senate) has not yet been elected. The Czech Republic has 80 municipalities (districts).

In 1996 the population was 10.3 million. The average population density is 131 per km^2; 65% of the population live in urban areas (1994); 13% of the population are aged $\geq$ 65 years and 18% aged 0–14 years (1996); and the dependency ratio is 46% (1996).

In 1994 the mean income per person was US $3200. The inflation rate is 10% and the unemployment rate 3% (1994); the lowest 10% of the population have a 5% share of income while the highest 10% have a 23% share (1994).

In 1996 the infant mortality rate was 7.6 per 1000 live births and average life expectancy at birth 73.3 years.

Total health expenditure accounts for 8.1% of estimated GDP.

The health care system in the Czech Republic is a contractual system with a clear separation between financing and provision. Several independent health insurance companies finance care. The Ministry of Health provides most care services.

Approach towards achieving health for all

The main causes of death include circulatory diseases (twice as high as the EU average) and malignant neoplasms (30% higher than the EU average). A long-term national health programme was drafted in 1995 and disseminated for consultation. The political leadership in the Ministry of Health has changed five times since 1989, which has disrupted the policy development process.

Several issue-specific policies reflect aspects of the WHO strategy for health for all. In 1993 a national plan was introduced to reduce the negative impact of disability, together with national programmes addressing cardiovascular diseases, cancer, aging, diabetes, perinatal care and mental health. In 1995 a programme was introduced to monitor the effect of the environment on health, as was a national environment policy.

The focus, however, has been on extensive health care reform. Some new institutions have been established. The National Institute of Public Health replaced the former Institute of Hygiene and Epidemiology, and the School of Public Health within the Postgraduate Medical School and an intersectoral commission to combat the use of illicit drugs were founded.

In 1991 a national programme for health restoration and promotion in the Czech Republic was drawn up; this was discussed by the Parliamentary Committee for Social Policy and Health and approved by the Government in 1992. The most notable changes were a dramatic liberalization of the health care system, characterized by the introduction of fees for service and a point system for financing health care delivery. A General Health Insurance Law was passed, marking the move to a compulsory insurance model, with limited market competition between insurers. A number of insurers (of which the General Health Insurance Company is the largest) finance health care providers on the basis of contracts.

Decentralization has also been attempted, largely through privatization; mass privatization of primary health care units has been one characteristic of this shift. So far it has not been possible to agree on privatization of secondary and tertiary care, with deep-seated mistrust of privatization among both politicians and the public. A number of the reforms adhere to the principles of health for all.

Focus on health outcomes and reorientation towards primary health care

Reorientation towards primary health care has been the basic philosophy underpinning the transformation of the health care delivery system. In 1995, the National Centre for Primary Care was established, comprising the Association for Home Care, the Association of General Practitioners, and the Association of Paediatricians and Practitioners for Adolescents. Primary health care physicians were previously under-used, a large part of their work being devoted to certifying absences from work. Financial incentives for primary health care physicians have somewhat broadened their scope, and one of the results of privatization has been the enhanced role of ambulatory care units, now considered to be the most efficient part of the health care delivery system. Initiatives in human resource development have aimed to support this reorientation, especially training in primary health care for nurses.

The Institute of Health Information and Statistics regularly monitors changes in the number and use of hospital beds. As a move towards health outcome orientation, the Institute regularly performs health surveys.

A hot debate on financial challenges, mainly the financing of large hospitals, started in 1994. Co-payments in hospitals were proposed when the crisis of financing health care deepened in 1995. In 1996, the first parliamentary elections held in the Czech Republic resulted in a coalition of three parties. According to opinion polls, measures pertaining to financing health care were the greatest failure of government policy. Reforms are planned to continue with the aim of reaching a higher level of efficiency while retaining equity.

Promotion of equity, public participation and intersectoral action

Equity

The state guarantees the health care system, which is now operating on the basis of compulsory health insurance, and pays premiums for children and elderly people. The insurance-based system may have compromised equity, however, by putting a ceiling on payments and allowing some insurers to be better funded than others and thus able to provide better services. In an attempt to ensure equity, the annual reports of the General Health Insurance Company for 1993, 1994 and 1995 dealt with the regional distribution of insurance funds. Groups such as immigrants and disabled people have been targeted for action to ensure appropriate care and to reduce the negative effects of disability. Sickness benefits are higher for people with lower income.

There are moves to promote a wider understanding of equity in health, including the translation into Czech of the WHO document *The concepts and principles of equity in health.*[a] On a practical level, laws on social security and mandatory employer insurance premiums for state employees and the acts on minimum subsistence and social need aim to guarantee an adequate income, which is one of the basic prerequisites for health. The Czech Republic is characterized by a relatively high level of social spending; coupled with low unemployment, this has played an important part in reducing poverty. The country has also adopted active labour-market policies, including measures to retrain workers and enhance labour mobility. It is also one of the few countries in central and eastern Europe that has begun to reform its pension system.

Public participation

Until now, users have had little say in health care decisions. Efforts to change that through extended programmes of health education and awareness-building have been initiated, and there has been a serious effort to keep people informed of progress and the reasons for change. This process begins at a young age. The national network of Health Promoting Schools aims to democratize decision-making in the health care sector and promote community participation among children. To encourage the development of organized interest groups, funding is provided to an association for promoting patients' rights.

Intersectoral action

The main aims of the reforms were to improve the efficiency of the health care system and to reduce health care expenditure. The functions of the National Centre for Health Promotion were transferred to the National Institute of Public Health in 1995. There have, however, been some attempts to link to other sectors such as the environment and to introduce legislation on lifestyle challenges, such as tobacco.

---

[a] WHITEHEAD, M. *The concepts and principles of equity in health.* Copenhagen, WHO Regional Office for Europe, 1990 (document number EUR/ICP/RPD 414).

Specific intersectoral initiatives include:

- research on the impact of environmental pollution, mainly in heavily industrialized areas;
- a "Quit and Win" series of television spots in accordance with the CINDI (countrywide integrated noncommunicable diseases intervention) programme, warning labels on cigarette packets and legislation on tobacco-free environments and tobacco advertising;
- maximum levels for vehicle emissions and periodic inspection of cars;
- consultation with social bodies in relation to rehabilitation and care of disabled people;
- training courses for teachers on sexual education and AIDS prevention organized by the National Centre for Health Promotion, and later by the National Institute of Public Health (training of teachers was organized by the former Centre); and
- legal measures to promote social support and cohesion on social security benefits, housing, maternity benefits and other prerequisites for health.

Denmark

Demography, policy environment and health care system

Denmark is bordered by the North Sea to the west, by the Skagerrak and Kattegat straits in the north and north-east (separating it from Norway and Sweden) and by Germany to the south. The *Folketing* (Parliament) has 179 members, and the legislative power lies with the Queen and the *Folketing* jointly. For administrative purposes Denmark is divided into 14 counties and 275 municipalities. Hospitals in the cities of Copenhagen and Frederiksberg are run by a special administrative body: the Copenhagen Hospital Corporation.

In 1997 the population was 5.3 million. The average population density is 123 per km^2; 85% of the population live in urban areas; and 13.3% of the population are aged $\geq$ 65 years and 18% aged 0–14 years (1997).

In 1994 the mean income per person was US $28 000. The inflation rate is 2% (1997) and the unemployment rate 9% (1996).

In 1995 the infant mortality rate was 5.3 per 1000 live births, and in 1994/1995 average life expectancy at birth was 72.6 years for men and 77.8 years for women.

The vast majority of health services are free of charge. Of the total expenditure on health care in 1995, public expenditure constituted 83% and private expenditure about 17%. Private health care expenditure mainly covers user payments for pharmaceuticals, dentistry and physiotherapy. The total public and private health care expenditure corresponds to about 6% of GNP. The system is characterized by extensive decentralization, with responsibility for health in the hands of regional and local government bodies (counties and municipalities). There are negotiated limits for expenditure by local government. The system is financed largely through taxation, with mainly public providers.

Approach towards achieving health for all

In 1989, the Government published *The health promotion programme of the Government of Denmark*, which gives priority to action against accidents, cancer, cardiovascular diseases, mental disorders and musculoskeletal diseases. This programme is still relevant, although there are plans to revise it. Health policies are formulated in close consultation with the counties, which are responsible for providing primary health care and hospital services. The municipalities are responsible for residential care and home nursing, which are very well developed.

To supplement the national plans, counties must prepare plans outlining their health objectives and how to achieve them. In 1993, each county was asked to formulate its own plan to promote health and to manage health services. These draft plans were discussed in late 1997 and will provide the basis for the development of an overall national health policy.

In 1984 Denmark decided to adopt WHO's health for all policy for the European Region and its 38 targets. Efforts will be made to enable people to live longer and healthier lives by reducing the numbers of premature deaths and of people in pain or with disabilities, and allowing more people to reach old age free of reduced mental or physical abilities. A comprehensive effort is specially needed in relation to vulnerable social groups. For example, there is a striking difference in health between the Danish and Swedish sides of the Øresund. On the Swedish side, on average 1158 men and 999 women per 100 000 inhabitants die every year, versus 1254 men and 1129 women on the Danish side. Further, life expectancy is longer in Sweden: 3 years longer for men and 3.5 years for women. This excess mortality also applies to those who are actively employed.

Specific programmes have been developed on tobacco, nutrition and alcohol. Nevertheless, Denmark still has higher levels of tobacco and alcohol consumption than many other European countries, and it can therefore be asked how successful these policies have been. The current tobacco consumption trends among women are especially worrying.

Focus on health outcomes and reorientation towards primary health care

The primary health care system is well developed; general practitioners generally play a gatekeeper role and refer patients for more specialized care when appropriate.

The Danish Institute of Clinical Epidemiology is responsible for research on health and health services. The National Research Council recently proposed strengthening research in health services, biochemistry and cardiovascular diseases and, in collaboration with scientific societies, to develop practice guidelines based on systematic reviews of evidence-based medicine.

Promotion of equity, public participation and intersectoral action

Equity
The *Health promotion programme of the Government of Denmark* does not refer explicitly to equity, but this is regarded as being implicit in all health care goals and objectives. Access to health services is only one element of a vast policy on health and wellbeing, based on clean living conditions, a healthy diet, good working conditions, pollution monitoring and an adequate welfare system. The entire population has equal and free access to almost all health services (there are user payments for dental treatment, some medicines and physiotherapy). The universal nature of the welfare system, based on a system of citizens' rights, means that inequities in health between lower and higher socioeconomic groups are not so

pronounced as in some other European countries. Health and social services cooperate closely in caring for such groups as elderly people. Plans for the future include further cooperation between the health and social services in targeting the needs of vulnerable groups.

The counties are responsible for hospitals and primary health care (except for home nursing services) and services are financed mainly through local taxes. To achieve more equitable distribution of resources, the counties receive government budget allocations to offset demographic and revenue differences. The level of local taxes is therefore a crucial political question in the county councils.

Although Denmark has less inequity than many other countries, the health care system is not without problems. Specific challenges for the future include the need to improve mental health services (both hospital and community services) and better health services for elderly people, including the establishment of geriatric units in each hospital.

Public participation

Since responsibility for both curative and preventive services is devolved to the regional and local levels, the national level can issue guidelines but must act through negotiation with the National Association of County Councils and the National Association of Local Authorities. The decision to develop a national health policy on the basis of county plans is an example of this bottom-up way of working. In recent years, local initiatives such as the Healthy Cities movement have been important in bringing about change. To promote the development of local action, the Ministry of Health has established a Health Project Fund for the initiation and evaluation of local health initiatives. In some instances, introducing an innovation first as a local initiative proves more acceptable than doing so at the national level. Many features of Denmark's system began locally but then quickly spread through the health system, such as 24-hour home nursing care, preventive visits by home nurses to elderly people, health promotion, and community mental health services. Each year the Ministry of Health identifies priority areas. A determining element in their success is the willingness of local bodies to provide co-financing and the long-term viability of the project after state assistance ends.

The Board of Patients' Complaints is intersectoral and includes people from outside the health sector, such as lawyers as well as health professionals.

Intersectoral action

Intersectoral bodies set up to promote health include the following.

• An interministerial committee formulated and followed up on the 1989 health promotion programme. Once the programme was formulated, the committee worked when there was a specific issue to be addressed. Due to difficulties in reaching consensus between conflicting agendas, and the loss of impetus once the plan had been formulated, the committee no longer meets.

- The Danish Council of Ethics has expertise in a wide range of areas, including legislation, culture, medicine, theology and sociology. Its role is largely consultative. Recent reports cover topics such as brain death and ethical questions surrounding reproduction.
- The Council on Health Promotion Policy is responsible for promoting health, both within the health sector and in other sectors of society, and for evaluating health promotion initiatives. It has the task of making health promotion a subject of public debate.
- The Danish Council on Smoking and Health is an independent board of experts whose main task is to limit the harmful effects of tobacco. An act on smoke-free environments has recently been passed, and trade unions and employers' organizations have been consulted as to its implementation.
- Special workplace health services have been set up with the aim of preventing work-related diseases and accidents; safety standards have been introduced in many factories and offices, and health promotion projects dealing with the issues of tobacco, nutrition, exercise and stress have been introduced in some workplaces.
- The Danish Veterinary and Food Administration and the National Board of Health aim to promote healthier food and nutrition through activities that include health education and awareness-building. The Administration cooperates with food producers, sometimes providing subsidies to companies that produce and promote healthy food.
- Within the past few years, the Government and health authorities have promoted efforts to ensure that health care is based on methods of proven scientific value (evidence-based medicine) and optimal use of available resources. A national strategy for evaluation of medical technology has been defined, and an institute for evaluation of medical technology has been created under the National Board of Heath. At the local level, a range of quality assurance programmes, including the setting up of standards for specific topics within health care, have been developed or will be forthcoming. Another focus is to identify and correct system malfunctioning within the delivery of health care services.

Estonia

Demography, policy environment and health care system

Estonia is bordered by the Baltic Sea to the north and west, by the Russian Federation to the east and by Latvia to the south. Estonia was annexed by the Soviet Union after 1940, but regained independence in 1991 and became a republic with a single-chamber elected assembly.

In 1995 the population was 1.5 million. The average population density is 33 per km^2 (1995); 70% of the population live in urban areas (1994); 13% of the population are aged $\geq$ 65 years (1995) and 20% aged 0–14 years (1994); and the dependency ratio is 55% (1996).

In 1993 the mean income per person was US $1200. The inflation rate is 16% (1996); the unemployment rate is 5% (1996); and the lowest 10% of population have a 3% share of income while the highest 10% have a 29% share (1996).

In 1995 the infant mortality rate was 14.8 per 1000 live births and average life expectancy at birth was 68 years.

In 1991, Estonia moved from a state-funded health insurance system to one consisting of a central fund and 17 regional funds, and from a centralized to a decentralized system. Decentralization has largely taken the form of deconcentration, whereby only administrative (and not political) responsibilities have been turned over to the county level. The process has been hampered by a failure to train staff to deal with new administrative procedures prior to their introduction, and the 15 counties and 17 sickness funds to which responsibility was transferred were too small for efficient planning and management.

Approach towards achieving health for all

The Estonian health policy concept is based on health for all. A draft document was disseminated for consultation with a number of groups and organizations, revised and finalized in 1995. Parliamentary discussion is not the usual process for such documents in Estonia, although the Government approved the health policy concept. The policy included several main areas for reform, including legislation, financing of health services, research and development, quality of care and an integrated approach to public health. The intention was to follow this up with a specific action plan, but the process has taken significantly longer than had been expected because of several changes of government.

Focus on health outcomes and reorientation towards primary health care

Primary and secondary care have been decentralized to the local administrative level in accordance with the Health Organization Law of 1994. The main principle is that primary care is organized around the general practitioner, who has a gatekeeper role in relation to specialized care. General practitioners are required to provide 24-hour continuity of care and a wide range of health promotion and preventive activities, such as health education, immunization, family planning or screening services to the population for which they are responsible. The shift to primary health care has been a gradual process, largely because physicians and nurses need to be retrained in these areas. Since 1991, Tartu University has provided two-year courses for retraining hospital specialists and practitioners currently working in ambulatories, and a Chair of General Practice has been established. An information network for family physicians has been established, and research is being conducted on the cost–effectiveness of the work of family physicians. Greater efforts are being made to integrate health promotion and disease prevention into health services, and there is more consultation and negotiation between the association of family physicians and the association of hospitals. Family physician centres are being established to help develop a family practice concept.

There is ongoing monitoring of health status, and this information has been used to set priorities for health education topics according to their level of importance for people's health, so that health outcome information becomes the basis for developing and implementing health promotion programmes and planning health services. The process of collecting information on health outcomes is also being monitored.

Promotion of equity, public participation and intersectoral action

Equity
Almost the entire population is covered by the health care system. Since the 1994 reforms, however, some people may be without coverage, mainly those who do not pay taxes or who are living illegally in the country. Fees were introduced for some services, but such groups as elderly people and children are exempt. Opting out of the public insurance scheme is not allowed, so there has been little opportunity for a private insurance system to develop. Some areas deserve particular attention, such as Narva, which is inhabited largely by ethnic Russians.

The amalgamation of the Ministry of Health and the Ministry of Social Welfare has facilitated a more integrated understanding of and approach to dealing with inequities. In April 1995, the Social Welfare Law defined social welfare broadly as providing assistance to individuals or families. Certain subsidies are also available for housing and children's allowances, and there have been changes in the treatment of some groups such as disabled people and ethnic minorities. Recent reforms in care for disabled people include education in vocational training and self-help, but access to services is limited due to a shortage of places in such schemes and a lack of appropriate institutions. Health education is now available in minority languages. Despite the legislation, there is a gap between what has been stated as a right and what can be implemented with the available resources. Nevertheless, social attitudes towards mental and physical disability and strategies to deal with vulnerable groups generally have changed markedly.

Public participation

Ensuring patients' rights has been a high priority. A draft Law on Patients' Rights was prepared in 1995 and presented to the Government. To encourage more active participation, the approach of promoting health in such settings as schools and workplaces has been found to be particularly successful, and the Health Promoting Schools project aims to encourage participation at a young age. Similar initiatives have been started up in the workplace. To achieve more participation from policy-makers working at the regional and local levels, training programmes have been introduced for key health decision-makers in county and municipal offices.

Intersectoral action

In 1993 the formerly separate Ministries of Health, Social Welfare, and Labour were merged to form a new Ministry of Social Affairs. Within the new Ministry, the Department of Public Health is responsible for coordinating activities between health bodies and relevant agencies (including other ministries). The Ministries of Education, the Interior and Sports were also consulted in preparing a health programme specifically for schoolchildren. In 1994 the establishment of the National Centre for Health Promotion and Education gave life to intersectoral action for health by establishing interdisciplinary teams to develop programmes for cardiovascular health and combating smoking. The most important initiative has been the establishment of a Health Promotion Fund that finances health promotion projects from different sectors. This fund, created in 1995, uses 1% of the budget of the sickness fund to finance local health promotion projects. A Chair of Health Promotion has also been established at the Medical Faculty of Tartu University.

Specific actions aimed at promoting intersectoral action include:

- joint research between the health and employment sectors on the effects of different working environments on workers' health and between the health and social welfare sectors on how best to coordinate care of mentally ill people;
- the use of different settings such as schools and work environments to promote health;
- educating employers to recognize the risk factors inherent in the work environment and establishing an intersectoral council to promote healthy work environments;
- campaigns against smoking and abuse of other substances and to promote healthy nutrition;
- legal measures such as a ban on tobacco advertising, health and safety objectives in the working environment and a law on social insurance;
- health training for teachers and training of occupational health workers; and
- monitoring changes in smoking habits.

Finland

Demography, policy environment and health care system

Finland is bordered by Norway to the north-west and north, by the Russia Federation to the east, by the Baltic Sea to the south and by Sweden to the west. Finland has been an independent republic since 1917. Parliament consists of one chamber of 200 members elected by direct and proportional representation. The country is divided into 15 electoral districts, but for administrative purposes comprises 5 provinces.

In 1996 the population was 5.1 million. The average population density is 17 per km^2; 65% of the population live in urban areas; 14% of the population are aged $\geq$ 65 years and 19% aged 0–14 years (1996); and the dependency ratio is 50% (1996).

In 1996 the mean income per person was US $22 300. The inflation rate is 0.6% (1996); the unemployment rate is 16% (1996); and the lowest 20% of the population have a 6% share of income while the highest 20% have a 17% share (1995).

In 1995 the infant mortality rate was 3.9 per 1000 live births. The average life expectancy at birth is 72.8 years for men and 80.2 years for women (1996).

In 1994, total health expenditure accounted for 8% of estimated GDP.

The Ministry of Social Affairs and Health supervises social and health services at the national level through information and by means of legislation, municipal self- government and administrative solutions and practices. Within the health care system, there is a statutory state sickness insurance scheme.

Approach towards achieving health for all

See the case study on Finland, page 27.

France

Demography, policy environment and health care system

France is bordered by Belgium and Luxembourg to the north-east, by the Rhine, Germany, Switzerland and Italy to the east, by the Mediterranean Sea to the south, by Andorra and Spain to the south-west and by the Atlantic Ocean to the west.

France is a republic and Parliament consists of the National Assembly and the Senate. The country is divided into 22 regions with 96 departments within the regions, each governed by a directly elected general council.

In 1993 the population was 57.3 million. The average population density is 104.5 per km^2 (1993); 73% of the population live in urban areas (1993); 15% of the population are aged $\geq$ 65 years and 19% aged 0–14 years (1992); and the dependency ratio is 52% (1993).

In 1994 the mean income per person was US $23 420. The inflation rate is 1.7% (1994) and the unemployment rate is 12.5% (1994); the poorest 20% of the population receives 6% of the income and the most affluent 20% receives 26% (1989).

In 1992 the infant mortality rate was 6.8 per 1000 live births and the life expectancy at birth 78 years.

In 1996 health care expenditure comprised 9.8% of GDP. This figure is among the highest in Europe, and has raised questions of whether the current levels of expenditure are sustainable. The French health care system set up from 1945 attempts to reconcile the principles of liberalism and solidarity with a collective system of funding. Health care is financed mainly by social insurance with mixed public and private providers.

Approach towards achieving health for all

The Haut Comité de la Santé Publique (High Committee on Public Health) was established in 1991 to advise the Ministry of Health on health issues. In 1994, the Committee produced a preliminary report entitled *La santé en France,* which defines priorities and identifies the main health issues for various population groups (cardiovascular diseases, cancer, mental health, suicide and AIDS). Strategies for reducing the number of deaths arising from illicit drugs, tobacco, alcohol, psychotropic medicines and environmental health are especially emphasized. It is not usual for Parliament to discuss general public health policy, unless it is a matter of legislation. In 1996, a major national health policy conference was held to discuss aspects of health care, especially rising costs. The report from the conference, which was attended mainly by representatives of the health professions and regional authorities, was submitted to Parliament as the background for the discussion on a proposed new law on health insurance.

Focus on health outcomes and reorientation towards primary health care

Patient care may be provided in ambulatory care outside or inside the hospital. Outpatient care is provided by general practitioners and practising specialists, who work individually (or increasingly in group practices) on a fee-for-service basis or in health centres established and managed by communes, voluntary societies and other organizations. The patient can choose between these types of service. Physicians are increasingly working as part of multidisciplinary teams along with other health professionals and social workers. General practitioners are cooperating more and more with the emergency departments of hospitals.

The assessment of the cost–effectiveness of various health actions has been growing in importance. The National Institute for Health and Medical Research (INSERM) especially emphasizes population-based research activities. At the national level, strategic planning is based on regional reports that focus on needs and on the capacity to respond to those needs. To facilitate the provision of appropriate quantitative and qualitative information, a National Network on Public Health was set up in 1992 to monitor infectious diseases and environmental risks and provide information on which to base policy decisions. An information system on hospital services has gradually been extended to cover all hospitals and is intended to allow a more equitable distribution of resources. Quantified targets have been set in a number of areas.

Promotion of equity, public participation and intersectoral action

Equity
France has a strong record in certain forms of medical treatment (organ transplants, cancer, cardiovascular and digestive surgery, etc.). Challenges remain in the areas of infant mortality, chronic diseases caused by an aging population, and psychological and social problems. A recent report from the Haut Comité identifies as one of its main objectives reducing geographical, socioeconomic and gender inequalities. The report emphasizes people's right to a decent quality of life (covering such aspects as housing and shelter, daily living needs and social integration) and improved access to medical and social services, especially for vulnerable groups. A number of measures are proposed to support vulnerable groups, such as improved access to dental services for people on low income, increased primary health care initiatives targeting low-income groups, and a more equitable geographical distribution of medical specialists.

Health insurance (one of the aspects of the social security system) was set up to ensure national solidarity and protect the population from a series of social risks. Almost the whole population is covered by sickness insurance that reimburses the fees paid by the patient. In addition to the cost of hospital treatment, people are fully or partly reimbursed for the cost of drugs. In 1992 the Law on Medical Aid allowed for the provision of a supplementary health benefit to vulnerable groups.

Although a reasonably high level of equity in health has been ensured so far, emerging trends and diminishing public resources could challenge this capacity. It is feared that people's chances to lead a meaningful life will be seriously challenged in the next century; technology may widen rather than narrow the gaps; cost constraints may put vulnerable groups at risk; and social exclusion, long-term unemployment and breakdown in the social fabric may pose serious challenges for health, solidarity and social cohesion.

Public participation

Since 1990, a concerted effort has been made to make individuals aware of their responsibility for their own health, largely through comprehensive preventive and health education activities. Participation in policy-making, however, still tends to be led by experts. More than 120 public health professionals were involved in formulating the current health policy. Working groups were set up to discuss the priority areas of concern and to define health objectives and the strategies to achieve them. The agreed objectives were later accepted by the Ministry of Health and became national priorities. Following publication of the report *La santé en France*, a series of regional conferences was held to discuss the priorities. The national priorities were used as a framework to develop regional objectives.

Intersectoral action

At national level, the Ministry of Social Affairs and the Ministry of Health share responsibility for health. Three directorates are especially involved: the Social Security Directorate, the Hospitals Directorate and the Health Directorate. At the regional level, regional health and social action directorates and departmental health and social action directorates have been established. The former deal with the more administrative aspects and the latter organize health care delivery, health promotion and preventive activities.

Other ministries that have responsibility for health include the Ministry of Finance, which allocates the budget, the Ministry of Education, the Ministry of Industry and Commerce (for setting the prices of drugs) and the Ministries of Environment, Agriculture and the Armed Forces.

According to the recent reform adopted at the end of 1995, Parliament determines health and financial aims based on the recommendations presented by the Haut Comité de la Santé Publique. Those recommendations are based on preliminary documents prepared by the Conference Nationale de Santé and the conferences régionales de santé.

In April 1996, regional hospital agencies were set up. These are the driving force of the Government's referral hospital policy and will approve contracts with public and private hospitals, setting out medium-term strategic aims and objectives going beyond the normal one-year time horizon. They will also supervise the distribution of regional funding and monitor the purchasing of public hospitals.

Various mechanisms have been established to promote intersectoral action. The Health Education Committee aims to build awareness of health risks arising from tobacco, alcohol dependence, lack of physical activity, poor nutrition and problems of social integration, and to encourage healthier lifestyles. Under the leadership of the Committee, these issues are then taken up at the local level in schools, workplaces and associations. The National Association for the Prevention of Alcoholism and the Committee to Combat Tobacco deal specifically with the challenges of alcohol and tobacco consumption. The National Agency for Accreditation and Evaluation in Health has responsibility for drawing up professional recommendations, arranging the accreditation of hospital services and assessing public health programmes.

Georgia

Demography, policy environment and health care system

Georgia is bordered by the Black Sea to the west, by the Russian Federation to the north and east and by Armenia, Azerbaijan and Turkey to the south. Georgia regained its independence in April 1991. The August 1995 Constitution defines Georgia as a presidential republic with federal elements. The Parliament has 225 members elected by a system combining 75 single-member districts with proportional representation based on party lists.

In 1996 the population was 5.3 million. The average population density is 77 per km^2 (1996); 55% of the population live in urban areas (1996); 9% of the population are aged $\geq$ 65 years and 25% aged 0–14 years (1990); and the dependency ratio is 53% (1990).

In 1996 GDP was only 30% of the level before 1991 and the inflation rate was 2.1% per month. The poorest 10% of the population receive 5% of the income and the most affluent 10% receive 48%.

In 1997 the infant mortality rate was 17 per 1000 live births, and in 1993 the average life expectancy at birth was 72.9 years.

In 1995 total health care expenditure accounted for 3.2% of GDP.

The health care system covers all parts of the country. Within each administrative district, a central district hospital and a polyclinic provide health services, supported by small branch facilities (ambulatories) in most of the villages. In the larger cities separate hospitals and polyclinics carry out the same function, specializing in services for children or adults.

Approach towards achieving health for all

Health care reform has been initiated as part of the broader programme for economic and social development, but severe internal conflicts in 1992 made it increasingly difficult to proceed with the reform process. The effect of war on the economic situation has dramatically worsened living conditions for the population, a situation reflected in deteriorating health status. Infant and maternal death rates increased in 1993 and 1994. Diphtheria and tuberculosis have continued to rise among children and adults, as have meningitis and rabies and deaths due to cardiovascular diseases and cancer. Re-emergence of previously eradicated diseases such as diphtheria, tuberculosis and malaria and the lack of vaccines make epidemics a very real risk. Natural disasters, such as the Racha earthquake or landslides in the Ajara and Lechkhumi regions, have also seriously affected people's health.

Deteriorating socioeconomic conditions have also adversely affected people's mental health, and psychiatric services are unable to cope with the additional burden. Increased levels of stress and stress-related behaviour have resulted in an increase in death rates, especially among men, and high rates of depression and suicide. Abuse of alcohol and drugs, especially the intravenous use of opium, is a growing problem and indicates that many people have a sense of despair about the future.

At present the economy is in a state of complex and heterogeneous transition from a centrally planned to a market system. The process of economic stabilization started in 1995 and is continuing today.

A new currency unit, the lari, was introduced in 1995 and is considered to be stable. Despite some success, the level of tax collection still remains unsatisfactory.

Focus on health outcomes and reorientation towards primary health care

In view of such basic health problems, the focus of health policy has largely been on disease prevention and quality of care. Despite serious obstacles, in 1995 the Government initiated reforms of the administration and financing of the health care system. Attempts were directed toward dismantling the huge administrative machinery, which consumed considerable resources. A system for registering all medical institutions was put in place, and plans were started to link this to a system of hospital accreditation and licensing of health facilities and medical staff. The plans for decentralization and moves to an insurance-based system have already started. Judicial institutions and enforcement mechanisms are being reformed. Parliament has adopted a health law.

The budget for state health programmes in 1997 amounted to about 49 million lari (about US $37 million). The state financed three main groups of programmes:

- preventive programmes: immunization, control of infectious diseases, health promotion, prevention of sexually transmitted diseases including AIDS, development of health information systems, prevention of goitre and a survey of radiation, prevention of drug abuse, and blood safety;
- medical insurance programmes: mental health, tuberculosis, safe motherhood, children under one year of age, and prevention and management of malignant diseases; and
- health care programmes: health care of the population in mountainous regions, people disabled in armed conflict, orphans, and people with diabetes.

The main objective of the reform is to improve the health of the entire population by designing and implementing a system based on primary care that emphasizes health promotion, disease prevention and health protection. In keeping with the move away from the perception of health as being limited to disease prevention, there are plans to develop a health promotion policy with special emphasis on substance abuse and drugs.

As in other newly independent states, Georgia inherited a strong health system from the Soviet period albeit with serious distortions leading to an excessive supply of hospital beds and specialist physicians and poor development of primary health care and health promotion. Long-term deficiencies in planning had reached crisis point, and overall funding was unable to keep up with needs. Efforts to contain costs have largely pre-empted the moves towards primary health care.

A World Bank project (Health I) was agreed in February 1996. Such objectives as reorientation of the health care system, modernization of public health services, healthy children and safe motherhood, development of human resources for health and rehabilitation of health facilities are now being implemented. A further project (Health II), aimed at promoting primary health care and modernizing the system of financing health, is being considered.

The previous health information system was not designed to highlight deficiencies and provide a basis for policy decisions. An objective of the reforms is to establish a comprehensive health information system and to put in place appropriate mechanisms for monitoring and evaluation.

Promotion of equity, public participation and intersectoral action

Equity
The current economic reforms are undermining the traditional social support system based on low prices for basic goods and services and guaranteed jobs. Almost all subsidies have been removed, which makes it essential to strengthen the social safety net, but this requires more money and more accurate information on poverty and income distribution. A system of bread subsidies aims at some redistribution from the rich to the poor, but the subsidies are frequently inadequate and can open up new opportunities for corruption. The real value of social assistance and benefits still needs to be improved. The resulting polarization of society is especially severe in urban areas, where people depend heavily on a cash economy.

People's diets have changed dramatically as food becomes increasingly unaffordable. Most people are not underfed, but many are poorly nourished in terms of calories or essential micronutrients, and the lack of money for basic food makes them more susceptible to certain illnesses. This situation causes deficiencies of iodine, iron and vitamins. Many people lack fuel for heating and cooking. Disadvantaged children are less likely to attend school, especially in winter, which perpetuates their disadvantaged state. Housing lacks basic utilities; electricity and water are often irregularly supplied and of poor quality. Aside from the physical effects of poverty, a degree of social exclusion is evident as people are unable to participate in normal life, including hosting and attending family celebrations. Since the extended family plays an important role in Georgia, those in need who have no family have a serious problem;

similarly, being unable to help another family member is a clear indicator of a difficult personal financial situation.

Now that the guaranteed flow of central funds to support development of the health system has ceased, many medical institutions are falling into chronic disrepair, levels of care are falling and even basic services such as inoculations and primary health care are not always provided. The introduction of user fees also means that the poor can no longer afford even the most basic services.

Public participation
Many countries in central and eastern Europe and the newly independent states have experienced difficulty in making the transition to democracy and its implications for policy development. The concept of transparency in decision-making in government has not been wholly taken up, making it difficult for ordinary citizens to become involved and to challenge policy developments. The pressing socioeconomic problems of survival also make it less likely that people will show active interest in policy decisions that might affect them. The Soviet system did not encourage people to be proactive; they are generally not accustomed to taking initiatives to improve their situation, and therefore remain passive and feel disempowered.

Intersectoral action
Many of Georgia's health problems originate in the wider socioeconomic determinants of health. There are also serious environmental problems, especially in the area surrounding the Black Sea. Transport services are poor and often expensive, with the result that those living in remote areas can become quite isolated, a situation exacerbated by the increasing trend towards rural depopulation. To counteract many of these problems, a comprehensive programme of macroeconomic stabilization and structural reforms has been designed with the assistance of international organizations such as the World Bank and International Monetary Fund.

Germany

Demography, policy environment and health care system

Germany is bordered by Denmark and the North and Baltic Seas to the north, by Poland to the east, by the Czech Republic to the east and south-east, by Austria to the south-east and south, by Switzerland to the south, and by Belgium, France, Luxembourg and the Netherlands to the west.

Germany is a federal republic comprising 16 *Länder* (states), divided into a total of 29 administrative regions (*Regierungsbezirke*). Legislative power is vested in both the *Bundestag* (Federal Assembly) with 672 members and the *Bundesrat* (Federal Council) with 79 members.

In 1995 the population was 82 million. The average population density is 279 per km^2 (1994); 86% of the population live in urban areas (1994); 15% of the population are aged $\geq$ 65 years and 16% aged 0–14 years (1994); and the dependency ratio is 45% (1994).

In 1993 the mean income per person was US $23 500 and the inflation rate 1.5%; in 1996 the unemployment rate was 9%.

In 1995 the infant mortality rate was 5 per 1000 live births, and in 1994 the average life expectancy at birth was 76.6 years.

In 1996 total health care expenditure accounted for 9.5% of GDP.

The *Länder* have the main responsibility for health policy. Health services are financed mainly by social insurance with mixed public and private providers. The health care system in Germany encompasses all institutions and people contributing to the health of the public. See also the case study for one *Land*, North Rhine-Westphalia, page 41.

Approach towards achieving health for all

Germany's federal nature means that the *Länder* develop health policies. The federal state, the *Länder*, the local authorities, the sickness insurance funds and the care providers share responsibility for protecting public health. The Constitution clearly defines the rights and responsibilities of the various levels. Although the power to legislate is shared, the *Länder* are in principle responsible for administering legislation. The federal state issues guidelines on forms of treatment by physicians; early recognition of disease; pregnancy and childbirth; new methods of diagnosis and treatment; prescription of drugs, hospital and home care; assessment of incapacity for work; and family planning. All the *Länder* have formulated health policies; some are explicitly based on the health for all approach and others simply bear the health for all principles in mind. The *Länder* coordinate their activities through the Conferences of Health Ministers and Labour and Social Ministers, which discuss all matters relevant to public health but cannot adopt binding resolutions.

Focus on health outcomes and reorientation towards primary health care

The whole population has access to primary health care, mainly provided by private practitioners. The first contact is either with a family practitioner or a specialist. Sickness insurance covers medical and dental outpatient care, hospital care, drugs, health products and other appliances, diagnostic tests, and assistance for mothers and pregnant women. Most screening programmes are also covered. To improve the quality of care, a family physician must follow three years of specialist training to obtain a licence to practise. There is a relatively sharp distinction between ambulatory care provided by physicians in their own practices and inpatient care. Hospitals give ambulatory care only on a limited scale, such as in emergencies.

In 1993, the Ministry of Health developed a mechanism for funding health-related evidence-based research. This focuses on topics related to the environment, nutrition, lifestyles and the health problems of vulnerable groups. The aim is to incorporate research results in ongoing health care programmes, thus ensuring greater effectiveness.

Promotion of equity, public participation and intersectoral action

Equity
The social insurance system is based on laws that date from 1883 and 1889 and that have been considerably revised since then. The health care system is based on the principles of solidarity and subsidiarity. Almost the entire population (including non-German citizens and their families) enjoys comprehensive protection under sickness insurance schemes. Most people are members of the statutory insurance scheme; a few are affiliated to private insurance funds. Insured people receive services without co-payment. The services include health promotion measures, medical and dental treatment, provision of pharmaceuticals, hospital treatment, long-term care and home care. The regulations of the statutory health insurance system ensure that no-one has to do without services covered by this system for financial reasons, and that no-one is unreasonably burdened financially. For example, no insured person has to pay more than 2% of his or her gross annual income in out-of-pocket expenses.

Public participation
Since the health care system is both federalistic and pluralistic, a multiplicity of planning and financing bodies participate in decision-making. The role of the sickness funds is quite important, and several

organizations of professionals with differing functions are involved in the process of formulating policies, as are numerous non-profit-making organizations.

The health care system strongly emphasizes the responsibility of individuals for their own health, and social justice and self-determination for individual people, including freedom to choose their physician. Information on health rights and entitlements is widely available, as is a wide range of mass media education related to health. Priority areas include health promotion during pregnancy, birth, infancy, early childhood and at school, support to chronically ill and disabled people and help them cope with their illness or disability, and health education on risk-taking behaviour. The Health Promoting Schools networks (both the European and national networks) are active in Germany and aim to invest young people with participatory decision-making skills.

Intersectoral action

Intersectoral action for health in Germany is facilitated by the involvement of three ministries, apart from the Ministry of Health, in health care matters.

The Federal Ministry of Labour and Social Affairs is responsible for social insurance (except for statutory health insurance), including social security pension insurance, statutory unemployment and accident insurance, occupational and social medicine, (including veterans' health care), rehabilitation services and the statutory protection of employees.

The Federal Ministry of the Environment, Nature Conservation and Nuclear Safety is responsible for issues related to protecting health in connection with environmental pollution, and deals with corresponding problems in the areas of air pollution control, water and soil conservation, foodstuffs, noise pollution control and radiation protection. Subordinate authorities support the Ministry and establish the scientific and technical groundwork for the decision-making process of the federal Government.

The Federal Ministry of Research and Technology promotes subjects relevant to health research, which are incorporated in various programmes and are not restricted to a particular field of responsibility. The federal Government's Health Research 2000 Programme includes research projects in such areas as preventive medicine, preventing and controlling diseases, and public health. Other programmes involve setting priorities in such areas as medical technology, health and the environment, and work and technology.

A number of institutions of the former Federal Health Office are responsible for:

- research into the safety of pharmaceuticals, consumer protection, monitoring environmental pollution and radiation levels, disease prevention and human and veterinary medicine;
- executive tasks in relation to various legal areas including pharmaceuticals and narcotics, epidemics, application of pesticides, and chemicals and gene technology; and

- scientific consultancy work for government and other institutions.

The Federal Centre for Health Education is responsible for promoting and maintaining the quality of public health by providing practical health education and informing the public on health matters. It establishes the basic policies and guidelines for the contents and methods of health promotion measures, which mainly emphasize drug and alcohol abuse, smoking, nutrition, exercise, advice on family planning and AIDS.

Greece

Demography, policy environment and health care system

Greece is bordered to the north by Albania, Bulgaria and the former Yugoslav Republic of Macedonia and to the east by Turkey. Greece is surrounded in the west by the Ionian Sea and in the east by the Aegean Sea. It is a presidential republic, and Parliament has 300 members.

In 1996 the population was 10.5 million. Some 59% of the population live in urban areas (1996), and 16% of the population are aged ≥ 65 years and 16% aged 0–14 years (1996).

In 1996 the mean income per person was US $11 500. The inflation rate is 4% (1996) and the unemployment rate is 10% (1996).

In 1996 the infant mortality rate was 7.2 per 1000 live births. The average life expectancy at birth is 75 years for men (1994) and 80 years for women (1996).

In 1996 total health care expenditure accounted for 8.5% of GDP.

Approach towards achieving health for all

According to Article 23 of the Greek Constitution of 1975, the state is responsible for providing health care services to all its citizens. The health care policy is formulated by the Ministry of Health and Welfare in close collaboration with other sectors of administrative and political life as well as with professional and social groups. During the last 15 years, the health care system has been reformed and modified. In 1983 a National Health System (NHS) was created and subsequently modified in 1992 and in 1997. The main axes of the NHS are: equity in access to public health care services, priority to primary health care (according to the principles of the Alma-Ata Declaration), promotion of health and prevention of disease, mental health reforms and the prevention of drug addiction.

Greece has not yet formulated a national policy for health for all. Nevertheless, the health for all approach, the implementation of the 38 European targets for health for all and determining new targets is a continuing procedure influenced by current social, economic and political conditions.

Focus on health outcomes and reorientation towards primary health care

Primary health care is provided by the 180 health care centres and satellite dispensaries as well as by outpatient hospital departments (mainly in urban areas) and by outpatient departments of social security institutions. The role of the general practitioner and family physician has been seriously reconsidered and reorganized during the last 10–15 years, occupying a continually upgraded position in the functioning of primary health care services. The goal is to have family physicians function as the cornerstones of the primary health care system to optimize primary care and reduce expensive, potentially useless, over-specialized outpatient care, either public or private.

Priority in preventing disease and promoting health is accorded to the major causes of mortality: cardiovascular diseases, cancer, chronic respiratory tract diseases and injuries.

Primary prevention focuses mainly on establishing healthy lifestyles and behavioural patterns, including nonsmoking behaviour, healthy nutritional habits, and safety in everyday life at home, at the workplace and in transport.

A Division of School Medicine has been created at the Ministry of Health and Welfare and a school physician has been appointed for each school, both public and private. Further, recent legislative texts confirm and clarify the rules for occupational safety and the role of occupational and other relevant control carried out by state and departmental authorities.

Another major concern is preventing communicable diseases. The main aims are the successful implementation of the national vaccination programme, food safety, quality of the water supply, and preventing disease in the most vulnerable social groups: children, elderly people and migrant populations.

Promotion of equity, public participation and intersectoral action

Equity

Social security is based on a social insurance system. The entire population has access to public health care services. Inpatient public hospital care is fully covered by social security. Primary health care in the public sector is free of charge, while outpatient hospital care requires a small individual co-payment. The social security system reimburses 75% of the cost of medicines contained in the national list of approved qualified pharmaceutical products published in April 1998. The individual co-payment is 10% for people with specific chronic or disabling diseases.

Disease prevention and health promotion programmes are being implemented and developed, mainly focusing on migrant populations. The immigrant population in Greece increased by 45% during the last decade. An effort is being made to reach those who are difficult to reach: the gypsy population and refugees as well as legal and illegal immigrants. The health authorities, mainly at the county level, are attempting to integrate these populations, both Greek and non-Greek citizens, in the existing health care system.

Mentally and physically disabled people are being actively rehabilitated and socially integrated. A national strategy for the home care of elderly and disabled people was launched in 1998, implemented and supported jointly by the national and municipal health care and welfare services.

Public participation

Since 1993 the county health and welfare divisions have been substantially decentralized, being financially and administratively autonomous from the central level (Ministry of Health). County health authorities are responsible for implementing health policies, controlling and preventing communicable diseases, controlling food and water safety, and general disease prevention and health promotion measures in their departments. Scientific societies and professional groups participate in and collaborate with this procedure at the local or national levels.

Intersectoral action

Intersectoral collaboration is implemented at the national level with the Ministries of Education, Commerce, Labour and Social Security, Economics and Justice and any other relevant authority. Intersectoral collaboration is also implemented at the local and county levels for food safety, water quality and preventing communicable diseases.

In collaboration with the education authorities, priority is accorded to ways of preventing disease and promoting health by creating health-promoting lifestyles among specific target groups: children of school age, adolescents and young adults.

Hungary

Demography, policy environment and health care system

Hungary is bordered by Slovakia to the north, Ukraine to the north-east, Romania to the east, Croatia and the Federal Republic of Yugoslavia to the south, and Austria and Slovenia to the west. Hungary is governed by a single-chamber National Assembly with 386 members. In October 1989 the National Assembly approved the Constitution establishing Hungary as an independent, democratic state. The country is administratively divided into 19 counties (*megyék*) plus the capital, Budapest.

In 1996 the population was 10.1 million. The average population density is 109 per km^2 (1966); 64% of the population live in urban areas (1993); 14% of the population are aged ≥ 65 years and 18% aged 0–14 years (1996); and the dependency ratio is 48% (1993).

In 1996 the mean income per person was US $4300. The inflation rate is 19% and the unemployment rate is 11% (1996). The lowest 10% of the population have a 4% share of income, while the highest 10% have a 23% share (1993).

In 1996 the infant mortality rate was 10.9 per 1000 live births. In 1995 the average life expectancy at birth was 69.8 years.

In 1996 total health expenditure accounted for 7% of estimated GDP.

The Ministry of Health and Social Affairs was reorganized in 1990 and renamed the Ministry of Welfare. The Act on Local Governments (1990) transferred the ownership of health care facilities and responsibility for health care provision exclusively to town, county and municipal governments.

Approach towards achieving health for all

See the case study on Hungary, page 64.

Iceland

Demography, policy environment and health care system

Iceland is an island of 103 000 km^2 in the North Atlantic Ocean, located close to the Arctic Circle. In December 1995, the country was divided into 170 communes of which 31 had the status of a town. The commune councils are supervised by the Ministry of Social Affairs.

In 1995 the population was 268 000. The average population density is 3 per km^2 and 92% of the population live in urban areas (1995); 11% of the population are aged $\geq$ 65 years and 25% aged 0–14 years (1994); and the dependency ratio is 52% (1993).

In 1996 the mean income per person was US $27 000.

In 1995 the infant mortality rate was 6.1 per 1000 live births and the average life expectancy at birth was 76.5 years for males and 80.6 years for females.

In 1995 total health expenditure accounted for 8% of estimated GDP (1995).

Approach towards achieving health for all

In 1986, the Government decided to develop a health for all policy. The framework and a consultation document were circulated in 1987 for comment, and the health plan was finally endorsed by a parliamentary resolution in 1991. In 1996 a committee was established to revise the health plan. The new plan will have a problem-oriented approach and its development is closely related to that of the revised European strategy for health for all.

The current policy covers elderly people, accidents, mental health, health promotion and disease prevention, alcohol, food and nutrition, water and sanitation, and the physical and working environments. The new health plan will focus on general strategies and specific measures concerning children and young people, adults, elderly people, and some minority groups such as handicapped people.

Focus on health outcomes and reorientation towards primary health care

The 1991 policy reinforced the role of the primary health care approach, stating that primary health care centres should be the cornerstone of care in cooperation with the outpatient clinics of hospitals and other specialized institutions. Primary health care services are available to all, and an objective in recent years has been to ensure uniformity in services throughout Iceland.

In an effort to decentralize some aspects of health care, in addition to the health for all policy, a parliamentary resolution stated that public health offices would be established in all regions with responsibility for planning and supervising health care services. In view of the moves to promote prevention, increasing skills and staff training in primary health care, prevention, health promotion and public health topics have gained an important place on the agenda.

Public health reports have been produced in Iceland for over 100 years. A system will be set up to monitor the activities of the primary health care centres, the hospitals and the work of health care personnel. Since the health for all policy was published, research on the relationship between different lifestyles and environment and health has been strengthened.

Promotion of equity, public participation and intersectoral action

Equity

Uniform health care services are available free of charge in Iceland in accordance with the Health Care Act of 1974. The main recent emphasis has been on reducing geographical inequalities in access to health care. Primary health care services have been set up in each district and information on personnel needs is being systematized. Human resource planning has been based on demographic trends to allow, for example, for more physicians specializing in care for elderly people.

The basic prerequisites for health such as food, housing, income and education are generally quite equitably distributed, although recent evidence has brought to light some economic inequalities. One area that requires more attention is the lack of data on perceived health, quality of life, social health and social support.

Public participation

Measures to increase the level of health education in schools have been stepped up as one means of increasing public participation and making young people aware that they can influence things. New legislation on patients' rights came into effect in July 1997, ensuring that all patients have equal access to health services of the same quality.

Intersectoral action

Various structures have been established to facilitate intersectoral action.

The Institute for Preventive Medicine and Health Promotion supervises activities relating to lifestyles, and works with other groups and sectors, such as the Icelandic Sports Federation in promoting physical activity. To discourage smoking, the price of tobacco products is to be raised more than the average level of price increases. A new law introduced in 1996 restricts areas where people can smoke and increases the legal age for purchasing cigarettes by two years. To provide more effective prevention and treatment of alcohol-related problems, cooperation between the health authorities and nongovernmental organizations dealing with substance abuse has been increased. The price of alcoholic beverages has also been raised more than the average level of price increases. It is proposed that the price of spirits be increased more than those of wine and beer.

The Ministries of Health and Agriculture have cooperated in developing food pricing guidelines. The future emphasis will be on producing and supplying healthy food. Healthy choices will be facilitated by making available easily understood consumer information.

The Ministries of Health and of Transport have set up the Accident Prevention Council.

The Ministries of Health and of Education have developed basic health promotion training and public health education for community health workers and hospital staff.

An Environmental Health Inspection Unit has been set up to monitor and control risk factors in the environment, particularly in relation to food safety. The emphasis on preventing exposure to the harmful effects of radiation. Efforts are also being made to reduce noise and the polluting effects of transport and industry, with emphasis on education and cooperation rather than directives from authorities. Other measures include the organization of urban planning so that people, especially older and handicapped people, can enjoy the environment, exercise and outdoor activities; and the development of a programme for occupational safety, noise control and reduction of the effects of hazardous substances in the workplace, with the cooperation of primary health care centres and workplaces.

The Ministries of Health and of Social Welfare have worked together to plan care and health services for elderly people.

Ireland

Demography, policy environment and health care system

Ireland lies in the Atlantic Ocean, separated from Great Britain by the Irish Sea to the east, and bordered to the north-east by Northern Ireland (United Kingdom). Ireland is a sovereign independent republic. Its Parliament exercises jurisdiction in 26 of the 32 counties of the island of Ireland.

In 1996 the population was 3.6 million. The average population density is 52 per km^2 (1996); 57% of the population live in urban areas (1993); 11.5% of the population are aged $\geq$ 65 years and 24% aged 0–14 years (1996); and the dependency ratio is 58% (1996).

In 1994 the mean income per person was US $13 530. In 1966 the inflation rate was 1.5% and the unemployment rate 11.9%.

In 1996 the infant mortality rate was 5.5 per 1000 live births, and in 1994 life expectancy at birth was 73.2 years for males and 78.7 years for females.

In 1994 health care expenditure comprised 6.9% of GDP.

The Government develops priorities for health and health care, which are then communicated through a devolved hierarchical system to local health boards or authorities. According to set criteria, residents with full eligibility for public health care (about one third of the population) are entitled to the whole range of public health and hospital services, free of charge for themselves and their dependants. Those with limited eligibility receive consultant care and hospital services free but are not entitled to general practitioner, dental or aural services.

Approach towards achieving health for all

A health strategy document, *Shaping a healthier future – a strategy for effective health care in the 1990s*, was approved by the Government and published in 1994. The main theme of the strategy is reorienting the system towards more effectiveness and efficiency by reshaping the way that health services are planned and delivered. The strategy is underpinned by the three principles of equity, quality of service and accountability.

Quantified targets are presented for reducing the risk factors associated with premature mortality and the incidence of cardiovascular diseases, cancer and accidents. Since the overall strategy was published,

issue-specific documents on health promotion, women's health and alcohol have also been published. There has also been a white paper on mental health; recommendations for a food and nutrition
policy; a national policy on breastfeeding; a national cancer strategy; a dental health action plan; a
report of a review group on health services for people with physical or mental disability; an
assessment of needs for services for people with a mental handicap; and a management development
strategy for health and personal services. The *Statement of strategy for the Department of Health*
published in 1997 is part of the continuing process first mapped out in *Shaping a healthier future* in
1994.

Focus on health outcomes and reorientation towards primary health care

The health strategy recognized that applying its principles of equity, quality of service and accountability
presupposes a comprehensive and high-quality database with information on needs, activities, costs and
outcomes. In this respect, the establishment of regional departments of public health, which are intended
to have a key role in the information area, is an important development. The establishment of these
departments, together with the ongoing development of the hospital inpatient enquiry and the Casemix
programme and the more recent developmental work on a public health information system, have laid the
foundation for a strong information base to assist in decision-making.

Consultants and general practitioners working together will undertake certain activities currently
undertaken by hospitals but more appropriate to the community setting. A number of group practices are
being established on a pilot basis, providing a range of primary health care services with close links to
hospital services. General practice units and departments of public health medicine are also being
established in each health board. Resources are to be made available on a phased basis to promote the
development of clinical audit and research, and the effectiveness of services will be monitored continually, taking both costs and outcomes into account.

Promotion of equity, public participation and intersectoral action

Equity
Numerous initiatives are promoting equity in health:

- the development of information systems, comprehensive population registers and demographic and
  health profiles to help identify needs;
- targeting health education programmes and community services to meet the needs of special groups
  such as travellers, and close monitoring of the impact of such programmes;
- uniform rules for eligibility and charges for services across Ireland;
- shorter waiting lists for public services to protect the most vulnerable groups;
- training programmes for those working with disadvantaged groups;
- the allocation of specific funds to reduce hospital waiting lists; and

- the enshrinement, in the Health Insurance Act 1994, of the principle of community rating, thereby safeguarding the right to private health insurance of those who are vulnerable through age or ill health.

Public participation

In preparing the strategy, account was taken of the submissions made through the formal consultative processes following the initial report of the Commission on Health Funding in 1989. Relevant groups were consulted regarding implementation of the action plan, which was an integral part of the strategy.

A number of measures have been introduced to encourage consumer participation, including:

- requiring all health authorities to put appropriate complaint procedures in place;
- developing charters for various client groups; and
- widely circulating a new guide entitled *Information guide to our health services.*

There is a comprehensive communication programme. Each health board has designated a health strategy coordinator to act as a contact during the implementation process. Advisory groups have been set up in each health authority area to provide input from the users of services. It is also planned to invest the boards of health authorities with a statutory function to channel to the ministers the views and concerns of their catchment populations. Until then, monitoring is restricted to reviewing the mechanisms to measure consumer satisfaction.

Intersectoral action

The Department of Health works with other sectors and groups such as:

- the Departments of Education and of the Environment in conjunction with community and statutory groups, to encourage participation in sports and to support the value of regular exercise;
- the Department of Education concerning nutrition in schools; and
- the Departments of Education, of Enterprise and of Employment to promote healthy lifestyles, the education and training of people with disabilities, and health and safety in the workplace.

Services for which the Departments of both Health and of Social Welfare are responsible will be improved and changes made to the organization of the Departments. Structures for health promotion have been revised, and a national consultative committee on health promotion has been established. Voluntary and professional organizations and self-help and mutual aid groups are involved in the process. A multisectoral approach towards accident prevention and a safer environment is being developed involving a wide range of agencies, and intersectoral coordination is in place to improve the investigation of child abuse. Regular interdepartmental meetings are held to ensure that the health implications of policies formulated by other public bodies are assessed fully.

Israel

Demography, policy environment and health care system

Israel became an independent democratic state in May 1948. The *Knesset* (Parliament) has 120 members. In 1995 there were 57 municipalities, 138 local councils and 54 regional councils.

In 1995 the population was 5.5 million. The average population density is 253 per km^2; 90% of the population live in urban areas (1995); 9% of the population are aged $\geq$ 65 years and 29% aged 0–14 years (1995); and the dependency ratio is 65% (1995).

In 1994 the mean income per person was US $14 500. The inflation rate is 10% and the unemployment rate 7% (1995). The lowest 10% of the population have a 5% share of income while the highest 10% have an 18% share (1994).

In 1995 the infant mortality rate was 6.8 per 1000 live births. In 1994 the average life expectancy at birth was 75.5 years for men and 79.4 years for women.

In 1993 total health expenditure accounted for 4% of estimated GDP.

Approach towards achieving health for all

Israel is currently formulating an overall health for all policy based on a draft document prepared in 1994. The preliminary draft has been revised several times. A women's health committee recently proposed that issues concerning elderly people and women's health should be expanded, and a revised policy is due to be presented to Parliament in the near future.

Focus on health outcomes and reorientation towards primary health care

According to the draft policy document, primary health care will include health promotion and protection, disease prevention, medical care and rehabilitation. It is recognized that reorienting towards primary health care will involve restructuring secondary and tertiary care. Incentives will be provided to encourage hospitals to support the other levels of the health care system. The Ministry of Health is also working with other groups and sectors such as the Society of Family Medicine to promote coordination between the primary health care sector and the secondary and tertiary levels.

Primary health care is provided through independent physician's practices and family health centres. The network of primary health care facilities has gradually widened. The reorientation to primary health care has been facilitated by the WHO CINDI (countrywide integrated noncommunicable diseases intervention) programme, which in 1995 focused on initiatives to control cardiovascular risk factors. Goals included the publication of guidelines on preventive practice, training of primary health care teams, programmes for the prevention of cardiovascular risk factors, lifestyle management of risk factors, and controlling hypertension without drugs.

Training and education in primary health care has been increased, and physicians and nurses from 120 primary care clinics have already been trained and are intended as role models. As part of this effort, a document on preventive practice was disseminated to all general practitioners.

Cost–effectiveness and improving efficiency are being emphasized more, although the development of information systems and use of health outcomes as a basis for planning the health care system do not yet appear to be the main priorities.

Promotion of equity, public participation and intersectoral action

Equity
The National Health Insurance Law of 1995 ensures equal access to health services for the entire population. Particular attention is devoted to ensuring a reduction in the gaps in health status between population groups such as immigrants, minority groups and those living in underprivileged areas. The current draft policy document makes specific reference to the wider socioeconomic determinants of health, such as housing, unemployment, income and education. Lack of formal education is highlighted as an important source of inequity. The document refers to the prevalence of certain behavioural patterns among certain population groups; for example, the level of smoking was found to be higher among Arabs.

Measures to promote equity in health include: consumer choice between sickness funds, criteria for allocating funds according to weighted capitation and decentralization of hospitals.

Public participation
The Patients' Rights Act of 1996 protects patients' interests (including confidentiality). The new policy refers to people's right to participate actively in health care decisions. It is proposed that the level of public debate in the mass media be increased to inform people of their rights.

Intersectoral action
The new policy has been drafted on the basis of a government agreement to foster coordinated action by all sectors. Government approval should ensure maximum support for implementation of the plan.

The policy focuses on lifestyles, especially on smoking cessation, nutrition and physical activity, avoiding overexposure to the sun, limiting alcohol intake and changing behaviour by increasing awareness and health education. The Ministries of Health and of Education will work together to implement health education programmes. Health promotion is seen to be the responsibility of everyone working within and outside the health sector, including the mass media. A Health Education Department has been established within the Ministry of Health, and training courses in community medicine and health promotion are being run for health professionals.

The new policy strongly emphasizes the use of such settings as schools, work environments, community centres and army bases to tackle such challenges as smoking and environmental protection. Legislative measures to promote healthier lifestyles include a ban on smoking in public places and workplaces and a warning label on cigarette packets. Environmental legislation (drawn up in consultation with the Ministry of the Environment) has been passed on the collection and recycling of waste, the wearing of safety belts in cars and the use of lead-free fuel.

Intersectoral bodies and mechanisms include:

- a committee with representatives from the Ministry of Health, the sickness funds and the Israeli Defence Force to promote healthy lifestyles, with special attention to immigrants' needs;
- district health and welfare centres consulting on the coordination of care of elderly people in the community;
- the Ministries of Agriculture, of Trade and of Industry consulting to ensure the availability of foods low in animal fat and obligatory food labelling; and
- the Ministries of the Environment and of Health collaborating in drafting environmental legislation.

Italy

Demography, policy environment and health care system

Italy is bordered by Austria and Switzerland to the north, by Slovenia and the Adriatic Sea to the east, by the Ionian Sea to the south-east, by the Mediterranean Sea to the south, by the Tyrrhenian and Ligurian Seas to the south-west and by France to the west. Italy is administratively divided into 20 autonomous regions (5 with special statute), subdivided into 94 provinces and 1230 municipalities.

In 1995 the population was 57 million. The average population density is 190 per km^2; 67% of the population live in urban areas (1993); 17% of the population are aged ≥ 65 years and 15% aged 0–14 years (1995); and the dependency ratio is 45% (1995).

In 1994 the mean income per person was US $19 500. The inflation rate is 2% and the unemployment rate 12% (1997). The lowest 20% of the population have a 7% share of income while the highest 20% have a 22% share (1986).

In 1993 the infant mortality rate was 7.3 per 1000 live births. In 1995 the average life expectancy at birth was 74.1 years for men and 80.5 years for women.

In 1995 total health expenditure accounted for 8% of estimated GDP.

The provision of health services through the Servizio Sanitario Nazionale (SSN) (National Health Service) is a regional responsibility, operationally managed at the local level by the local health authorities, with funding set and distributed by the Government. Health care provided by the SSN is financed mainly through contributions (53% in 1995) and general taxation (40%). SSN providers are mainly public: 87% of 1994 hospital expenditure went to public providers, as well as 67% of expenditure for diagnostic tests and 40% of expenditure for specialist care. General practitioners, paediatricians and pharmacies are under contract to SSN.

Approach towards achieving health for all

In Italy, a formal national health planning system was installed at the same time as the SSN was established in 1978. It was intended that a strategic health plan would be produced every three years and presented to Parliament, providing a framework for the development of regional and local plans. Due to a lack of parliamentary consensus on health policy directions, however, the process was delayed and the first national health plan was first agreed in 1993, following major restructuring of the political system and reform of the SSN. The new plan identifies a number of priority areas and sets basic standards of health care that must be met in all regions. Priority areas set in the National Health Plan for 1994–1996 included maternal and child health, care of the elderly, mental health, cancer prevention and treatment, organ transplants and chronic kidney disease.

Focus on health outcomes and reorientation towards primary health care

Primary health care services are well established in Italy. General practice and paediatric services are available to all, free of charge and/or by co-payment, either at the practice or at home.

Allocation of financial resources to regions is based on a per person quota according to uniform levels of service for any person in any part of Italy. Regions can provide services above these standards, but must pay any additional expenditure from their own resources. Public health reporting is used to define objectives and to assign resources on a regional basis. The effectiveness of different clinical interventions is being increasingly measured, and the results form the basis for policy decisions.

Promotion of equity, public participation and intersectoral action

Equity

The SSN guarantees equal access to health services. It aims to eliminate territorial differences and to establish uniform health care services throughout Italy. Establishment of the SSN has helped to eradicate inequalities under the previous system whereby the former health insurance bodies maintained different standards according to the various classes of insured workers. General practitioner and paediatrician consultations and hospital care are free, whereas prescribed drugs (since 1998), specialist consultations (since 1986) and laboratory and radiological diagnosis services (since 1982) are subject to co-payment.

Public participation

Public awareness has been growing since 1994 of health risks and problems and intensive information campaigns involving the mass media have been launched at the national level to promote health. In 1992, legislation was introduced endorsing the promotion of community participation and the safeguarding of citizens' rights. Italy is represented in the WHO European Network of Health Promoting Schools, which supports children developing skills of participatory decision-making and consensus- building from a young age. Since 1986, people's awareness of environmental health has increased greatly, as demonstrated by the rising number of nongovernmental organizations focusing on such issues. National referenda have been called on a number of issues, including the peaceful use of nuclear energy, the use of pesticides in agriculture and the separation of local environmental services from local health services. The latter has resulted in extensive reorganization of these sectors.

Intersectoral action

Following some initial institutional difficulties, which were successfully overcome, the health-promoting schools project is implemented jointly by the Ministries of Health and of Education.

Population-based education campaigns have been initiated in environment and health, lifestyles (tobacco and drug use, AIDS and nutrition), health protection at work and the prevention of infectious diseases. A health promotion unit has been set up within the Department of Health to promote healthy behaviour in all these areas.

The establishment of the Ministry of the Environment in 1986 was a turning point for the development of environmental policy. The Ministry of the Environment was given lead responsibility for most environmental health issues, whereas the Ministry for Health maintained the lead role in relation to drinking-water and bathing water. An intersectoral committee for the environment was also established, which led eventually to increased resources for environmental health, updating of regulations, development of plans and programmes, and reorganization of the structures responsible for the environment at the local level. The national budget for environmental health increased, although this decreased again in 1993 as a result of economic crisis. The areas in which regulations have been updated since 1986 include water protection, waste disposal, air pollution, noise, environmental health impact assessment, industrial risks and soil protection.

Economic measures to promote a healthier environment include a tax on waste production and disposal, fees on refuse collection and on refuse bags, and lower prices for unleaded fuel. The Ministry of the Environment is working with regional bodies in the areas of soil reclamation; establishment of parks and marine reserves; support for local communities to build wastewater treatment and waste disposal plants; improved monitoring of pollutants; and technological research on risk factors. Monitoring is also carried out in relation to health and hygiene in homes, schools and workplaces; prevention of diseases of animal origin; and health and hygiene as it relates to food and drink at all stages of production.

Finally, in 1994 the Italian National Environmental Protection Agency was established. Challenges for the future include air pollution; the shortage of high-quality drinking-water; the shortage of waste disposal plants; industrial risks; traffic accidents; radon in homes; and chemical contaminants.

Kazakhstan

Demography, policy environment and health care system

Kazakhstan is bordered to the west by the Caspian Sea, by the Russian Federation to the north and west, by China to the east, and Kyrgyzstan and Uzbekistan to the south. Kazakhstan gained full independence in December 1991, and a new Constitution was adopted in January 1993. Parliament consists of a Senate with 47 members. The country is divided into 14 provinces. There are 82 towns, 197 urban settlements and 221 rural districts.

In 1997 the population was 16.4 million. The average population density is 6 per km^2; 56% of the population live in urban areas; and 7% of the population are aged $\geq$ 65 years and 30% aged 0–14 years (1997).

In 1994 the mean income per person was US $561. The inflation rate is 24% (1996) and the unemployment rate is 1% (1993). The poorest 10% of the population receive 3% of the income while the most affluent 10% receive 25% of the income.

In 1997 the infant mortality rate was 25.3 per 1000 live births, while in 1995 life expectancy at birth was 65 years.

In 1991 health care expenditure comprised 4.4% of GDP.

Kazakhstan has a centralized health care system in which the state owns and funds all health services. The health administration is organized around the 14 provinces. In 1993, the Law on Local Authorities attempted to decentralize power to the local authorities, but this was not successful, and efforts are being made to recentralize power to the central Government again.

Approach towards achieving health for all

Kazakhstan does not yet have an overall policy for health for all, but the process of social and economic development has emphasized broad policies for health care. As part of this initiative, a draft programme for reforming the health care system has been prepared. Consultation on the document is not planned, nor is it usual for the Senate to discuss such documents. Plans for an insurance-based system have been delayed because of inadequate training of health authorities and health personnel, and of difficulties in reorganization and in reducing the existing number of hospital beds.

Focus on health outcomes and reorientation towards primary health care

Previously, central funds financed large-scale construction of hospitals and the training of physicians and other health professionals. Financing of care was based on such factors as the number of beds and length of stay, with the result that hospitals tried to increase the number of beds beyond what was needed, leading to a structural distortion away from primary health care. As in most countries in the first stages of economic transition towards a market economy, the revenue available to finance existing health services has declined. One of the main tasks of health care reform is to redress the structural imbalance between primary and secondary care, but plans are still in the very early stages, with some districts initiating the process by first shifting to a general practitioner system.

There is no real tradition of orientation towards health outcome, but plans to strengthen the information system and to establish a school of public health are expected to facilitate moves in this direction.

Promotion of equity, public participation and intersectoral action

Equity

Under the previous Soviet model, relatively good health care was available to the entire population. Since the sector was well financed, efficient distribution of resources seemed less pressing. The present growth of such diseases as tuberculosis, diphtheria, dysentery and sexually transmitted diseases is linked to the numerous prevalent socioeconomic problems. The collapse of the social support system and the decline in real income pose a serious challenge to people's health. Consistently high levels of mortality in the northern provinces require particular attention. The state pays a special allowance to large families (those with four or more children), but this generally inadequate to meet basic needs.

Plans to introduce compulsory health insurance and fee-for-service medicine could also endanger access to health services, although an equalization fund will be established to provide additional resources to poorer provinces with the 1995 Health Insurance Law.

Public participation

Adequate information is a vital prerequisite for empowering people to make decisions affecting their health and wellbeing. Among the earliest laws passed, therefore, was the Law on the Press, which prohibited government control over the mass media. Since then, the independent press and television has developed rapidly, although progress has been hampered by the fact that broadcasting equipment tends to be outdated. In 1993, recognition of the International Bill of Human Rights granted Kazakh citizens economic, social, cultural, civil and political rights. This has become an important part of the social fabric, although the initial dream that democracy would solve many burning issues has given way to more practical concerns of basic survival.

Intersectoral action

Some of the most pressing challenges stem from health-damaging behaviour. Smoking and alcohol use are serious risk factors, especially for men, and about 16% of the population are overweight. Under the WHO CINDI (countrywide integrated noncommunicable diseases intervention) programme, screening has been introduced in pilot districts to assess the prevalence of noncommunicable diseases and their risk factors. The results will be used as the basis for a new health care model.

Environmental problems also pose a serious challenge. In the past, large industrial complexes were developed without regard for their effect on the environment, and today more than one third do not have standard protective zones. Supplies of safe drinking-water and wastewater disposal systems are inadequate. Certain heavily polluted areas have higher rates of disease. A number of international bodies have recently begun to address the problems, and in 1993 the International Fund for Saving the Aral Sea was founded. Nuclear testing in the Semipalatinsk region has also given cause for grave concern. In an attempt to clean up the environment, in 1991 the Government passed the Law on Environmental Conservation, and the Commission on the Conservation of Biological Diversity was established.

Present economic difficulties have given rise to a poor food supply system, resulting in restricted access to many basic foods. Poor hygiene and unsanitary conditions in the food-processing industry and public catering enterprises result in contaminated products; many dairies are bacterially contaminated. The number of state-financed dwellings has declined, and the private sector is not sufficiently well established to satisfy the growing demand for housing. The situation is especially serious for young families.

To help reduce growing levels of crime, the Law on State Support for Entrepreneurship for Youth was introduced to encourage business opportunities for young people by offering tax concessions and loans for businesses, housing, transportation and credits for education. Nevertheless, the implementation of the law has been postponed because of the economic crisis.

Kyrgyzstan

Demography, policy environment and health care system

Kyrgyzstan is situated in the Tienshan mountains, bordered to the north by Kazakhstan, to the west by Kazakhstan and Uzbekistan, to the south by Tajikistan and to the east by China. Kyrgyzstan gained independence in 1991. The country is divided into six *oblasts* (provinces), each having several *rayons* (districts), beneath which are the village administrations. Kyrgyzstan has a multiethnic population (about 53% Kyrgyz, 21% Russian and 26% others).

In 1994 the population was 4.4 million. The average population density is 22 per km^2 (1995); 39% of the population live in urban areas (1994); 6% of the population are aged ≥ 65 years and 38% aged 0–14 years (1995); and the dependency ratio is 75% (1995).

In 1994 the mean income per person was US $630. The inflation rate is 284% (1994). The poorest 40% of the population have a 10% share of income while the most affluent 20% have a 57% share (1994).

In 1995 the infant mortality rate was 27.7 per 1000 live births and the average life expectancy at birth is 65.4 years.

The main actors involved in managing health services are the Ministry of Health, the Ministry of Finance and the *oblast* health administrations. The main source of funding is taxation, as it was under the previous Soviet system. Severe economic difficulties have reduced the health care budget to about 10–15% of what it was under the Soviet system. There are plans to introduce a social insurance system once the economic situation has stabilized.

Approach towards achieving health for all

The economic potential of the country is low and industry has only recently started to develop. Many basic commodities and services are inadequate. Despite the serious problems caused by transition from a centrally planned to a market economy an overall health policy document, *State programme for a healthy nation (1994–2000)*, has been published. The document clearly states that health policy needs to be integrated into overall socioeconomic policy and outlines the following key principles:

- equity, participation, cooperation and partnerships at all levels;
- intersectorality and pragmatism, taking account of limited resources and the need to set priorities;

- maintenance of a degree of continuity with past achievements; and
- adoption of and adherence to international norms.

A number of priority areas have been agreed on, including the family, maternal and child health, the environment, safe drinking-water and healthy lifestyles, and targets have been set in these areas. The document defines the agencies responsible for implementing the policy measures, sets time frames for their implementation, and defines sources of funding. The policy is a long-term initiative; however, other medium- to short-term initiatives have been developed to help achieve those objectives. These include health care reforms, policy documents on immunoprophylaxis and drugs, and a national environmental health action plan.

Focus on health outcomes and reorientation towards primary health care

One of the medium-term initiatives is the MANAS health care reform programme, which has been drawn up according to the principles of health for all and is to guide health care reforms, bringing together health and health care personnel, the major donors (the World Bank, the Turkish International Development Agency, Overseas Development Assistance of Japan, UNDP, UNICEF and the US Agency for International Development) and others to coordinate the work. Decisive reforms often come about as a result of action by key people, and political leaders in Kyrgyzstan have played an important role in promoting health care issues.

Under the Soviet system, a sizeable health care budget was used to carry out large- scale construction of hospitals and to train large numbers of workers, physicians and other health professionals. The system of financing led to a structural distortion in the balance of care, with hospitals favoured over primary care. One of the main tasks of the current reforms is to redress this structural imbalance and to strengthen primary health care facilities through such measures as:

- reducing the number of hospital referrals;
- introducing a formula for geographical allocation of resources;
- reimbursing primary health care facilities based on capitation;
- introducing comprehensive primary health care training for health personnel and retraining of existing specialists as general practitioners; and
- establishing a system of family physicians.

There is no real tradition of orientation towards health outcome, but strengthening the epidemiological information for policy-makers should lead to some improvements. The curricula for medical education will focus on this more in the future.

Promotion of equity, public participation and intersectoral action

Equity
Under the previous comparatively well funded system, relatively good health care was available to the entire population. In 1993, a new Constitution was adopted that states that "Citizens of Kyrgyzstan shall

enjoy the right to protection of health and shall benefit freely from the network of state public health institutions". Diminishing resources, however, have necessitated the introduction of fees for some services. In 1994, a Ministry of Health order introduced user fees at health facilities; the same order identifies vulnerable groups who are exempted from paying fees. In terms of the broader socioeconomic determinants of health, legislation defining a minimum wage exists but is not enforced in practice. Similarly, the *State programme for a healthy nation (1994–2000)* outlined a number of measures to promote greater equity in health, including:

- providing low-income families with a minimum health care package;
- reducing inequitable distribution by establishing regional primary health care services; and
- providing food and clothing for groups of lower socioeconomic status.

Nevertheless, the poor economic situation means that many initiatives never move beyond good intentions. The MANAS plan will attempt to redress some of the inequities inherited from the Soviet system and differences in the levels of services between urban and rural areas. The impact of the new reforms on equity will be monitored.

Public participation

Under the Soviet system, public participation was not very common. Professional and voluntary organizations are relatively new and have not been traditionally involved in policy-making. An inherent weakness of the recent document on health policy is the failure to describe the process by which policy is to be adopted by the population, health professionals and other sectors. The policy was developed by high-level officials, but the process was not extended to field-level personnel who should have the most active role in its implementation. The MANAS initiative plans to introduce consumer satisfaction surveys as one means of monitoring and evaluating the health care reforms. Increasing the role of professional associations and, in the longer term, users in hospital management is also planned.

Intersectoral action

An intersectoral commission was set up to oversee the initial formulation of the health policy document, the Cabinet of Ministers (also intersectoral) discussed the proposed legislation and plans, and a coordination board was established (headed by the Deputy Prime Minister and consisting of the Ministries of Finance, Economics, Environment, Media, Trade Unions and Health) to oversee its implementation. The policy document itself outlines a number of initiatives aimed at improving health status that require collaboration with other sectors to be successful, such as environmental controls or initiatives aimed at promoting safe conditions at work and preventing accidents, which can best be achieved with the help of employers' organizations and trade unions. It is not clear, however, how this intersectoral collaboration is to be achieved and who has responsibility for the overall coordination.

In general terms, the Ministry of Health is restricted by the fact that the Ministry of Finance has sole responsibility for budgeting and resource allocation. The Ministry of Health has the main responsibility for health, but it is not involved in the budgetary process, and this can sometimes lead to discrepancies between the goals and priorities sets by the two ministries.

Latvia

Demography, policy environment and health care system

Latvia is located on the eastern Baltic coast, bordered by Estonia to the north, the Russian Federation to the east, Lithuania to the south and Belarus to the south-west. Latvia regained independence from the Soviet Union in 1991. The Parliament (*Saeima*) has 100 members elected for a three-year term. Since 1993, power has been decentralized to 33 municipal councils, all local self-governing units.

In 1995 the population was 2.5 million. The average population density is 40 per km^2 and about 72% of the population live in urban areas (1994); 13% of the population are aged $\geq$ 65 years (1994) and 21% aged 0–14 years (1995); and the dependency ratio is 51% (1995).

In 1993 the mean income per person was US $1765. The inflation rate is 36% and the unemployment rate 6.5% (1994). The poorest 10% of the population receive 4% of the income, and the most affluent 10% receive 22% (1993).

In 1995 the infant mortality rate was 15.7 per 1000 live births and life expectancy at birth was 65.4 years.

The health care system consists of primary and secondary health care provided by local government (the Basic Care Programme) and specialized tertiary care provided by the state (the State Programme of Medical Care).

Approach towards achieving health for all

Latvia has one of the shortest life expectancies at birth in Europe for both men and women. Infant mortality reached alarming proportions in 1993, and there are rising levels of alcoholism, suicide (especially among men) and communicable diseases, especially tuberculosis caused by poor socioeconomic conditions. Rates of sexually transmitted diseases also increased dramatically between 1990 and 1993. In 1993, the Council of Ministers passed a decree declaring maternal and child health, cancer, mental illness, respiratory illness, cardiovascular and infectious diseases, AIDS, diabetes and accident prevention as priorities. In 1994, the objectives of a new health policy were established during the conference Better Living, Better Latvia - a Strategy for Health and Social Care Development. The principles underlying the policy document generally reflect health for all objectives and principles. An action plan is being prepared.

A number of issue-specific policies have been developed in maternal and child care, alcohol and tobacco consumption, AIDS, communicable diseases, mental health, rehabilitation services, tuberculosis, chronic renal failure, cancer, cardiovascular diseases and stroke prevention. Plans are under way for the development of a national programme on family planning and sexual health.

Focus on health outcomes and reorientation towards primary health care

The main objective of Better Living, Better Latvia was to reorient health care services towards primary health care, marking a shift from a previously medically oriented system to one more focused on health.

Measures aimed at reorienting towards primary health care services include:

- the offer of a choice of family physician;
- training in primary health care for general practitioners; and
- introduction of the community health nurse responsible for health care and health promotion at the municipal level, working with community groups and other nongovernmental as well as governmental organizations.

It is planned to move Latvia towards an insurance-based health care system. Currently each district has a choice of two models. Physicians are paid fees for services or through a system of capitation. Future plans include promoting a gatekeeper role for general practitioners and primary health care based on a contracted individual or group practice model and an expanded range of services, but progress has been hampered by economic and political instability.

Promotion of equity, public participation and intersectoral action

Equity
The transition to a market economy has had serious repercussions, with high levels of inflation and unemployment and rising poverty. The Government has therefore exempted low-income groups from taxes and, within budgetary constraints, pension funds, unemployment benefits and other social benefits have been made available. All Latvian citizens and permanent residents are entitled to free health care. Others, such as illegal immigrants, are only eligible for emergency care.

Access to care is equal in theory and according to law. In practice it cannot be guaranteed, largely because different local governments have different levels of resources. To counteract this, the Equalization Fund for Local Self-Government has been set up, but this not adequate to cover all the differences. Although free choice of physician is guaranteed under the new law, in practice only those living in cities have this choice, since there are too few to choose from in rural areas. Similarly, modern hospital equipment tends to be located in central areas. Therefore, the state as a whole supports services based in Riga that are not accessible to the rest of the population. High co-payments exacerbate inequity. There have been few attempts to use such policy instruments as health education or research and development to target inequity or to monitor population health status according to socioeconomic group.

Public participation
The Ministry of Welfare drafted, finalized and disseminated an overall health policy document to a number of interest groups for consultation. It was not discussed in Parliament, although it was presented to a ministerial cabinet as is usual in Latvia.

The health care reforms were largely initiated by the Latvian Physicians' Association, which was re-established in 1988 and played a major part in initiating changes in the wider social environment. Users of health care have not yet played much of a role. Since 1993, the Government has implemented some essential mechanisms for moving to a more democratic system, including decentralizing power to local governments, which are taking more responsibility for the health of their populations. People are also being encouraged to take more responsibility for their own health, and a programme to inform citizens of their rights has been established. The mass media are being used to develop campaigns on health promotion and disease prevention. There have been some efforts to train groups of health professionals so that they have the skills necessary to respond appropriately to the needs of certain groups, such as training social workers in dealing with mentally ill people. The Ministry of Welfare has been broadening its horizons in terms of participation from the traditional actors to groups outside the health care sector. Nongovernmental organizations play an important role in providing assistance to those who are socially and economically disadvantaged, but involvement tends to be in implementation rather than in policy formulation, and as charities rather than representatives of patients' interests.

Intersectoral action
In 1993, the Ministries of Health, of Labour and of Social Welfare merged to become the Ministry of Welfare, the objective being to promote intersectoral cooperation and avoid bureaucratic barriers. The Ministry of Welfare has four departments dealing with health, environmental health, pharmaceuticals and narcotics and aims to take an integrative approach to health issues. Environmental pollution is a serious problem and has been cited as one of the key causes of cancer of the digestive tract and intestines. The air is polluted, drinking-water is insufficiently purified (about 20% of the population do not have access to clean drinking-water), pesticides and fertilizers are used inappropriately, and the quality of food products has been adversely affected by soil contamination. Serious measures to control food quality are required.

The Environmental Health Department is responsible for controlling communicable diseases. A national integrated programme on environment and health is being developed that includes communicable diseases. A national environment health action plan is being developed. The Ministry of Welfare has also been cooperating with other sectors, including setting standards for advertising alcohol and tobacco products, involving consultation with the Ministry of Finance; monitoring alcohol consumption through the state programme for alcohol, drug and tobacco abuse; and planning the social care and health care budget with the Department of Welfare and Social Affairs.

Lithuania

Demography, policy environment and health care system

Lithuania is situated on the eastern Baltic coast. It is bordered by Belarus to the east, by Latvia to the north and by Poland and the Kaliningrad exclave to the south. In March 1990 Lithuania declared its independence from the Soviet Union. There are 56 local self-governing councils elected every two years, and 10 district advisory councils comprising the mayors of the local councils.

In 1995 the population was 3.7 million. The average population density is 56.9 per km^2 and 68.1% of the population live in urban areas (1994). In 1995 12.43% of the population was aged $\geq$ 65 years and 21.24% aged 0–14 years, and the dependency ratio was 51.3%.

In 1993 the mean income per person was US $1162. The inflation rate is 13.1% and the unemployment rate is 6.2% (1996). The poorest 10% of the population receive 3.4% of the income, and the most affluent 10% receive 28% of the income (1993).

In 1996 the infant mortality rate was 10 per 1000 live births and life expectancy at birth was 70.6 years.

In 1996 health care expenditure comprised 4.3% of GDP.

Statutory health insurance was introduced on 1 July 1997 and is administered by one state health insurance company and 10 regional companies. As an additional service, there are many voluntary health insurance companies. There is social insurance, which is administered by the State Social Insurance Agency and supervised by a tripartite council consisting of representatives of the Government, the trade unions and employer organizations.

Approach towards achieving health for all

See the case study on Lithuania, page 82.

Luxembourg

Demography, policy environment and health care system

Luxembourg is bordered to the west by Belgium, to the south by France and to the east by Germany. This relatively small country is a constitutional monarchy administratively divided into four electoral districts. The Chamber of Deputies (Parliament) has 60 members.

In 1995 the population was 410 000. The average population density is 157 per km^2; 89% of the population live in urban areas (1994); and 14% of the population are aged $\geq$ 65 years and 18.4% aged 0–14 years (1995).

In 1994 the mean income per person was US $39 850. In 1995 the inflation rate is 1.4% and the unemployment rate is 3%.

In 1995 the infant mortality rate was 5.5 per 1000 live births and the life expectancy at birth was 77.4 years.

In 1993 health care expenditure comprised 6.9% of GDP.

The health care system is financed mainly through social insurance, with mixed public and private providers.

Approach towards achieving health for all

Luxembourg's approach towards health for all is encapsulated in an overall policy for health, *Santé pour tous*, published in 1994, which proposes integrated and multisectoral action for health. *Santé pour tous* presents the main health problems and risk factors and addresses a number of priorities, especially reducing cardiovascular diseases and cancer. The strategy aims to reduce premature and avoidable deaths and improve the health status of the population, and sets precise objectives and targets.

Focus on health outcomes and reorientation towards primary health care

In Luxembourg, preventive medicine is on a relatively sound footing and was established formally in the early 1980s. Primary health care services are well established and accessible to everyone. The orientation to health outcomes is not quite so well grounded, but research on health status is increasingly being used to direct policy decisions. Moreover, the focus is no longer just on disease but also on the effect of other factors such as quality of life and psychosocial environment, as *Santé pour tous* demonstrates.

Promotion of equity, public participation and intersectoral action

Equity
The entire population has access to primary, secondary and tertiary care, either through compulsory membership of the health insurance scheme as employees or co-insured persons, through voluntary insurance, or through compulsory insurance as part of the guaranteed minimum income (under the Act of 26 July 1986 on combating poverty). There is little information on differences in health status according to socioeconomic group. The health information system is being developed to compile this type of information.

Public participation
Wide consultation was carried out in preparing *Santé pour tous*, involving discussions with a parliamentary committee, a working group and a multidisciplinary task force. Nevertheless, despite the involvement of many professional groups in formulating the policy, no concerted effort was made to involve the public. In Luxembourg, representation generally (not just for health for all) tends to be quite formal, such as through the sickness funds. This type of formal participation is facilitated by the fact that representatives of policy-holders, employers and trade unions sit together on management committees of health insurance funds. Joint programmes have been developed between the health insurance organizations and the Department of Health (under the Ministry of Health) that involve employers in developing prevention programmes they will then support. Trade unions are an important partner in the policy-making process in Luxembourg and, as such, are a vehicle for representing the interests of consumers. Government subsidies to consumer groups aim to promote a wider expression of health interests.

Intersectoral action
The Ministry of Health and the Ministry of Social Security are responsible for health. Other ministries are also involved in health care decisions: the Ministries of Finance, Education (training of health professionals), Economic Affairs (determination of prices), the Interior (public health and emergency aid) and Family Welfare (services for elderly people and handicapped people).

In Luxembourg, policy-makers have drawn on a wide variety of policy instruments to support intersectoral action. Legislative measures include controls on environmental pollution, quality control on foodstuffs, vehicular speed limits and restrictions on alcohol both in relation to driving and at the workplace. Special occupational health legislation has been introduced, and workplaces must comply with EU Directive 89/391 on health and safety at work and the provision of occupational health services.

Attention is focused on risk factors arising from lifestyles and links to cardiovascular diseases, the nutritional status of the population, physical exercise, population groups at risk of suicide, ultraviolet light and skin cancer, causes of accidents and workers most at risk, and the risks posed by dangerous products.

A settings approach has been adopted to promote healthy lifestyles. Various guidelines have been produced on lifestyle issues, and such institutions as schools, hospitals and workplaces are encouraged to adopt these guidelines.

The Ministry of Health has consulted with a number of other ministries on programmes for elderly people, workers, young people and women, and with groups outside the health care sector such as food manufacturers to promote healthy foods (for example, low-fat dairy products and whole-grain breads). The National Advisory Committee on Ethics for the Life and Health Sciences has been set up within the Ministry of State but depends administratively on the Ministry of Culture. This government body advises on the ethical aspects of the life and health sciences as well as solutions and measures to be implemented.

Financial measures have mainly been directed at reducing smoking and promoting health generally. This has meant specific allocation of funds towards health promotion and increasing taxes on tobacco. The impact of nutrition policies is also being evaluated.

Malta

Demography, policy environment and health care system

The three Maltese islands and minor islets lie in the Mediterranean Sea 93 km (at the nearest point) south of Sicily and 288 km east of Tunisia. Malta became independent in September 1964. The Constitution provides for a President and House of Representatives. The country is divided into 67 local councils.

In 1996 the population was 370 000. The average population density is 1183 per km^2 (1996); there is no real distinction between urban and rural areas. In 1996 12% of the population were aged $\geq$ 65 years and 22% aged 0–14 years, and the dependency ratio was 46%.

In 1996 the mean income per person was US $6800, the inflation rate was 2.5% and the unemployment rate was 4.3%.

In 1996 the infant mortality rate was 10.7 per 1000 live births (the national figures include all registrations, even when birth weight is below 500 g) and average life expectancy at birth was 74.9 years for men and 80 years for females.

Total health expenditure accounts for 10.3% of estimated GDP.

The Government provides comprehensive health services, funded by general taxation, that are free of charge at the point of delivery. All residents have access to preventive, investigative, curative and rehabilitative services in government health centres and hospitals. People with low income are entitled to free pharmaceuticals. Moreover, people who suffer from one or more of a number of chronic diseases are entitled to free treatment, irrespective of financial means. Private health services exist in addition to the government service.

Approach towards achieving health for all

See the case study on Malta, page 94.

Monaco

Demography, policy environment and health care system

The Principality of Monaco comprises 195 hectares located in the extreme south-east of France. The coastline is 4.1 km long. The Principality is a hereditary and constitutional monarchy, the Prince embodying the Monegasque State both abroad and within the country. He represents the Principality in its relations with foreign powers. Government functions are exercised by a Minister of State, who represents the Prince and is assisted by a Government Council. The National Council – the elected assembly – consists of 18 members elected for five years by direct universal suffrage. It adopts the national budget and legislation.

In 1990 the population was 30 000. The average population density is 15 800 per km^2 (1990); 22% of the population are aged $\geq$ 65 years and 12% aged 0–14 years (1990).

In 1996 the inflation rate was 1.7% and the unemployment rate 2.6%.

In 1996 the infant mortality rate was zero and average life expectancy at birth was 82 years.

Approach towards achieving health for all

The main categories of disease affecting the population are similar to those found in neighbouring countries: cardiovascular diseasess (40%) and malignant neoplasms (28%). Among communicable diseases, AIDS is a public health priority: the decline in the number of AIDS cases, which began in 1996, continued in 1997, owing in particular to the new treatments available in France and now also provided in Monaco.

Focus on health outcomes and reorientation towards primary health care

Hospital physicians collaborate in biomedical research initiated abroad, notably in France.

Monaco's health policy is mainly focused on prevention

- The 6000 schoolchildren in the Principality are given a medical and dental check-up each year.
- Health education is a priority in schools, with information campaigns regularly organized on AIDS, smoking and other topics. As from 1998, the health education and drug abuse control programme is being strengthened through the establishment of networks, etc.

- Child psychiatrists and paramedics provide services free of charge to schoolchildren with behavioural disorders.
- A centre for sports medicine offers free, regular check-ups to people who want to practise sport and take part in competitions.
- The 32 000 salaried employees have to undergo a check of their fitness for work before they are taken on; each salaried employee is given an annual medical check-up, with additional examinations as required.
- The Directorate of Health and Social Work organizes hygiene training courses for people working in the food sector. These courses, leading to a certificate, are entirely paid for by the state.
- The population is served by an anonymous and free AIDS case-finding centre, which monitors the health status of HIV-positive people at their request.
- A non-profit-making association carries out free screening for breast cancer for women aged 40–70 years.
- A unit for preventive health and social work ensures outpatient follow-up of people in difficulty who are affected by alcohol or drug abuse. This unit is responsible for administering methadone to drug addicts.

Promotion of equity, public participation and intersectoral action

Equity
Working or retired people have access to care in Monaco or France via the health insurance system, which is financed solely by contributions from employers. The patient's co-payment is always 20% regardless of the service provided. Insured people have a free choice of health service doctor.

People without insurance coverage are taken care of by a welfare organization that provides for their health care and gives them a monthly allowance. The budget allocated by the state to this public body is 9.12% of government expenditure.

Intersectoral action
Responsibilities in the social sector are shared between the Department of Public Works and Social Affairs (which oversees social security issues) and the Department of the Interior, under which comes the Directorate of Health and Social Work. The latter, in addition to its own activities in the health and social spheres, represents the Government in various other public health and social organizations such as hospitals, private clinics, homes for adolescents and social welfare institutions.

The work undertaken by the Directorate of Health and Social Work is in general organized in collaboration with the Director of National Education, Youth and Sports, especially concerning measures for young people or anti-doping measures in sport.

This Directorate also works with the Environment Service, which is responsible for urban hygiene. Particular attention is paid to the bacteriological quality of bathing water, to noise pollution of all kinds and to the quality of drinking-water. Facilities for the incineration of household refuse are equipped with a high-performance smoke filtration system.

Netherlands

Demography, policy environment and health care system

The Netherlands is bordered to the north and west by the North Sea, to the south by Belgium and to the east by Germany. The Netherlands is a constitutional and hereditary monarchy. The central executive power of the state rests with the Crown, while the central legislative power is vested in the Crown and Parliament. The country is divided into 12 provinces and 572 municipalities.

In 1997 the population was 15.6 million. The average population density is 457 per km^2; 82% of the population live in urban areas (1996); and 13% of the population are aged $\geq$ 65 years (1996) and 18% aged 0–14 years (1995).

In 1995 the mean income per person was US $17 500. The inflation rate is 2% and the unemployment rate is 7% (1996). The poorest 20% of the population have a 6% share of income while the most affluent 20% have a 38% share (1995).

In 1995 the infant mortality rate was 5.3 per 1000 live births and the average life expectancy at birth was 74.6 years for men and 80.3 years for women.

In 1996 total health expenditure accounted for 8% of estimated GDP.

The health care system in the Netherlands is characterized by a mix of public and private elements. The Government has a strong role in regulating the health care system, and private organizations are almost completely responsible for providing health care.

Approach towards achieving health for all

See the case study on the Netherlands, page 110.

Norway

Demography, policy environment and health care system

Norway is bordered by the Arctic Ocean to the north, by Finland, the Russian Federation and Sweden to the east, by the Skagerrak Straits to the south and by the North Sea to the west. Norway is a constitutional and hereditary monarchy. There are 19 counties divided into 435 municipalities.

In 1994 the population was 4.3 million. The average population density is 13 per km^2 and 73% of the population live in urban areas (1994); 16% of the population are aged ≥ 65 years and 19% aged 0–14 years (1994); and the dependency ratio is 54% (1994).

In 1993 the mean income per person was US $24 000. The inflation rate is 1% and the unemployment rate 5% (1994). The poorest 20% of the population have a 6% share of income while the most affluent 20% have a 37% share (1990).

In 1994 the infant mortality rate was 5.9 per 1000 live births and average life expectancy at birth was 78 years.

In 1993 total health expenditure accounted for 8% of estimated GDP.

The county councils are responsible for developing health plans, for managing hospitals and specialist and dental services and for granting funds for the treatment of drug and alcohol addiction. The municipalities are responsible for managing primary health care and social services (including nursing homes and care for elderly people) and allocating funds for health and social services.

Approach towards achieving health for all

In 1985, the Norwegian Government endorsed the European strategy for health for all. Since then, Norwegian health policies have been in line with the concepts and principles of health for all. In 1987, *Helse for alle i Norge?* [Health for all in Norway?] outlined 38 targets related to lifestyles, environment and health care. Responsibility for achieving these targets is spread across the national, regional and local levels. A parliamentary white paper, *Health policy towards the year 2000* (1987–1988), highlighted preventive health as one of the most important areas for the future. Action areas include health promotion, disease prevention, care and medical rehabilitation, and monitoring and evaluation. As the basis for developing a more comprehensive and active prevention policy, it was decided to prepare the strategy document *Fler gode leveår for alle – forebygningsstrategier* [Adding life to years – on strategies for prevention].

These documents incorporate the three areas of responsibility that come under the Ministry of Health and Social Affairs: health, social affairs and social security. The preventive interventions proposed cut across district boundaries, public and private areas of responsibility and administrative lines.

Other documents prepared by the Ministry of Health and Social Affairs and presented to Parliament include the Norwegian social insurance scheme.

Focus on health outcomes and reorientation towards primary health care

One of the main objectives is to divert more resources to primary health care services and to curb the growth of health care institutions. The Municipal Health Services Act (1984) assigned to municipalities the administrative responsibility for primary health care, which includes all services by general practitioners, nurses and physiotherapists. Other primary health care responsibilities include environmental health care and care of groups with special needs, such as the establishment of mother and child clinics. The county councils are responsible for hospital and other specialist health institutions, but debate has been increasing on whether responsibility should be shifted to the national level or to the municipal level, or whether a regional system based on the amalgamation of four or five counties should be established.

In recent years, Norway has increased primary health care training and joint education and training for health and non-health professionals, mostly those working in social care. The Ministry of Health and Social Affairs and the Ministry of Education and Research have cooperated in preparing these programmes. Advanced training of certain groups such as nurses' assistants has also been introduced, especially in care of elderly people and psychiatric services.

Norway was one of the first countries in the European Region of WHO to establish criteria for setting priorities. Increasing attention has been given to the effective use of resources and the use of health outcomes to allocate resources. Information on rates of disease and injury is also being used to define priorities and focus action. The Norwegian Institute of Public Health is the main body responsible for evidence-based research and effectiveness measures.

Promotion of equity, public participation and intersectoral action

Equity

The interpretation of equity in health is wide, encompassing not just access to health care services (to which everyone is legally entitled) but broader determinants such as education, income and housing. Health and welfare are seen to be very closely linked with the Norwegian social security scheme, providing a comprehensive social safety net in case of illness, unemployment and other conditions affecting people's opportunity to work and receive an adequate income. Since the social system is well developed, inequity is not as pronounced as in other countries but is still an issue of concern. Policy measures to promote equity include monitoring various types of inequity, financial intervention and training.

Special attention is being paid to gender inequity and a special committee has been established to oversee the development of health services for women. Research is being carried out on the implications of unemployment for health; the main focus, however, is currently on inequity according to urban or rural residence and on the health risks faced by children living in cities. New indicators are being developed to monitor changes in health status and the standard of living.

Concern about whether the welfare state can be sustained has led to reductions in social benefits, such as disability benefits. The range of diagnoses that justify payment of sickness benefit has been reduced and criteria for eligibility have been tightened. The number of disability pensioners declined slightly in 1992. It is too early to assess the results of these changes. Recent efforts have focused on levelling out resources (including personnel, places of treatment and costs) between municipalities and counties. Block grant allocations to county and municipal health services seem to have created a more equitable geographical distribution of resources.

Education and training for health personnel in the care of immigrants have been increased, and psychosocial teams are being established to deal with the needs of immigrants.

Public participation
There is a long tradition of community participation, linked to the great importance attached to health education. Various nongovernmental organizations, such as the Association of Patients, the Consumers' Council and those concerning specific diseases, receive government subsidies and are consulted regularly. In 1997, legislation to protect patients' rights was introduced. Ministries dealing with human rights, health, finance and the local community have been responsible for developing mechanisms to protect patients' rights.

Intersectoral action
The existence of one Ministry of Health and Social Affairs facilitates an intersectoral approach. The Municipal Health Services Act (1994) defines environmental health care as "all the factors known at any time to have a direct or indirect effect on health". Each municipality is responsible for public health and wellbeing and for creating supportive social and environmental conditions for health. Good examples of cooperation exist in accident prevention, nutrition policy and family health, but intersectoral action has largely been restricted to the traditional areas of lifestyles, environment and the social sector.

In 1993, three specific targets related to mental illness and psychosocial problems, musculoskeletal disease and accidents were adopted because they represent problems that are multicausal, originating between people and their environment. Strengthening social networks, local communities, schools and workplaces and the physical environment were emphasized to reduce the prevalence of risk factors for these diseases.

Other measures to promote intersectoral action include:

- research on health status and living conditions, risk factors, injuries, and the relationships between illness and social problems and between poor health and the working environment;
- monitoring and evaluating the impact of living conditions on health and quality of life and developing measures specifically for evaluating preventive activities;
- human resource development and training using a policy book on health for all in Norway, a textbook used in training most health professionals;
- consultation between relevant ministries to develop a safety culture and to reduce the number of injuries from accidents; the Labour Inspection Act ensures, for example, that the Ministry of Local Government monitors working environments;
- increasing the possibility of making healthy choices, limiting the availability of health-threatening factors such as tobacco and drugs and creating supportive health and social conditions as a means of preventing unnecessary stress and mental health, with special emphasis on gender differences;
- reducing socioeconomic, geographical and gender inequity by ensuring that people's basic financial needs are met;
- passing legislation to promote health: enforcing smoke-free environments, placing health warning labels on cigarette packets, banning the advertising of spirits, table wine and beer on television, radio, printed media and billboards, and raising the real price of alcohol since 1989–1994; and
- ensuring shared responsibility for some social services, such as care of the elderly and mental health services.

The health and social sectors have collaborated in providing home nursing and care in the community. In the early 1990s, health and social welfare clinics were integrated on an experimental basis. Services (mainly paying out pensions and unemployment benefit) were administered from the same building under common management. The experiment failed, however, as some elderly people were intimidated by having to attend the same premises as people addicted to drugs or alcohol.

Poland

Demography, policy environment and health care system

Poland is bordered by the Russian Federation and the Baltic Sea to the north, by Belarus, Lithuania and Ukraine to the east, by the Czech Republic and Slovakia to the south and by Germany to the west. The country is divided into 49 voivodships, and these in turn are divided into 845 towns and 2465 wards. In 1989, a democratic Government was elected.

In 1993 the population was 39 million. The average population density is 123 per km^2 and 64% of the population live in urban areas (1993). In 1993 11% of the population were aged $\geq$ 65 years and 23% aged 0–14 years and the dependency ratio was 53%.

In 1994 the mean income per person was US $2400. The inflation rate is 19% (1996) and the unemployment rate is 16% (1994). The poorest 10% of the population have a 4% share of income while the most affluent 10% have a 22% share (1992).

In 1995 the infant mortality rate was 13.6 per 1000 live births and the average life expectancy at birth was 72 years.

In 1993 total health expenditure accounted for 5% of estimated GDP.

The Ministry of Health and Welfare has the main responsibility for developing health policies, for monitoring health and pollution and providing medical and social services, for the clinical aspects of medical education and for research.

Approach towards achieving health for all

In 1983 Poland produced one of the first documents related to health for all in central and eastern Europe: *Health for all by the year 2000 — Polish strategy and targets*. Following the collapse of the Soviet Union, a new national health programme was accepted by the Government and approved in 1991 by the socioeconomic committee of the Council of Ministers. Major reforms ensued in an attempt to devolve power from the centre. The provincial authorities (voivodships) acquired substantial power for planning health services and allocating funds. In 1993, power was further devolved from the provincial to the local level, to increase the strategic management functions of the Ministry of Health and Welfare and to reduce its involvement in the operation of health care.

In 1991 the Health Care Institution Act provided for market-led initiatives. This was modified following consultation with health care employees, trade unions and professional associations. Local government bodies can now purchase clinical and non-clinical services through competitive contracting. Examples of where the market has gained include the privatization of sanitoria and hospital catering services and the contracting out of emergency services.

The Strategy for Health (1994) is part of the Government's programme for economic and social reform, and the national health programme for the years 1996–2005 was revised and approved in 1996. Rapid changes and a more pluralistic environment (increasing numbers of nongovernmental organizations, local councils and trade unions) demanded new ways of collaborating. Consequently, the revised strategy was prepared by a team of experts together with an interministerial coordinating team. The strategy has three main objectives:

- creating conditions that support and develop people's motivation, knowledge and skills in choosing healthy lifestyles and undertaking actions for improving their own health and the health of others;
- creating environments supportive to health, work and education; and
- reducing inequalities in health and in access to health services.

A number of operational targets are included to achieve these objectives. The document was disseminated for consultation, revised on the basis of comments, and discussed in the Parliament.

There is also a document on the management of health care services, but frequent changes in central, provincial and local authorities have tended to destabilize the system and lead to conflicts, so that good managers are often discouraged from remaining in the health care system.

In February 1997, Parliament passed the Comprehensive Health Insurance Act, which were subsequently signed by the President. This Act is the basic legal document regulating the problems of transforming health care and its financing.

Focus on health outcomes and reorientation towards primary health care

Financing of health care was previously based on such criteria as the number of beds and length of patient stay, which led to a structural distortion favouring hospitals. Reforms to redress this include:

- the use of foreign aid to equip primary health care facilities and decentralizing primary health care to the community level;
- reducing the number of hospital referrals;
- introducing a new formula for geographical allocation of resources;
- primary health care facilities to be paid on a capitation basis (experimental phase);
- comprehensive primary health care training and retraining of existing specialists as general practitioners;

- a system of family health services centred around newly trained family physicians who will act as independent contractors; and
- establishing self-governing hospitals.

Poland is currently reorienting its health information system to monitor health outcomes for planning, management, contracting and evaluation purposes. Outcome targets have been set, but mainly only in relation to mortality. Resource allocation will increasingly be based on indicators collected within a centralized information system. The use of health outcomes is being emphasized more in the training of medical staff. Interdisciplinary hospital committees have been set up to develop systems for quality improvement, including the setting of criteria and standards of medical care. A hospital accreditation programme has been put in place by the National Centre of Health System Management, which is responsible for the analysis, evaluation and quality of care.

Promotion of equity, public participation and intersectoral action

Equity

The state ensures universal access to health care services. The previous emphasis on hospital care led to services being mainly located in cities, and geographical inequities were common. These regional inequities were reinforced by allocating resources on a historical basis rather than targeting need. The new strategy aims to eliminate regional, urban and rural disparities in the quality of and access to health care services. Resource allocation will be based on demographic data and mortality indicators. Units are being established in voivodships to collect and analyse the necessary information.

So far, Poland has avoided the worst elements of market-led policies. Co-payments and private practice have been introduced but fees for service are capped. Legislation provides a framework allowing the private sector to grow and the establishment of a split between the purchasers and providers of health care without destabilizing existing services. The level of co-payments will be closely monitored and their impact evaluated. Initiatives to target the causes of inequity and poverty include the introduction of unemployment benefits, and housing provided by the state to people with low income.

Public participation

Fortunately, Poland maintained close links with western Europe and retained people with a memory of participatory decision-making and a keen sense of solidarity who could help to rebuild democratic institutions. The large number of voluntary organizations and groups and their growing importance in the policy-making environment is partly explained by this long tradition. The People's Councils and Territorial Self-government Act (1983) aimed to ensure the involvement of local authorities and communities in solving health-related problems. Today, research is being conducted on involving people less formally in decisions concerning their own health, for example, by strengthening the role of the family and other social groups in promoting positive health behaviour. Other measures include health education in such settings as schools and workplaces and targeted at certain groups, and legislation such as the Health Care Institution Act, which partly covers the rights of patients.

Intersectoral action

Until recently, the main objective was to minimize costs in the health services, and the potential for contributing to objectives in other sectors was not really explored. Changing this way of thinking takes time, and since 1990 the Government has worked hard to promote an intersectoral approach. This endeavour is now paying off with participation from an interministerial coordination team in the formulation of the health strategy.

There are a number of multisectoral initiatives to improve living, environmental and recreational conditions. For example, the Occupational Medicine Services Law will regulate working conditions and ensure occupational medical services. The ILO Occupational Health Services Convention (C161) has also been ratified.

Various intersectoral bodies have been established such as:

- the Institute of Occupational Medicine and Institute of Rural Medicine, responsible for coordinating worksite initiatives;
- the Health Promotion Council, set up following the first national conference on health promotion; and
- an interdisciplinary team of architects, sociologists, health professionals, ecologists, construction engineers and others responsible for a programme on healthy housing.

Portugal

Demography, policy environment and health care system

Mainland Portugal is bordered to the north and east by Spain and to the south and west by the Atlantic Ocean. It is divided into 18 districts and 305 municipal councils subdivided into 4209 parishes. The Atlantic archipelagos of the Azores and Madeira are autonomous regions.

In 1996 the population was 9.9 million. The average population density is 108 per km^2 and 48% of the population live in urban areas (1996).

In 1995 the mean income per person was US $10 060. The inflation rate is 2% (1997) and the unemployment rate 7% (1996).

In 1995 the infant mortality rate was 6.8 per 1000 live births and in 1996 the average life expectancy at birth was 75 years.

In 1996 total health care expenditure accounted for 8% of GDP.

The health care system is financed mainly by taxation. The Portuguese National Health Service is under the responsibility of the Minister of Health, a central administration and five regional administrations. It provides a very considerable part of the health care delivered in Portugal.

Approach towards achieving health for all

A Portuguese health strategy for the turn of the century (1998–2002) was initiated in 1996, adopted in 1997 and adjusted and reinforced in 1998. The strategy is centred on five main goals: targeted health gains, developing local health care systems, reviewing human resources development, a new model of financing health care, and adopting a European dimension in health policy.

On issues related to the life cycle and family health, the focus is on safe motherhood, on growing up healthy, on family-related violence and abuse and on healthy aging (equity being an important concern). In lifestyles and risk factors for disease, the main emphasis is on active living, substance abuse and accidents. Concerning specific diseases, the main focus is on tuberculosis, hepatitis, HIV infection and AIDS, antibiotic resistance, diabetes, depression, stroke and other diseases of the circulatory system, and certain forms of cancer. Environmental health very strongly emphasizes intersectoral cooperation, and the main priorities are carrying out a specific environmental health policy (including an action plan on hospital waste), reinforcing intersectoral mechanisms for food safety, and a new impetus on health-promoting schools and healthier urban living.

Targets for ten and five years and immediate (one-year) objectives have been established in these priority areas. Mechanisms for informing the public and promoting public participation have also been targeted.

Focus on health outcomes and reorientation towards primary health care

The main trends in health care reform in Portugal are:

- the implementation of five regional contracting agencies to ensure that resources are allocated according to health needs and the preferences of citizens;
- changing the management of hospital and health centres to promote decentralization and focus on performance, quality, outcome and efficiency gains;
- progressive implementation of local health systems emphasizing health gain, better access to health care, equity, community involvement and intersectoral cooperation;
- setting priorities within high-technology medical networks on cardiovascular interventions, oncology and chronic renal diseases; and
- testing new remuneration systems for health professionals.

Promotion of equity, public participation and intersectoral action

It is considered necessary to reinforce the quantitative and qualitative output of nursing schools (considerably) and of medical schools (moderately). Continual professional training is an important priority.

A proposal for a more sustainable model of health care financing is now under discussion that improves health gain, assures sustainability and solidarity in health system development, and considers people's preferences in funding health care providers. Regional allocation is also being reviewed.

A European dimension in the Portuguese health strategy is being adopted related to the policies of the EU and WHO and enhancing cooperation with Portuguese-speaking countries. The European dimension mainly includes the following:

- stronger participation in EU health programmes;
- preparation for the EU Presidency, for which Portugal is responsible for the first six months of the year 2000;
- participation in the WHO European strategy for health for all; and
- enhanced cooperation programmes with Portuguese-speaking countries in Africa.

Republic of Moldova

Demography, policy environment and health care system

The Republic of Moldova borders Romania and Ukraine. From 1918 to 1940 it was part of Romania, and from 1940 to 1992 a republic within the Soviet Union. It declared independence in 1992.

In 1997 the population was 4.3 million. The average population density is 129 per km^2 (1997); 51% of the population live in urban areas (1997); 26% of the population are aged $\geq$ 65 years and 10% aged 0–14 years (1996); and the dependency ratio is 75% (1993).

In 1993 the mean income per person was US $1000. The inflation rate is 500% (1994) and the unemployment rate 2% (1996). The poorest 10% of the population have a 3% share of income while the most affluent 10% have a 26% share (1992).

In 1996 the infant mortality rate was 20.2 per 1000 live births, and in 1995 the average life expectancy at birth was 66 years.

In 1993 total health expenditure accounts for 5% of estimated GDP.

The Basic Health Care Law, which was adopted by Parliament in 1995, regulates the organizational structure of the health care system.

Approach towards achieving health for all

The Republic of Moldova has not yet formulated an overall health policy. Nevertheless, the Ministry of Health is committed to the objectives of health for all, and current health care sector reforms take account of health for all principles. The Government has developed a number of issue-specific policies, resulting in the Basic Health Care Law (1995); a pharmaceuticals policy (1993); programmes on maternal and child health (1992), the rights of children (1995) and sanitary and epidemiological surveillance (1993); the Law on Preventive Activity on HIV/AIDS (1993); a bill on health insurance; and programmes on cancer, tuberculosis, diabetes, psychiatry and mental health, health care reform and alcoholism. The health care system is to be decentralized; district or municipal governments will have the opportunity to define health care priorities for their local populations.

Focus on health outcomes and reorientation towards primary health care

In the past, the allocation of resources tended to favour hospitals over primary health care. In towns of more than 3000 people, polyclinics are theoretically responsible for primary health care. Operated like small hospitals, polyclinics derive their funding from hospital budgets and are staffed by specialists. Priority tends to be given to more advanced secondary care, although a number of measures to promote primary health care are under way:

- research on management, financing and quality of primary health care services, especially in rural areas;
- a pilot project on new ways of administering and financing primary health care institutions;
- negotiating with scientists, medical associations and health care professionals on proposed changes in the role and responsibilities of general practitioners, including that of gatekeeper, although a lack of trained general practitioners is delaying this (previously, people were entitled to a wide range of specialist services, and resistance to change may pose a challenge);
- separating inpatient and outpatient facilities to counter the bias towards hospital care, closing a number of small rural hospitals and reducing the number of beds;
- shifting finances from hospitals to outpatient and primary health care;
- financing health services based on capitation rather than bed-days;
- postgraduate training in general practice for physicians; and
- primary health care training for nurses.

Routine health statistics and other information have been insufficiently used in planning and policy decisions. In the future, it is proposed to introduce legislation to require an orientation towards health outcome as part of the planning process.

Promotion of equity, public participation and intersectoral action

Equity
According to the Constitution, equal access to health services is guaranteed by the state. People are entitled to a basic minimum income according to law. In 1992, the Law on Health Assistance through Health Insurance was adopted, paving the way for moves to an insurance-based system. The Ministry of Health has developed a basic package of services to be provided free of charge, including separate financing for vulnerable population categories. The Ministry of Health is also carrying out research into inequity, especially in relation to the nutrition of pregnant women, infants and low-income groups. There are no long-term care institutions such as nursing homes or day care centres for chronically or mentally ill people; they are treated in ordinary hospitals. In the forthcoming reforms, it is hoped that long-term care can be established for special groups.

Public participation
There is a high level of consultation, with all major decisions being referred to trade unions and professional health associations for comment. Legislation on patients' rights is being developed. A

number of patient organizations and other associations have been established recently, extending decision-making in health to the wider community. More use is also being made of the mass media to analyse current conditions within the health services and the perspectives of forthcoming changes, such as insurance and co-payments in relation to new forms of management and financing. It is planned to subsidize these organizations in the future.

Intersectoral action

Prior to independence, various ministries were responsible for the health care of employees within their sector (the Ministries of Transport, of Internal Affairs and of Defence and Security, the trade union associations and the treatment and hygiene services provide primary and secondary care services). This feature remains today, and these services duplicate those offered by the Ministry of Health. The Ministry of Finance funds the services, and the Ministry of Health is responsible for monitoring standards and training staff.

Several studies on lifestyles are being carried out in relation to nutrition, HIV infection, drug use and sexual behaviour. The state programme on combating alcoholism supports a variety of measures to control the quality of alcohol and restrict its advertising and sale. Taxes on tobacco and alcohol were introduced by special decree in 1995. The Ministries of Health and of Education have agreed on health promotion initiatives in schools and other teaching institutions and on the provision of undergraduate medical education. The Ministries of Health, of Welfare and of Labour and Social Protection are responsible for the joint planning and management of orphanages and homes for handicapped children.

An intersectoral body, the State Committee on Environmental Protection, was created in 1994 with representatives of several ministries. A series of studies dealt with the impact of pesticides on the health of workers in rural areas, and requirements for standards in the physical and working environment have been formulated in policy documents concerning the health of women and children. Health professionals are also being trained in occupational health.

Romania

Demography, policy environment and health care system

Romania is situated in the south-eastern part of central Europe. It is bordered by the Black Sea and the Republic of Moldova to the east, by Ukraine to the north, by Hungary and the Federal Republic of Yugoslavia to the west and by Bulgaria to the south. Romania is a republic led by a President and governed by a two-chamber National Assembly comprising a Senate and a Chamber of Deputies. The district is the basic administrative unit of Romania. There are 41 districts with an average population of 555 000. Towns and wards are smaller administrative units.

In 1996 the population was 22.6 million. The average population density is 91.2 per km^2 and 55% of the population live in urban areas (1997). Some 12.4% of the population are aged $\geq$ 65 years and 20% aged 0–14 years and the dependency ratio is 47.1% (1996).

In 1997 the mean income per person was US $4130. The inflation rate is 139% (1996) and the unemployment rate 9.5% (1995). The poorest 10% of the population receive 4% of the income and the most affluent 10% receive 25% of the income (1992).

In 1996 the infant mortality rate was 22.3 per 1000 live births and in 1995 life expectancy at birth was 69.4 years.

In 1996 health care expenditure comprised 3.0% of GDP.

The health care system is almost entirely owned by the state and is coordinated by the Ministry of Health through 41 district health directorates and the Bucharest Health Directorate. Health services are financed through a mixture of national and local taxation, private payments, co-payments for drugs and external credits. Other sectors own smaller networks of health facilities, including the Ministries of Defence, of the Interior and of Labour and Social Welfare, and the Romanian Intelligence Service.

Approach towards achieving health for all

Romania faces poor socioeconomic conditions and a comparatively high rate of infant mortality. It is agreed that health is a priority and, although Romania has no overall health policy document, discussions have been taking place, mainly between professional organizations and the Ministry of Health, on the possible development of such a policy. A situation analysis carried out by WHO in 1989 forms the basis of collaboration with the World Bank, the EU and United Nations agencies. WHO is now involved in a number of programmes in the priority areas of drug supply and renovation of medical equipment, primary health care, maternal and child care (including family planning, which did not exist under the previous regime), nursing, mental health, AIDS and health management. Issue-specific policy documents have been produced in relation to tobacco, drugs and alcohol.

Focus on health outcomes and reorientation towards primary health care

In 1991, Romania received a World Bank loan of US $150 million to facilitate shifts away from hospital care to primary health care and from curative to preventive medicine, to support major restructuring of health sector financing and to help reform the health care system. This was seen to be the way forward, ensuring a sustainable, cost-effective health care system in the medium term. Until now, hospitals have controlled the funds for primary and secondary care, with the result that primary health care has been neglected in favour of more specialized medical care.

A project to decentralize health care management and improve resource allocation was introduced in eight pilot districts in 1994 and extended to four more districts in 1995. Responsibility for health care has moved from hospitals to local health authorities. Other features include:

- contracting of general practitioner services and introduction of a capitation-based payment system combined with fee-for-service;
- freedom for people to choose their general practitioner;
- accreditation of physicians; and
- the transformation of workplace health services into family practices or occupational hygiene services.

Access to hospitals and outpatient care now requires referral by general practitioners. So far, however, although referrals have fallen, hospital admissions and emergencies have not decreased.

Initiatives to support the development of primary health care include:

- research on the proportion of resources spent on primary health care and the development of an information network for primary health care;
- integration of health promotion and disease prevention into primary health care services;
- consultation with medical associations and between general practitioners and district health authorities;
- establishment and development of primary health care centres and training programmes for general practitioners; and
- monitoring the changes in the number and use of hospital beds.

The information system is being developed to better reflect the general level of health. Specific indicators have been developed for planning purposes, and training programmes are being organized to teach health care managers how to use them.

Promotion of equity, public participation and intersectoral action

Equity

In theory, the Constitution guarantees equal access to health care irrespective of income, but the actual degree of equity is difficult to assess. The impact of the parallel health care systems operated by other ministries can only be guessed at. Rural areas are generally poorly served by primary health care. Health care budgets are allocated between primary and secondary care and between districts on a historical basis.

As a cornerstone of health care reform, a major change in health care financing started in 1997, after the National Assembly approved the Law on Social Health Insurance. This will change the structure of the health care system from a tax-based to a premium-based (compulsory) system. The new financing mechanism will be introduced in two stages. In 1998 district health directorates and the Ministry of Health were due to begin contracting services with public and private providers, using funds collected by the Ministry of Finance as a separate contribution for health care of employers and employees. In 1999, autonomous insurance funds, governed by representatives of employers, employees and other insured parties and operating at the district level, will start administering the health insurance scheme, including both the contracting of services and the collection of funds.

Although the new system will be based on premiums, universal coverage will be assured. The system will improve the transparency and stability of health care financing, introduce competition between providers, increase efficiency, support the growth of private providers and introduce free choice of health care provider.

Measures to promote equity in health include:

- the development of a national information system to reveal possible inequities; and
- education and training programmes for health managers and specialists in public health to promote the needs of various socioeconomic groups.

Public participation

In deciding the priority areas for action, the Government involved all key actors in discussing the various strategies. Before the pilot programme was launched, a mass media campaign was initiated to inform the public. Close contact was also established with health care professionals, many of whom were frustrated with poor salaries and working conditions, to ensure their support. Consultation with medical associations was important in developing the health insurance bill. At the government level, a special Health Committee has been established that monitors progress. A Health Reform Coordination Committee was also set up in 1993. Nongovernmental organizations play an important role such as in liaising with outside experts.

To ascertain the views of the users of health care, various institutions supervised by the Ministry of Health conduct professional and user satisfaction surveys. A participatory approach should be inculcated from a young age, and the Health Promoting Schools project is one way of instilling children with the spirit of participatory decision-making and consensus-building. Health care professionals are also being trained in communication skills to help them to empower patients to make choices. Informed consent is mandatory for major medical procedures.

Intersectoral policy

Romania does not have a strong tradition of intersectoral action, although the high number of nongovernmental organizations has led to increased activity between sectors generally. A National Centre for Health Promotion and Health Education has been set up and allocated special funds. In each district, a Health Promotion Laboratory within the Inspectorate of Sanitary Police and Preventive Medicine has also been set up. Attention is focused on lifestyle challenges, including research on factors influencing lifestyle and health education programmes on smoking, alcohol and drugs. Smoking habits are being monitored at the national level. Changing attitudes and behaviour in relation to food has been somewhat more difficult, because obtaining certain types of food was difficult under the previous regime.

Specific intersectoral actions to promote health include a tax on tobacco and alcohol and a ban on tobacco advertising on television (although health warnings are not included on cigarette packages), a polluter-pays policy and maximum levels for vehicular emissions. Part of the Ministry of Labour and Social Welfare's budget is allocated to health. Teachers have been trained as part of the Health Promoting Schools project and in relation to HIV infection and AIDS prevention and health education and promotion. The Ministry of the Environment has developed training programmes in environmental health.

Russian Federation

Demography, policy environment and health care system

The Russian Federation occupies 17 075 400 km^2 from the far north to the Black Sea in the south and from the far east to Kaliningrad in the west. The Russian Soviet Federal Socialist Republic adopted a Constitution in April 1978. In June 1990, pending the promulgation of a new Constitution (in 1993), it adopted a declaration of republican sovereignty and became a founding member of the Commonwealth of Independent States in December 1991 under the name Russian Federation. There are 1852 regions, 1059 towns, 339 urban districts, 2066 urban settlements and 23 976 rural settlements.

In 1997 the population was 147 million. The average population density is 9 per km^2 and 73% of the population live in urban areas (1997).

In 1993 the mean income per person was US $2200. The inflation rate is 300% and the unemployment rate 1% (1994). The poorest 10% of population have a 1% share of income while the most affluent 10% have a 39% share (1993).

In 1995 the infant mortality rate was 17.1 per 1000 live births and average life expectancy at birth was 64.6 years.

In 1992 total health expenditure accounted for 2% of estimated GDP.

Until 1991, the key administrative body was the All-Union Ministry of Health. In November 1991, this ceased to exist, and was re-established as the Ministry of Health of the Russian Federation.

Approach towards achieving health for all

In 1991 the Law of the Russian Soviet Federal Socialist Republic on Health Insurance was passed. Voluntary health insurance was permitted from autumn 1991. From 1992 a federal insurance fund was established, as were regional compulsory health insurance funds. In 1993 the Basic Law of the Federation on the Promotion of Health of Citizens was passed.

The Russian Federation does not yet have an overall policy for health, but plans are being initiated for the development of a policy for health for all, with WHO support. The major causes of death are cardiovascular disease, cancer, accidents and poisoning, and respiratory and digestive diseases. There were increases in the prevalence of diphtheria, tuberculosis, viral hepatitis and sexually transmitted diseases, especially syphilis, in the early to mid–1990s.

Focus on health outcomes and reorientation towards primary health care

In 1992, the Ministry of Health issued a ministerial order on the phased transition to primary health care based on the principle of the general practitioner (family physician). In 1996, the Government approved a federal programme to improve primary health care for the population, and a detailed plan for its implementation was finalized in May 1997.

The information system is being revised to ensure greater comparability with indicators of health for all. More attention is also being paid to reporting on health outcomes and the needs of socially disadvantaged groups. Separate registers have been established to monitor the needs of disabled people and families with children.

Promotion of equity, public participation and intersectoral action

Equity

Equity concerns have not received sufficient attention during the transition. The redistribution of state-owned productive assets has polarized the population in terms of wealth and income. New economic opportunities have been generated on a smaller scale than originally anticipated and have been rapidly monopolized by existing groups, creating a situation in which fewer and fewer people can genuinely benefit from new economic opportunities. Social pressures caused by poor socio-economic conditions have adversely affected the levels of crime, suicide, alcoholism and family stability. Poverty has reached critical levels, especially for families with children, single mothers and unemployed people. Certain groups such as children are being targeted for special attention.

Under the former system, people had access to high quality health care services. In the transition process, the coverage, quality and role of state financing have declined. Laws aimed at improving the health of disadvantaged groups include the code of labour laws (1971), the Act on State Pensions in the RSFSR (1992), the Act on Employment in the Russian Federation (1995) and the Act on Government Allowances to Citizens with Children (1995). Special allowances are also granted to refugees, people with incomes below an established minimum level, elderly people, people disabled as a result of military conflict and people who have served as clean-up personnel for the Chernobyl disaster.

A number of programmes are being implemented in the areas of maternal and child health, job creation and social and economic development in disadvantaged regions and cities, incorporating initiatives in health protection, ecology, nutrition and the supply of medical equipment.

Public participation

Responsibility for the provision of health services has now been devolved from central to local government, which means that a more pluralistic system is slowly evolving. To promote more active community participation, health initiatives are especially targeting young people, mainly through health promotion in schools. Legislation has been drafted on patients' rights.

Intersectoral action

The strategic objectives, priorities and main directions of developing an integrated intersectoral policy for the promotion of healthy lifestyles remain unchanged. All branches of legislative and executive authority support health promotion activities. Although the Russian Federation has not yet formulated a national policy for health for all and strategies and mechanisms for its implementation, practical experience in intersectoral cooperation has been gathered through efforts to improve health status, especially among women, unemployed people and the homeless.

Various intersectoral bodies have been established, including the Intersectoral Commission on the Protection of the Health of Citizens and interdepartmental commissions on health care and environmental safety.

Monitoring the formulation and implementation of public policies to promote health is being revised. The main problem has been inadequate legislative and administrative support and insufficient investment in health promotion and research.

The CINDI (countrywide integrated noncommunicable diseases intervention) programme has been quite active in developing a framework through family medicine, the prevention of cardiovascular diseases (focusing on complications in people with diabetes), prevention programmes for children, workplace programmes and nutrition projects. Education became one of the main priorities in 1995, one of the main components of which is the Complex Essential Medical Education Needed Training (CEMENT) programme, which targets those involved in health promotion and disease prevention, such as physicians and other health care professionals, as well as patients.

Legislation has been introduced to reinforce state control over the sale of alcohol, drugs, the environment, town planning and food safety. An intersectoral approach is also being taken towards food policy, emphasizing urban and rural agriculture to improve the supply of home-produced foods. Federal programmes on ecological security in the Russian Federation and the rehabilitation of people and territories exposed to radiation are currently in operation.

San Marino

Demography, policy environment and health care system

San Marino is the oldest republic in Europe, founded in 301, and is situated in the north-eastern part of Italy. The land area comprises 61 km^2. The Great and General Council (Parliament) consists of 60 elected members and the executive power is vested in the Congress of State, comprising 11 ministers selected from among Members of the Parliament. There are two heads of state, called Captains Regent, designated from the two parties of the Government coalition. They stay in power for six months, and are appointed every six months (1 April and 1 October).

In 1996 the population was 25 058. The average population density is 409 per km^2 and 89% of the population live in urban areas (1996). In 1996 15% of the population were aged $\geq$ 65 years and 14% aged 0–14 years, the dependency ratio was 43%.

In 1996 the inflation rate was 3.9% and the unemployment rate 5.1%.

In 1996 the infant mortality rate was 10 per 1000 live births and the average life expectancy at birth was 74 years.

The main causes of death are cardiovascular diseases, which are responsible for 46.2% of all deaths, followed by cerebrovascular diseases and cancer.

Approach towards achieving health for all

In 1994 and 1996, San Marino signed an agreement with WHO to strengthen cooperation, with the aim of achieving the 38 European targets for health for all. The agreement focuses on preventing and reducing the causes of chronic diseases, promoting healthy lifestyles and combating the use of harmful substances such as tobacco and alcohol. San Marino signed the Saint Vincent Declaration related to reducing the causes and effects of diabetes.

Focus on health outcomes and reorientation towards primary health care

A database on cardiovascular diseases has been established, and evidence now available shows that the prevalence rates of ischaemic, cardiac and myocardial disease have been reduced. A system for collecting data on cancer was initiated recently.

Health programmes mainly focus on primary health care services, with a strong emphasis on prevention. A current initiative to prevent and control disorders of fat metabolism is being coordinated via national programmes to monitor and control the levels of cholesterol and hypertension in the population. A healthy lifestyles programme has been launched with monitoring, treatment and rehabilitation for people with myocardial infarction. Programmes for the prevention of communicable diseases such as AIDS and HIV infection, as well as blood transfusion control programmes, are carried out at the national level. The Centre for Autoimmune Diseases was established in 1994 to diagnose and treat chronic diseases.

Promotion of equity, public participation and intersectoral action

Equity
Equity is one of the main principles underpinning the health care system; the entire population has access to health care and to social welfare. Efforts to improve the quality of life have targeted certain groups such as elderly people.

Public participation
The Ministry of Health is responsible for health care programmes, although decisions are adopted either by the Congress of State or by the Great and General Council.

Intersectoral action
Environmental health is part of the overall health programme, and particular emphasis is given to:

- water pollution
- food quality control
- hygiene in the workplace
- control of dangerous and toxic wastes and substances.

A database has also been established on toxic substances and their implications for health and is available on the Internet.

A number of campaigns related to improving lifestyles are conducted at the national level and implemented at such settings as schools and hospitals.

Slovakia

Demography, policy environment and health care system

Slovakia is located in the heart of Europe, bordered by the Czech Republic to the north-west, by Poland to the north, by Ukraine to the east, by Hungary to the south and by Austria to the south-west. Slovakia was constitutionally founded in 1993. The National Council (Parliament) has a single chamber and a total of 150 deputies. Slovakia is divided into 8 administrative regions comprising 79 districts. Regional and district offices carry out state administration in local areas.

In 1996 the population was 5.4 million. The average population density is 109 per km^2 and 58% of the population live in urban areas (1994). In 1995 11% of the population were aged ≥ 65 years and 23% aged 0–14 years, and the dependency ratio was 53%.

In 1996 the mean income per person was US $3 200, the inflation rate 6% and the unemployment rate 13%.

In 1995 the infant mortality rate was 11 per 1000 live births and the average life expectancy at birth 72.5 years.

In 1996 total health expenditure accounted for 7% of estimated GDP.

The Ministry of Health is the main body responsible for health care along with regional and district state physicians, who have been delegated some tasks. Several ministries run specialized health care facilities for their employees. Health insurance companies finance contracted health care services. Professional associations and voluntary organizations are independent and monitor professional ethics and quality, and provide some advisory functions to the Ministry of Health.

Approach towards achieving health for all

Following the dissolution of Czechoslovakia in November 1989, Slovakia embarked on a series of sweeping changes. Despite several changes of government, the main thrust of the reforms has been maintained, indicating a high degree of political consensus. The new health care system is based on universal and compulsory health insurance delivered by a number of agencies.

In 1991 the National Council adopted the National Health Promotion Programme, based on the WHO European strategy for health for all, and in 1992 the National Health Promotion Centre was established.

In 1995 the Government approved a new national health for all policy, which has created a solid basis for action in health care services, disease prevention, health promotion, and health and the environment. In the same year, the Government adopted the updated National Health Promotion Programme, focusing on six priorities, to facilitate the implementation of the main health promotion and disease prevention actions. In 1996, the Government approved a document on the ongoing transformation of health care, together with the Action Plan on Environment and Health in January 1997.

Reforms in Slovakia have largely been driven by politicians in consultation with expert groups, based strictly on new legislation. The original Law on Population Health (from 1966) has been repealed and three new laws introduced in its place: the Law on Health Care, the Law on Protection of Human Health and the Law on Health Insurance. Under these laws, the previous hygiene services have been transformed into state health institutes in each district with a broader range of responsibilities, including health promotion and disease prevention. Former budgetary health care financing shifted completely to a health insurance scheme. The state health care facilities have been privatized, resulting in a mix of state and non-state providers. This has democratized the health care sector.

The National Council and the Government are strongly committed to improving the health status of the population. Thus, the Government approved the strategy, principles and priorities of the state environmental policy in 1993, and the National Council adopted the Act on Advertising and the Act on Protection of Nonsmokers in 1996. Other important health policy legislation is being prepared, including the Psychotropic and Narcotic Drugs Act and the Act on Drugs.

The updated National Health Promotion Programme accommodates the WHO settings approach to promoting health. WHO networks such as Healthy Cities, Health Promoting Schools and CINDI (countrywide integrated noncommunicable diseases intervention) counselling centres have been firmly endorsed.

Focus on health outcomes and reorientation towards primary health care

Primary care services were recently privatized, enabling physicians to leave the state system and work as independent contractors (general practitioners and gynaecologists are paid partly through capitation and partly through fee-for-service; dentists are paid through fee-for-service). Primary health care physicians, comprising general practitioners for adults, general practitioners for children, gynaecologists and dentists, have a gatekeeping role, but patients may refer themselves to certain specialists as regulated by law. Much preparatory work has been carried out, including home care, for the shift from hospital to primary care. The reimbursement system for hospital care is to be changed to encourage shorter inpatient stays. Measures to promote primary health care include:

* efforts to introduce health education, health promotion and disease prevention services into the health insurance scheme;

- establishment of an information system for general practitioners on aspects of primary health care, a database for insurance statistics and a research database;
- reinforcing better cooperation between the state health institutes and primary health care physicians;
- health promotion campaigns through the mass media, encouraging people to seek early health assessment; and
- consultation with the medical association on training physicians as general practitioners and training health care workers to embrace a primary health care approach.

Monitoring population health status is the first step in becoming oriented towards health outcome. The monitoring of selected indicators is being used as a basis for planning and financing health services. Other initiatives designed to promote an orientation towards health outcome include:

- building awareness of the use of health outcomes among health educators; and
- communicating the function of health outcomes to other sectors.

Promotion of equity, public participation and intersectoral action

Equity
The principle of equity has always been perceived in Slovakia as being anchored firmly in national legislation. Equal access to health care has been maintained under the new system, and people are entitled to a wide range of services. The same applies to the financing of health care services, as the principles of solidarity, equity and non-profit are followed strictly. Equity in health includes:

- the right to health protection under the law;
- the right and duty to obtain free-of-charge vaccination against the main communicable diseases;
- the prevention of common diseases in vulnerable groups through targeted programmes;
- free health insurance for economically inactive people; and
- equitable access to education for all population groups.

Public participation
Efforts to increase participation have been pursued on a number of levels. A medical quiz published in the newspapers aimed to assess people's awareness of policy issues. Comments on the draft policy document were also published in the mass media to stimulate discussion of health challenges. Young people are being introduced to participatory decision-making processes through the Health Promoting Schools project. Efforts to engage patients include encouraging patient representation on hospital councils, subsidizing patient organizations and publishing documents on patients' rights in the mass media. Training health professionals on how to communicate with and listen to patients is felt to be an important part of promoting more active participation. Greater attention is also being paid to increasing the involvement of trade unions, medical associations and parliamentary representatives, some of whom have been invited to participate on the National Board of Health and Social Affairs.

Intersectoral action

The Government established the Coordination Board headed by the Minister of Health to reinforce the implementation of the updated National Health Promotion Programme. Almost all sectors, including nongovernmental organizations, have members. The Ministry of Health cooperates closely with the Ministry of the Environment on issues of environmental health. Many measures have been undertaken to improve environmental health, including research and surveys. One area being heavily promoted is the recycling of materials such as paper and glass. Collaboration with the Ministry of Agriculture has resulted in the national Codex Alimentarius. The state supervision on safety and quality of foods is provided jointly by the Slovak Agriculture and Food Inspectorate and the Slovak Trading Inspectorate. Research is being carried out in a number of areas involving other sectors, such as health impact assessment of exposure to nitrates and nitrites and other chemicals contained in food.

The Council of Ministers to Combat Drug and other Substance Abuse was established in 1996. The Council coordinates all activities on these and related problems. Research is being carried out on certain vulnerable groups and how their behaviour has implications for health (annual research on drug abusers and campaigns against smoking and other substance abuse). A massive increase in the importation and advertising of health-damaging products has created new threats to people's health and evoked appropriate measures, including legislation (see above). Advertising of tobacco and alcohol and sponsorship by tobacco companies are not permitted.

The Ministry of Health and the Ministry of Labour, Social Affairs and the Family cooperate closely in social security. According to the law, health insurance companies pay for health care services and the Social Insurance Institution pays for social care, including sickness leave and various social benefits. Care for elderly and disabled people is also being improved by more efficient links between health and social care. The number of long-term facilities is being increased slowly. The social sector provides many facilities such as nursing homes, pensioners' houses and supportive home services. The beneficiaries must pay in part for these services. Both sectors have worked closely on a document on the state family policy, which aims to improve the living conditions of young families.

The state health institutes are the key to facilitating cooperation among various sectors. They initiate many intersectoral activities, carry out health education and training activities, and evaluate the effectiveness of health promotion interventions and other activities in accordance with the strategy for health for all.

Slovenia

Demography, policy environment and health care system

Slovenia lies in the southern part of central Europe with Italy to the west, Austria to the north, Hungary to the north-east, Croatia to the east and south and the Adriatic Sea to the south-west. Slovenia was formerly one of the republics of Yugoslavia. It declared its independence in June 1991. The Slovenian Parliament is composed of an assembly with 90 members and a state council with 40 members.

In 1996 the population was 2 million and the average population density was 100 per km^2.

In 1996 the mean income per person was US $9300. The inflation rate is 9% (1996) and the unemployment rate 14% (1994). The poorest 10% of population have a 4% share of income while the most affluent 10% have a 24% share (1996).

In 1996 the infant mortality rate was 4.7 per 1000 live births in 1996 and the average life expectancy at birth was 70.8 years for men and 78.3 years for women.

In 1996 total health expenditure accounted for 8% of estimated GDP.

Under legislation introduced in early 1992, both compulsory and voluntary health insurance systems were established. The legislation describes in detail the responsibilities of individuals, communities and the state in health and health care.

Approach towards achieving health for all

In 1992 the Government embarked on a process of radical reform, primarily to mobilize funds for health care and to bring costs under control. In 1996 it prepared an overall policy document on the national health care programme. The draft document was disseminated for consultation and will be revised accordingly. Current health legislation requires that Parliament ratify such programmes, and various parliamentary bodies have already studied the draft. Legislation has been passed on health care and health insurance (1992), health care services (1992), pharmacists (1992), investment in health (1994), communicable diseases (1995), medicinal products (1996), the use of tobacco products (1996) and bioethics (1997). Laws on genetics and biotechnology and on physicians and their role in health care are still under review, as is the national health care programme.

Focus on health outcomes and reorientation towards primary health care

One of the main elements of the reform was the privatization of physician practices in primary health care. Privatization was envisaged within the existing network of services, to reduce the risk of creating a two-tier system. It was hoped that efficiency would improve as privatized physicians competed with each other and with the public system for contracts with the National Health Insurance Institute. The quantity of privatized health services is still too small to say whether the system will yield the anticipated gains.

Research is currently being carried out on the possibility of shifting the focus to primary health care, and a health information system is being developed for this purpose. Other plans include:

- developing health promotion programmes aimed at high-risk groups;
- initiating preventive screening for adults (through hospitals and family physicians);
- screening of high risk groups, such as expectant mothers, newborn children and young people;
- regular meetings between primary care physicians and hospital doctors to transfer knowledge between the primary, secondary and tertiary levels;
- increasing the share of funds from basic health insurance allocated to primary level care;
- introducing specialized training for physicians in general family medicine; and
- training for nurses in health education and health promotion with special emphasis on approaches for children and adults.

Legislation on health protection, health insurance and medical practice provides the basis for negotiations between the primary, secondary and tertiary sectors, defines the functions and obligations of each and gives priority to primary health care institutions.

Routinely collected information provides details on health status and the quality of life. Surveys of certain groups are also carried out. On this basis, proposals are made to various health departments and agencies on possible policy interventions. Educational and training programmes are being upgraded to focus on health outcomes. WHO health for all indicators are also used to compare performance with other countries. The results of this exercise are available to all interested parties.

Promotion of equity, public participation and intersectoral action

Equity

In moving to a health insurance system, the Government sought to maintain equity and the provision of a comprehensive range of services. One of the fears about the new system is that wealthier people will have access to more and better quality services through their ability to pay out-of-pocket payments, or to better coverage through voluntary insurance. This would compromise the equity guaranteed under the former system. Equity may also be threatened if private physicians are well integrated into the publicly operated network, and direct their services toward a wealthier clientele, leaving the public network to take care of the rest.

To promote equity in health, the Government has introduced a number of interventions:

- routine statistical research and analysis of regional differences in health status and the quality of health services;
- incorporation of health education in the school curriculum:
- financial assistance to nongovernmental organizations;
- planning of human resources according to need, providing appropriate levels of medical staff in areas that are demographically threatened, and developing standards for these areas; and
- providing medical services without co-payment for vulnerable groups, disabled people, welfare recipients and people older than 75 years.

Public participation
Surveys are being carried out to determine public opinion on health issues. The Ministry of Health is financing health education programmes undertaken by nongovernmental organizations to involve the public more actively in health care issues. Progress reports are issued annually on the impact of programmes. More consultation is being carried out with consumer associations, trade unions and medical and other groups.

Intersectoral action
The Ministry of Health collaborates with the Ministries of Education, of Labour and of Social Affairs in providing social care for such groups as children and elderly people. Intersectoral initiatives are being developed in research and information. An environmental health information system examines the adverse effects of poor environmental control on vulnerable groups. Research is being carried out in health promotion, for example in relation to drug abuse and sexual behaviour among young people. Programmes are being developed to prepare young people for living a life free of tobacco and drugs and to promote healthy food and physical activity. Some ministries are carrying out joint research; for example, the Ministry of Health and the Ministry of Social Affairs are researching home services for elderly people.

Efforts are being made to make people more aware of factors that affect their health, including campaigns related to environmental issues and among workers concerning occupational health threats, such as dangerous technologies. Different settings are being used to promote health among certain groups (healthy schools, child care institutions and hospitals).

Various intersectoral bodies have been set up, such as an interdepartmental body to discuss health issues, a centre for health and environmental studies, a government Health Care Council and an intersectoral consultation body for health promotion.

Consultation is being carried out with educational bodies and with the Ministries of Finance and of Agriculture regarding changes in tax and government subsidy policies. In some cases taxes have been levied as a punitive measure such, as those on tobacco, alcohol and unhealthy foods. Part of that tax is used for health promotion.

Legal measures include those related to prohibiting smoking in certain areas, placing health warnings on cigarette packets, banning the sale of cigarettes to minors and promoting safety at work.

Regarding human resource development and training, health promotion is included in programmes at vocational schools and teacher training courses. The medical curriculum is to include subjects related to the environment and health economics, and medical staff (especially those working in industry and agriculture) are to be trained in environmental health.

Intersectoral monitoring and evaluation includes monitoring of drinking-water, soil, animals and air for pollutants, assessing the threats and measures for eliminating the hazards, and monitoring and evaluation of interdepartmental cooperation.

Spain

Demography, policy environment and health care system

Spain is bordered to the north by the Bay of Biscay and the Pyrenees, to the east and south by the Mediterranean Sea and the Straits of Gibraltar, to the west and south-west by the Atlantic Ocean and to the west by Portugal. Spain is a parliamentary monarchy. The country is divided into 17 regions (autonomous communities) with their respective governments and parliaments, two cities with a statute of autonomy (Ceuta and Melilla), 50 provinces and almost 8000 municipalities.

In 1992 the population was 39 million. The average population density is 77 per km^2 and 76% of the population live in urban areas (1993).

In 1993 the mean income per person was US $12 210. The inflation rate is 1% (1996/1997) and the unemployment rate is 21% (1997). The poorest 10% of the population have an 8% share of income while the most affluent 10% have a 22% share (1988).

In 1993 the infant mortality rate was 7 per 1000 live births and the average life expectancy at birth was 78 years.

In 1993 total health expenditure accounted for 7.3 % of estimated GDP.

Health care and social security are shared areas of responsibility. Thus, the health care system is planned and managed based on the need for fundamental consensus between the different political powers, the region-based administration and the central state.

Approach towards achieving health for all

Following major reform of the health care system in 1986, Spain passed the General Health Care Act. The Act ensured the right to public health care for the entire population, set out the national health planning system and brought all public health services under one umbrella. Prior to this, provision of services was fragmented, with responsibility shared between the Ministry of Labour, central government and local corporations. The health care sector was reformed concomitantly with decentralization of health services to the autonomous communities. As a result, hospitals from the various coexisting health care networks have been integrated within the domain of regional health services, and common objectives have been set. Autonomous communities are responsible for developing their own individual health plans according to the principles set out in the general health plan. At a later stage, a national health plan will be developed as an aggregation of regional plans. An interterritorial council acts as the coordinating body for the state and the autonomous communities in the area of health. Although 16 autonomous communities have now approved regional plans, a complete planning cycle involving all organizational tiers and regions has yet to take place.

Focus on health outcomes and reorientation towards primary health care

Reforms in the primary health care sector began in the 1980s with the establishment of health centres throughout Spain. Tackling health problems on an integrated basis called for the combined skills of a team of health care professionals including physicians (general practitioners and paediatricians) nurses and other health professions. Today, primary health care is supplied on both a traditional and a team basis: the traditional model involves an individual practitioner who provides curative functions on a capitation basis, and the team model is based on group practice with payment on a salary basis, with wider functions covering both preventive and curative services. In recent years the team-based model has taken precedence over the individual model. This may be explained by the growing importance being given to preventive medicine, which is now included in the basic package of health benefits.

Health outcome orientation is an area of growing importance in Spain. Research mainly focuses on effectiveness measures. Analysis of hospital admissions according to age and sex is facilitating the setting of health priorities and the identification of vulnerable groups. Funds are increasingly being allocated on the basis of health outcomes, and increased attention is being given to training professionals in health outcome measures. Protocols and clinical guidelines are being developed and distributed to health professionals to ensure more efficiency.

Promotion of equity, public participation and intersectoral action

Equity

Prior to the General Health Care Act (1986), the Spanish health care system had a number of problems. The variety of health care networks and range of bodies to whom they were responsible led to poor coordination and inadequate organization. Primary health care and preventive care were inadequately emphasized. Universal coverage was not guaranteed for the entire population. The General Health Care Act was the first step in ensuring a more equitable health care system. In 1989, switching funding from social insurance to general taxation ensured that coverage was extended on a noncontributory basis to people with insufficient resources, ending the previously charity-based health care system. In 1995 a basic benefit package was established to be provided by the national health system, and today a variety of measures are used to promote equity in health:

- monitoring based on WHO's 38 regional targets for health for all;
- health education and awareness-building for vulnerable groups;
- legislation including the General Health Care Act and the Royal Decree of Benefits Order; and
- provision of information about health entitlements to people with insufficient resources.

Devolution of responsibility to the regional level allows for more equitable allocation of resources in accordance with the sociodemographic and cultural characteristics of each region and, ultimately, to a more balanced development of Spain's health services.

Public participation

The health care reforms aimed to increase patient satisfaction (by reducing waiting times for both inpatient and specialized outpatient care and by introducing more choice of providers) and to promote greater participation by the public. Surveys of user satisfaction with the health care system have been carried out to determine the public perception of standards of care. Information on health rights and entitlements is also being made available more systematically than previously. Several of the schools in Spain are participating very actively in the European and/or national networks of Health Promoting Schools; this invests young people with participatory decision-making skills. A decentralized system increases the potential for wider participation in health care decisions, but the increased power of regional authorities can be problematic since it tends to undermine the legitimacy of the national authorities. Efforts have been made to increase organized participation by establishing district health councils involving citizens, trade unions and employers in health care decisions.

Intersectoral action

Spain has established priorities in lifestyles, environment and health care. Health promotion emphasizes tobacco, exercise, alcohol abuse and nutrition. Research is being conducted on lifestyles and the risk factors that influence physical and mental health. National action plans have been developed for alcohol and drugs.

Environmental health emphasizes biological, physical, chemical and work-related risks. The quality of air and water is monitored regularly. To promote health at work, special efforts are being made to increase training in occupational health, and guidelines on occupational health have been issued to health authorities. On a more general level, a national plan and strategy for highway safety and legislation on accident prevention have been prepared.

The health care system emphasizes public health, primary care, maternal and child care, oral hygiene and rehabilitation. Particular attention is being paid to intersectoral collaboration in training health educators and targeting certain population groups. Individual plans have been developed for the health of infants and adolescents and of elderly people, and for promoting equal opportunity for women.

The autonomous communities have authority to initiate intersectoral action in environmental control, health education and legislation limiting cigarette and alcohol advertising and consumption in public places. For some types of action, responsibility is shared with the national level such as food production, safety of industrial products, health and safety at work, road safety and governmental action against illegal drug trafficking. The national level has total responsibility for taxation policy on tobacco and alcohol, legislation on the trafficking and consumption of illegal drugs and social security.

The most successful area for intersectoral cooperation has been between health and social services in the provision of care for elderly people. The issue of elderly people requiring continual care has not yet been resolved satisfactorily, and practices vary considerably between autonomous communities. In many cases, home care is being expanded, but coordination with medical care is still inadequate.

Sweden

Demography, policy environment and health care system

Sweden is situated in the eastern part of the Scandinavian peninsula. It is bordered to the west and north-west by Norway, to the east by Finland and the Gulf of Bothnia, to the south-east by the Baltic Sea and to the south-west by the Kattegat. Sweden is a parliamentary monarchy; Parliament has 349 seats. The country is divided into 26 counties, which are mainly responsible for financing and providing health care.

In 1996 the population was 8.8 million. The average population density is 19 per km^2 and 84% of the population live in urban areas (1995); 17% of the population are aged $\approx$ 65 years (1996) and 19% aged 0–14 years (1993); and the dependency ratio is 57% (1996).

In 1996 the mean income per person was US $28 300, the inflation rate 0.8% and the unemployment rate 8%. The poorest 20% of population have a 9% share of income while the most affluent 20% have a 35% share (1995).

In 1996 the infant mortality rate was 4 per 1000 live births and the average life expectancy at birth was 79 years.

In 1994 total health expenditure accounted for 8% of estimated GDP.

The state is obliged to provide good health and other social services to all residents of Sweden. An advanced and extensive system of social security provides universal benefits for sickness, maternity and unemployment, children, elderly people and disabled people. Health care is publicly provided and financed.

Approach towards achieving health for all

See the case studies on pages 147, 161 and 185.

Switzerland

Demography, policy environment and health care system

Switzerland is bordered to the west and north-west by France, to the north by Germany, to the east by Austria and to the south by Italy. It is a federal state of 26 cantons. The Federal Assembly (Parliament) is composed of two chambers: the National Council (200 members) and the Council of States (46 members). The federal Government has seven members elected by the Federal Assembly, and each year one of the seven is elected President of the Swiss Confederation.

In 1995 the population was 7.1 million. The average population density is 171 per km^2 and 68% of the population live in urban areas (1995); 15% of the population are aged $\geq$ 65 years and 23% aged 0–14 years (1995); and the dependency ratio is 62% (1995).

In 1996 the mean income per person was US $31 400, the inflation rate 1% and the unemployment rate 5%.

In 1995 the infant mortality rate was 7 per 1000 live births and the average life expectancy at birth was 81.7 years.

In 1993 total health expenditure accounted for 9% of estimated GDP.

The Swiss health care system is based on a federalistic structure characterized by a complex division of responsibilities between the federal and cantonal authorities on the one hand and the private sector on the other. There is no Ministry of Health at federal level. The Federal Office of Public Health and the Federal Social Insurance Office are part of the Federal Department (Ministry) of the Interior.

Approach towards achieving health for all

Responsibility for health policy development lies with the cantons, there being no overall national health policy. In 1993, a survey of cantonal authorities revealed that 80% of cantons had heard of WHO's 38 European targets for health for all but only one third had referred to them in official documents.

Two cantons (Vaud and Ticino) are members of the WHO Regions for Health Network (Geneva was previously a member). In 1989, these three cantons agreed to develop a joint health strategy and to adopt the WHO recommendations for health for all. The group identified four topics of common interest: developing a shared information system; drawing up a single programme for health promotion and disease prevention; applying methods to make health systems more effective; and defining a joint position on environment and health. The Ministers of Health from the three cantons prepared and signed a declaration of intent based on these areas of interest. The declaration was later submitted to the Swiss Conference of Ministers of Health. Following this, a number of other cantons also committed themselves to developing their policies in accordance with the principles of health for all. The new intercantonal group established various working groups to draw up practical plans for attaining the selected health objectives. These plans were later submitted to the governing bodies of the cantons. This was the first time that Switzerland had introduced joint action for health at the cantonal level.

Focus on health outcomes and reorientation towards primary health care

The whole population has access to primary health care, which includes preventive action, health education and home treatment of chronically sick and elderly people. Primary health care is highly developed in some cantons; in others, public health nurses (who sometimes belong to voluntary bodies) provide care. Specialized services are generally obtained at polyclinics attached to large hospitals.

One of the areas of concern to the intercantonal group was the development of a shared information system. This involved setting up a health indicators project to measure differences in health status between regions and to secure an information base for decision-making.

Promotion of equity, public participation and intersectoral action

Equity

Social security is based on a comprehensive social insurance system. The population has equal access to health services and is provided with the minimum requirements for basic living. Compared with other countries, overall health status is very good but there are differences between the sexes and between various age and social groups. Specific measures or programmes to promote equity for defined population groups include:

- AIDS prevention programmes for immigrants, with federal support;
- monitoring of geographical inequalities between the cantons, differences in risk factors by socio-economic groups and the consequences for health of long-term unemployment; and
- current debates on defining criteria for access to medical intervention if resources are limited (such as a limited supply of organs donated for transplantation).

Public participation

Switzerland's federal structure lends itself to a high degree of community participation at the cantonal and community levels, as does the decentralized system of health services. Various mechanisms facilitate population intervention at all levels, so that the public ultimately takes basic health policy decisions. Specific groups, such as people with AIDS, receive federal funding and are consulted on decisions concerning them.

Intersectoral action

Federal authorities are responsible for the control of communicable diseases; the regulation of certain drugs and other poisonous substances; food safety and radiation protection; and laws governing the environment and the training of certain health sector professions. In 1980, an attempt was made to include health promotion as part of federal responsibilities. The draft law was rejected by nearly all cantons, which considered it a threat to their autonomy. Intersectoral initiatives to promote health have mainly been restricted to the more traditional aspects of lifestyles (alcohol and tobacco use and cancer prevention) and a healthy environment, including:

- establishment of the Swiss Society for Social and Preventive Medicine, which produced a guide (1986) on health promotion and prevention in Switzerland;
- establishment of the Swiss Foundation for Health Promotion (1989) through which various public authorities and nongovernmental organizations agreed on a national strategy for 1993–1997, giving priority to health promotion in the workplace and among young people and to cancer prevention;
- provision by the Swiss Foundation for Health Education of courses and information material on its objectives, and of health education for young people on AIDS and drugs;
- targeting of specific groups such as women and children by establishing mother and child clinics and providing school health services for all children of compulsory school age;
- a basic environmental health law (1986) based on the principles of anticipatory prevention, the polluter-pays principle, and cooperation at all levels; reduced vehicular speed limits; introduction of lead-free petrol; reducing the emission of pollutants from industrial plants; and a legal obligation for government to inform and advise the public about environmental concerns;
- the Alpine initiative: no through roads may be built or extended in the Alps, and by 2005 all freight in transit through Switzerland must be transported by rail;
- monitoring and controlling of air pollution; and
- consultation and negotiation: a whole range of interdepartmental working groups are responsible for coordinating activities within the federal administration.

Tajikistan

Demography, policy environment and health care system

Tajikistan is located in the south-eastern part of central Asia, bordered to the south by Afghanistan, to the east by China, to the west by Uzbekistan and to the north by Kyrgyzstan and Uzbekistan. The state system includes the legislative, executive and judicial power. The country has a modern presidential form of government. The administrative and territorial structure includes one autonomous region, two regions, 51 rural districts and 22 cities.

In 1997 the population was 6 million. The average population density is 42 per km^2 and 27% of the population live in urban areas (1997); 7% of the population are aged $\geq$ 65 years and 46% aged 0–14 years (1997); and the dependency ratio was 112% (1997).

In 1997 the unemployment rate was 3%.

In 1997 the infant mortality rate was 30.7 per 1000 live births and the average life expectancy at birth was 68 years.

Approach towards achieving health for all

Tajikistan is undergoing multi-faceted economic and social transition. In the long term it is hoped that this will increase choice and wellbeing. In connection with the transition period to a market economy and the development of small businesses and various forms of enterprise, important changes are taking place in the structure of the population's employment and the forms of property ownership.

The first part of the transition period led to reduced industrial and agricultural production and increased inflation, affecting the health and wellbeing of the population. Tajikistan continues to struggle to overcome the consequences of the ongoing civil war that started in 1992.

A national policy for health for all has been formulated in accordance with WHO recommendations. At the beginning of 1997 a political document was developed on a strategy for promoting the health of the population up to the year 2005. Four key areas were defined: improving health, preventing disease, protecting the environment and improving the efficiency of health care. These were reflected in 29 qualitative and quantitative targets. The draft of this document was developed jointly with 40 experts and was discussed in meetings with representatives of WHO and another international organizations. Specialists from the WHO Regional Office for Europe examined the document, and their comments were combined and used to create a final version of the health for all policy, foreseeing the transition to a comprehensive long-term policy on health care that would ensure equitable access to health care and prolong life expectancy.

In 1997 a law on health care promotion was passed. This law foresaw a health care system with both public and private elements, including pluralism in financing public health care.

The Ministry of Health has a programme of reforming health care for the period up to 2001. The programme reflects the above policy, foreseeing measures for changing the financing of public health care, improving organization and management, developing staff, improving and developing technology, organizing medical and sanitary care and changing drug policy. In accordance with a reform of medical and pharmaceutical education started in 1996, a three-level system of staff education was introduced, as well as a two-level system of educating specialists in nursing, including physician assistants, midwives and nurses.

The changes in staff policy are intended to reduce various kinds of existing imbalance and excessive specialization and to develop the education of general practitioners and specialists in nursing.

The report on the population's health has not clearly identified the problems or defined their severity and influence on the population's health. Tajikistan is reinforcing the information system in health care, taking into consideration this problem. Successful development of existing health policy requires external support.

Focus on health outcomes and reorientation towards primary health care

During the Soviet period primary health care was not supported sufficiently. Most funds were allocated to developing more expensive kinds of medical services, especially in hospital care (hospital beds). The purpose of the new strategy is to change this balance, reduce the number of hospital beds and redistribute resources in favour of primary health care. Other measures include creating educational programmes explaining to the population the advantages of primary health care. The weaknesses of the information system are similar to those in other countries in the eastern part of the Region. The current plan is to improve the system without making such radical changes that the old system falls apart.

Promotion of equity, public participation and intersectoral action

Equity

Tajikistan has the lowest per capita income in the European Region, and poverty has had a profoundly negative effect on health. The number of patients that can be treated in polyclinics and hospitals has been reduced because of the social and economic problems of the transition to a market economy and the financial capacity of hospitals. Elderly people suffer especially severely from the breakdown of medical and social services and are more likely to be impoverished than younger people. This should be improved in the near future. Local clubs for retired and elderly people are being organized, and special transport is available to reach those who are disabled, living in remote areas or unable to afford transport to receive essential services. The Ministries of Health and of Social Protection plan to work with other ministries and with regional city councils to find ways of integrating mentally disabled people into the workforce.

There is serious inequity between rural and urban areas. Rural areas have poorer infrastructure, fewer hospitals, clinics and schools and poorer access to water. Rural residents in general have lower incomes and poorer nutrition. Some areas are totally inaccessible except in summer. Rural areas in the south have suffered many deaths and extensive damage in the civil war. Development programmes will be implemented for such geographically disadvantaged areas.

Women are also vulnerable, having less educational and employment opportunities than men and a higher propensity to suffer from poor nutrition and anaemia. Maternal and infant mortality is high. Work is needed to control anaemia among women and children, to improve reproductive health and family planning and to increase the social status of women. The Ministry of Health is planning work with other ministries and agencies to develop a national plan on women's health.

A basic diet is beyond the reach of many families, and the diet of women and children is estimated to be less adequate than that of men. Information on rational nutrition and preventing diseases connected with poor nutrition should be widely disseminated.

There is still little reliable information on the impact of such factors as the level of education and income of certain social groups that have come about as a result of economic and social change.

Public participation
The establishment of a constitutional democracy in 1993 laid the basis for a comprehensive reform of institutions and legislation, although there remains considerable uncertainty in all areas of civil society. Democratic processes take time to evolve, and specific measures must be introduced if people are to be engaged in decisions that concern them. In relation to the overall health for all strategy, apart from the over 40 experts involved, an interagency conference was held and an association of health for all development was set up to include participation by various ministries, state committees, trade unions, nongovernmental organizations, the mass media and regional councils.

Intersectoral action
The new strategy refers to the need for healthy public policies in all sectors and the mobilization of partners at all levels. Research is being undertaken in relation to iodine deficiency, and a National Centre for Control of Iodine Deficiency Diseases has been established to conduct the research. A Centre for the Prevention of Noncommunicable Diseases has also been established at the Research Institute of Preventive Medicine, and the effects of damage due to harmful products, such as tobacco and alcohol, are

being explored. A reproductive health centre, centres to combat diarrhoeal diseases and acute respiratory infections, centres to combat AIDS and other sexually transmitted diseases and tropical diseases and centres on breastfeeding and immunization have been created.

Various studies have been conducted on the impact of environmental problems on health, with special attention being paid to the working environment. A database on work-related diseases has been set up, and policies to address occupational hygiene and health and safety are being developed.

The Ministry of Health has begun to collaborate closely with the Ministry of Culture and Information, arranging regular television and radio programmes on family planning and healthy living. The Ministry also works with the Ministry of Education to promote healthy eating and physical exercise and to highlight in schools the dangers of tobacco and alcohol consumption. A population-wide campaign has been launched against smoking and chewing tobacco.

Various intersectoral bodies have been established to promote health, including the Coordination Committee for the Control of Sexually Transmitted Diseases, an interregional Committee on Healthy Living, an interministerial committee on drug, alcohol and tobacco control, national and local bodies to develop and implement accident prevention programmes, and a committee to oversee the development of a national environmental programme.

National and regional centres for health promotion have been set up, and the Ministry of Health is consulting other ministries and bodies such as:

- the Ministry of Environment, in planning residential areas;
- the National Housing Committee on safe management of water resources;
- the Ministry of Transport on switching all motor vehicles to lead-free petrol;
- the State Committee on Industry and the Committee on Agriculture and Construction on creating sanitary zones around industrial areas;
- the Ministry of Agriculture, together with regional, district and city councils, on the possibility of draining water reservoirs that are not needed and organizing national irrigation of fields to prevent salt deposits on land and breeding sites for mosquitoes;
- the veterinary and sanitary epidemiological sectors on early detection of tuberculosis in cattle at state and private farms;
- nongovernmental organizations and other agencies, to develop a national plan aimed at ensuring the survival and development of children; and
- the Ministries of Agriculture and of Industry on issues of trade, food processing and food storage.

Various legal measures have been introduced to ensure people's right to a safe environment, including laws on safe housing, environmental protection, healthy air, labour protection, water quality, forestry and soil. A draft law is being elaborated to prohibit the sale of non-iodized salt.

Legal measures aim at promoting a healthier environment. Cooperation with the Ministry of Agriculture has been instigated to enforce rules banning the use of prohibited chemicals.

Intersectoral training has largely been confined to those working in the sale and production of food and occupational health and safety. Monitoring has focused on evaluating environmental health risks and monitoring levels of air pollutants such as sulfur dioxide, nitrogen oxide and lead.

The former Yugoslav Republic of Macedonia

Demography, policy environment and health care system

The former Yugoslav Republic of Macedonia is bordered to the north by the Federal Republic of Yugoslavia, to the east by Bulgaria, to the south by Greece and to the west by Albania.

The country proclaimed its independence in 1991 and is administratively divided into 123 municipalities. The National Assembly has 120 members.

In 1994 the population was 1.9 million. In 1994 the average population density was 76 per km^2, 60% of the population lived in urban areas, and 8% of the population were aged $\geq$ 65 years and 25% aged 0–14 years.

In 1994 the mean income per person was US $1600. The inflation rate is 16% and the unemployment rate 36% (1995).

In 1996 the infant mortality rate was 16.4 per 1000 live births and the average life expectancy at birth was 73 years.

In 1994 total health care expenditure accounted for 5% of GDP.

Approach towards achieving health for all

Health care in the former Yugoslav Republic of Macedonia is based on a combination of preventive and curative measures (diagnosis, treatment and rehabilitation) and the principles of accessibility and continuity. Health care is provided by public and private providers and consists of primary, secondary and tertiary health care services.

Under the Health Care Law, which applies the principles of compulsory insurance, solidarity and reciprocity, all citizens are entitled to health care. Services are provided free to the following categories of citizen: children and young people up to age 18 years or up to 27 years if attending school, pregnant women (includes family planning), and people affected by certain diseases (such as contagious diseases, rheumatic fever, malignant neoplasms, cerebral palsy and multiple sclerosis). Compulsory health insurance ensures that insured people and family members have access to health services in primary care, specialist and consulting services and hospital treatment. Co-payments are collected for the services provided. This co-payment (except for treatment abroad) is not required for the following categories of the population: children up to 14 years of age, pregnant women, perinatal and postnatal care and family planning, people suffering from work-related injuries and occupational diseases, people receiving public social welfare benefits, people affected by certain severe diseases, blood donors who have donated more than ten times, and people older than 65 years of age. Nevertheless, for drugs the co-payment for these categories of people is 5% of the price of the drug.

Focus on health outcomes and reorientation towards primary health care

As part of the transition process, reform of the health care system has aimed to achieve cost-effective preventive and curative primary health care services as the sound basis of the health care system. A step towards this has been the establishment of a family physician system. This will give people the right to choose their practitioner, which will ensure better protection of their health and better relationships between patients and primary health care practitioners.

Promotion of equity, public participation and intersectoral action

Equity

Health care is clearly defined as a constitutional right. Each citizen is legally guaranteed the right to health care and to primary, secondary and tertiary health care through compulsory membership of the health insurance scheme as an employee or as a co-insured family member of the employed person.

The preventive health care measures outlined in the annual programmes adopted by the Government continue to be applied. Since 1993, the Institutes of Public Health have provided preventive care within eight programmes on:

- compulsory immunization against certain contagious diseases;
- active health care of mother and child;
- blood donation;
- regular health examination of pupils and students;
- research, prevention and control of brucellosis;
- preventive measures for tuberculosis;
- providing resources for dialysis treatment of patients, drugs for patients with transplanted organs, cytostatics, insulin and growth hormone; and
- AIDS prevention.

The Government has adopted these programmes and finances them through the state budget.

Public participation

The former Yugoslav Republic of Macedonia adopted a national programme on the implementation of the strategy for health for all by the year 2000, which encompasses the main priorities of the Government and activities in health. It was prepared with participation from a multidisciplinary task force, involving such professional groups as those in health, education, science, financial policy and economics. Government and parliamentary commissions and the National Assembly reviewed the programme.

Regarding health promotion, besides the activities of the health care sector, the activities of other sectors such as education and certain nongovernmental organizations have been included in the plan.

The Ministry of Health cooperates with numerous international organizations and associations. Several projects supported by WHO and UNICEF, such as the Expanded Programme on Immunization and the programmes on health care for mothers and children, breastfeeding, cardiovascular diseases and mental health, have been implemented.

Intersectoral action
The Ministry of Health takes responsibility for the health of the population within a framework defined by national legislation. Other ministries are also involved in health care decisions, such as the Ministries of Finance, of Education, of Science, of Development and of the Interior. In terms of regulatory measures, legislation on controlling environmental pollution and quality control on foodstuffs and water has been adopted. The Ministry of Health has established various national committees around specific health challenges such as biomedical ethics, iodine deficiency, breastfeeding and the eradication of poliomyelitis, communicable diseases, brucellosis and AIDS.

Turkey

Demography, policy environment and health care system

Turkey is bounded to the west by Greece and the Aegean Sea, to the north by Bulgaria and the Black Sea, to the east by Armenia, Georgia and the Islamic Republic of Iran and to the south by Iraq, Syria and the Mediterranean Sea. The political system of Turkey is parliamentary democracy. The country is administratively divided into 80 provinces; the governor of each province is appointed by the Council of Ministers on the recommendation of the Ministry of the Interior and is responsible to all central government ministries.

In 1995 the population was 62.2 million. The average population density is 73 per km^2 (1990); 59% of the population live in urban areas (1993); 8% of the population are aged ≥ 65 years and 58% aged 0–14 years (1990); and the dependency ratio is 65% (1990).

In 1995 the mean income per person was US $3000. The inflation rate is 106% (1994) and the unemployment rate 9% (1996). The poorest 20% of the population have a 5% share of income while the most affluent 20% have a 55% share.

In 1996 the infant mortality rate was 42.2 per 1000 live births and the average life expectancy at birth was 65.7 years for males and 70.3 years for females.

In 1995 total health expenditure accounted for 5% of estimated GDP.

The Ministry of Health is the major provider of hospital and primary care and the only provider of preventive health services. At the national level, the Ministry of Health is responsible for Turkey's health policy and health services. At the provincial level, provincial health directorates accountable to the provincial governors administer health services.

Approach towards achieving health for all

See the case study on Turkey, page 194.

Turkmenistan

Demography, policy environment and health care system

Turkmenistan lies in the southernmost part of the former Soviet Union, bordered to the north by Kazakhstan, to the south by Afghanistan and Iran, to the east by Uzbekistan and to the west by the Caspian Sea. Turkmenistan gained independence in 1991, and the Constitution adopted in 1992 established a President (as head of state) and a Cabinet of Ministers. The capital is Ashgabat. The country is divided into five administrative–economic regions (*velayats*) comprising 46 districts and 20 towns.

In 1995 the population was 6 million. The average population density is 9 per km^2 and 45% of the population live in urban areas (1995); 4% of the population are aged ≥ 65 years and 40% aged 0–14 years (1994); and the dependency ratio is 50% (1994).

In 1996 the mean income per person was US $1270 and the inflation rate was 50%.

In 1995 the infant mortality rate was 42.2 per 1000 live births and the average life expectancy at birth was 63.9 years.

According to unofficial figures provided by the Ministry of Health, the total health expenditure accounts for 2% of estimated GDP (1995).

The Ministry of Health and the *hakimlik* (administration) in each *velayat* have the main responsibility for providing health services. The Ministry of Health and the national health services operate 33 national health care institutions. Although the *hakimlik* finances the health care institutions in each *velayat,* the institutions report to the Ministry of Health for technical matters.

Approach towards achieving health for all

In 1994, Turkmenistan embarked on a radical process of economic and social development, focusing mainly on enhancing production. The health care system is undergoing a process of reform in accordance with the presidential health programme declared in 1995. The main objectives of this programme are: shifting to a family physician system (strengthening of primary health care); reducing the number of hospital beds and rationalizing the structure of medical institutions; introducing a medical insurance system; developing a domestic pharmaceutical industry; reforming health care financing; and improving legislation.

Focus on health outcomes and reorientation towards primary health care

As in other former Soviet republics, the supply of hospitals and medical specialization are excessive and primary health care is underemphasized. Health services are fragmented, physicians are inadequately trained and managerial expertise is insufficient to implement reforms. The number of hospital beds will be reduced by 40–45% by 2000, and preventive services will be developed.

A family physician system has been introduced throughout Turkmenistan. The main tasks of family physicians are prevention, screening, diagnostic and ambulatory care, emergency services and health education. Difficulties in functioning of the new system include a shortage of properly trained staff and of equipment, lack of transport and training materials, and obsolete educational programmes in medical institutes and medical schools.

Several long-term primary health care initiatives are in operation, including the promotion of breastfeeding, reproductive health of the family, control of acute diarrhoeal diseases and health education of school-children. Immunization, especially of children, has been accelerated to deal with re-emerging diseases such as poliomyelitis, diphtheria and tuberculosis.

Promotion of equity, public participation and intersectoral action

Equity

Turkmenistan has suffered greatly in moving from strong dependence on the former Soviet Union to dependence on market forces and international prices for determining trade flows. During the Soviet period, the level of industrial development in Turkmenistan was very low; this problem is being solved. Turkmenistan has large reserves of natural gas, but several former Soviet republics cannot pay for gas imports, leading to a growing external debt and declining gas output. Problems in the transition period have reduced the standard of living of the population. As a result, health problems have increased and the capacity to deal with them has been reduced.

The 1992 Constitution (Article 33) guarantees free health services to all citizens provided by publicly owned facilities but also provides for payment for services. The public financing of the system predominantly comprises general state revenues. In 1996, a voluntary insurance system was introduced, but the income from premiums appears to be too low to meet the demands on the insurance system. From 1998 a compulsory insurance system is planned to be introduced.

The ratio of physicians to population will be reduced, but the health care authorities will attempt to make the geographical distribution of specialists more equitable. New research is planned on the relationship between social problems and people's health needs and status.

Public participation

Turkmenistan is moving to a market economy and a more democratic system of governance. The Government has decided, however, that the economic model chosen requires the maintenance of strong state power if the planned reforms are to be achieved. For this reason, power may be decentralized more slowly than in other economies in transition.

Intersectoral action

Under the Soviet system, little attention was paid to preventive measures, such as keeping people well through healthier environments, public health programmes and changes in lifestyles. These are some of the main areas in which changes are now being initiated. Research is being carried out to assess the level of preventive activities taking place. Working groups are to be set up to plan future preventive activities. Cooperation will be encouraged between various sectors in implementing a general national plan of action on preventive activities. Current health promotion activities include a ban on smoking in public buildings and plans to tax imported alcoholic beverages. Other challenges that will be addressed include alcohol, smoking, drug abuse, iodine insufficiency and nutritional anaemia. A presidential decree has been drafted banning advertising of all types of alcohol. In an effort to use certain settings to promote health, health promotion is to be included as part of the school curriculum, focusing on healthy lifestyles and improved nutrition.

A proportion of the income allocated for preventive services is planned to be used to upgrade water supplies and sewerage systems.

Ukraine

Demography, policy environment and health care system

Ukraine is bordered to the east by the Russian Federation, to the north by Belarus, to the west by Hungary, Poland, the Republic of Moldova, Romania and Slovakia, and to the south by the Black Sea and the Sea of Azov. Ukraine declared its independence in December 1991, and the new Constitution was adopted in 1996. The Parliament (the Supreme Council) has 450 seats. The country is divided into 24 provinces and the Crimea, which has a degree of autonomy. There are also councils subordinate to the provincial authorities.

In 1996 the population was 51 million. The average population density is 86 per km^2 and 68% of the population live in urban areas (1994); 14% of the population are aged $\geq$ 65 years and 22% aged 0–14 years (1994); and the dependency ratio is 52% (1994).

In 1994 the mean income per person was US $1900. The inflation rate is 282% and the unemployment rate is 0.5% (1995). The poorest 10% of the population have a 4% share of income while the most affluent 10% have a 21% share (1992).

In 1996 the infant mortality rate was 14.3 per 1000 live births and in 1994 the average life expectancy at birth was 68 years.

In 1995 total health expenditure accounted for 5.0% of estimated GDP.

Basic health services are organized under the Ministry of Health at four levels: national, regional (25 regions), district (447 districts) and local. There are several parallel administrations, and only the general public health care system operates under the Ministry of Health. Military personnel, transport workers and various enterprises run their own health systems as a kind of fringe benefit. These parallel systems duplicate services, making the overall health sector inefficient and creating unequal access to services.

Approach towards achieving health for all

Ukraine does not have an explicit policy on health for all. In the context of its medium-term cooperation with the WHO Regional Office for Europe, however, the following priority areas of concern have been agreed:

- support to health care reform (improving health care policies, health care delivery and building competence);

- strengthening national capacity to use available health information for planning, management and monitoring;
- preventing and controlling communicable diseases in accordance with the WHO European target for health for all;
- technical assistance to the national family planning programme;
- thyroid cancer among radiation sickness victims after the 1986 Chernobyl accident;
- ensuring the quality of drinking-water and recreational waters, tourism and health; and
- the countrywide integrated noncommunicable diseases intervention (CINDI) programme.

Focus on health outcomes and reorientation towards primary health care

Ukraine inherited a system of health care similar to that of other countries in central and eastern Europe, with high ratios of specialized medical personnel and a tendency towards hospital care rather than primary health care. Growing budget restrictions have encouraged more efficient use of resources with more emphasis on outpatient care. Following parliamentary discussions, Ukraine is now undergoing health care reform. The new concept is heavily focused on the development of primary health care. During 1995 and 1996, the number of hospital beds has been reduced, and the concept of the family physician has gained ground. It is planned to increase the number of general practitioners, and training for this has been incorporated in medical training institutions. This will help to precipitate a shift towards primary health care, although the plans are still in the very early stages.

Promotion of equity, public participation and intersectoral action

Equity
Article 49 of the Constitution grants everyone the right to health protection, medical care and medical insurance. State institutions provide medical care free of charge, and the state is responsible for developing and maintaining medical institutions. Nevertheless, long-term economic problems have made this objective difficult to achieve in practice. A large proportion of health expenditure goes towards paying the salaries of medical professionals. The Ministry of Health has recently developed a draft law on social medical insurance, which has been submitted to the Government for consideration.

An important part of the overall programme of economic reform has been to ensure that people still have access to basic services such as health care, housing and education. The value of incomes and pensions has fallen in real terms as prices have risen sharply. Thus, people spend more on food than they did under the Soviet system but many families find it increasingly difficult to afford an adequate and balanced diet. Certain food subsidies are available.

The three basic components of the social support system are pensions, unemployment compensation, and assistance to families with children. Most people are eligible to receive benefits based on their participation in the workforce, although all Ukrainian citizens are entitled to receive a minimum income.

Apart from these benefits, the 1993 Law on State Assistance for Families with Children guarantees a minimum level of income support for all families with children. The legislation was developed jointly by the Ministries of Social Protection, of Labour and of Finance. Nevertheless, the rapid increase in prices has substantially reduced the real value of these benefits.

Public participation

The declaration of a republic in 1990 made a commitment to the development of a civil society. In reality, the delay in agreeing to a new Constitution and ambiguous election laws held up the development of mechanisms that would enable people to participate in political decision making processes, which also has implications for decisions taken in relation to health. However, one of the first laws passed after independence was the Law on Public Associations. A large number of public organizations and political parties have now been registered with the Ministry of Justice. Numerous regional and local nongovernmental organizations have also been established, some of which are engaged in the task of improving people's health. In June 1996 the Constitution was drawn up to guarantee human rights and freedoms.

Intersectoral action

According to the Constitution, everyone has the right to a safe environment and to compensation for damage inflicted through the violation of this right. Everyone is guaranteed the right of free access to information about the state of the environment and the quality of food and consumer goods, and the right to disseminate such information.

The storage and processing of food continues to be inadequate, leading to substantial losses, waste and low quality products. Special attention is being paid to the quality of food (especially because of the effects of the 1986 Chernobyl accident). A system has been set up to control foodstuffs in the contaminated zones to ensure food quality in these areas.

The main focus of the CINDI programme in Ukraine in 1995 was fighting high serum cholesterol levels. This was done by:

- informing the public about the causes of high cholesterol levels and the associated risks to health;
- providing physicians with the latest information on lipid metabolism;
- establishing a centre to examine specifically the topic of lipids;
- surveying the national diet and the latest developments in fat metabolism;
- transmitting television programmes on hypercholesterolaemia; and
- establishing screening centres for high cholesterol levels.

United Kingdom

Demography, policy environment and health care system

The United Kingdom comprises England, Wales, Scotland and Northern Ireland, and each is subdivided into a number of local authorities. Each local authority is represented by one or more elected members of parliament who sit in the House of Commons, the main legislative body. The United Kingdom is governed centrally, although some legislative, fiscal and other powers have been devolved to separate Scottish and Welsh assemblies.

In 1995 the population was 59 million. The average population density is 238 per km^2 and 89% of the population live in urban areas (1995).

In 1995 the mean income per person was US $18 300. The inflation rate is 2.5% (1994) and the unemployment rate 8% (1995). The poorest 40% of the population have a 15% share of income while the most affluent 20% have a 44% share (1994).

In 1995 the infant mortality rate was 6 per 1000 live births and the average life expectancy at birth was 77 years.

Total health expenditure accounts for 7% of estimated GDP.

The health care system is financed primarily through taxation. Central government priorities for health and health care are communicated through a hierarchical system to the National Health Service (NHS) Executive, its regional offices and district health authorities.

The management and organization of health services differ between England, Wales, Scotland and Northern Ireland, although the separation between the purchasers and providers of health services, introduced under the health care reforms of 1990, is common throughout the United Kingdom at present. These reforms gave district health authorities a role as commissioners of health care, negotiating contracts with health care providers to meet the needs of their local populations. Similarly, general practitioners were able to become "fundholders". This system has recently been reviewed and a White Paper was published in late 1997. It proposes the removal of the internal market in the health service through a process of evolutionary change. The separation of planning and provision will be retained but there will be a new emphasis on partnership between health authorities, health service providers, general practitioners and other organizations, including local authorities. Health authorities will have responsibility for developing "health improvement programmes", backed by a duty of partnership, and "primary care groups" (most of which are expected to be led by general practitioners) which will commission and monitor health services for geographically defined local populations. The primary care groups will replace fundholding.

Approach towards achieving health for all

Policy on health and health services is broadly determined by the central Government, although each of the four countries has developed its own health policy. A ministerial-level subcommittee on health strategy, with representatives from the health departments of all four countries and from a range of other government ministries, coordinated these policies. The new administration has established a similar Cabinet subcommittee to oversee the development and implementation of revised health strategies.

Focus on health outcomes and reorientation towards primary health care

All four policies have objectives or targets related to health outcomes, as well as to process and other interim indicators of health status. Progress towards the objectives and targets is monitored routinely, and the chief medical officer of each country reports annually on the health status of the population.

In recent years the NHS has increased its sharp focus on health outcomes and on the effectiveness of clinical interventions to make better use of limited resources. A national research and development strategy seeks to ensure that the content and delivery of care in the NHS is based on high-quality research, and a Health Outcomes Unit has been established alongside the Cochrane Collaboration Centre to monitor the effectiveness of interventions and to disseminate information about them. A public health common data set has been developed, as have health service indicators incorporating health status.

The United Kingdom has a long tradition of health care based on general practice. General practitioners have acted as gatekeepers to specialist services, and since the 1960s general practitioner services have increasingly been provided in health centres as a base for multidisciplinary primary health care teams. More recently, the role of general practitioners has broadened, and payments have been introduced as an incentive to undertake more health promotion and disease prevention activities. Institutional care for elderly people, people with mental health problems and people with physical or learning disabilities has been a move away from institutional care towards care in the community. The "New NHS" White Paper introduces the development of primary care groups, which will have responsibility for all aspects of the health of local communities as well as providing primary care and integrating it with community services.

Promotion of equity, public participation and intersectoral action

Equity
The United Kingdom has a relatively high overall health status, but substantial evidence demonstrates inequalities and inequities between different population groups. In particular, on the basis of a number of

measures, the gap between people in social classes I and II (higher) and those in social classes IV and V (lower) has been widening since at least the early 1980s. The Government is now working to address health inequity and social exclusion in all areas of policy, including health and health services. For example, inequalities are a major theme running throughout *Our healthier nation*, the new health strategy for England.

The NHS maintains an important underlying principle of equal access to health care for equal need, with most services being free at the point of delivery, but the use of services varies between population groups. The health policies of all four countries attempt to redress this imbalance and inequities in health status. In Northern Ireland, for example, one of the main themes of the health policy is to promote equity in health and social wellbeing. In England there is a recent report on differences in health status, and funds have been set aside for research on interventions that promote equity in health and in resource allocation between district health authorities. Capitation payments for general practitioners are already based on socioeconomic variables within their catchment areas.

The many ethnic groups in the United Kingdom merit specific attention, and a number of interventions have been introduced. For example, health education material is published in the languages of ethnic minorities, an ethnic minority unit has been established within the Department of Health and, from April 1993, the NHS has been asked to monitor the delivery of health services to communities with substantial ethnic minorities in each district.

Public participation

Wide-ranging consultation has been a feature of the development of all four health policies, and the policies have been disseminated widely. In Northern Ireland there have been explicit efforts to involve local people in decisions about service provision, and the strategy for Wales aims at a people-centred service. A patient's charter that sets minimum standards to be expected by those using the health services has also raised public awareness of health service issues throughout the United Kingdom.

Intersectoral action

Health policy in the United Kingdom encompasses far more wide-ranging issues than those normally covered by the departments of health. At the national level, this is reflected in the Cabinet sub-committee on health, with membership spanning 12 different departments. At the local level across the United Kingdom, intersectoral action is being encouraged through the promotion of alliances and the development of health improvement programmes, and by focusing on specific settings for promoting health.

See also the case studies on pages 209 and 236.

Uzbekistan

Demography, policy environment and health care system

Uzbekistan is located in the heart of central Asia between the region's two main rivers, the Amu Darya and Syr Darya. It is bordered to the north by Kazakhstan, to the east by Kyrgyzstan and Tajikistan, to the south by Afghanistan and to the west by Turkmenistan. Uzbekistan declared independence in December 1991, and the Olij Majlis (Parliament) has 250 seats. There are 120 towns, 114 urban settlements and 163 rural districts. Local authorities are appointed by the President of the Republic and confirmed by Parliament.

In 1995 the population was 23.5 million. The average population density is 52.4 per km^2 and 38% of the population live in urban areas (1996); 41% of the population are aged 0–14 years and 4% are aged ≥ 65 years (1995); and the dependency ratio is 81% (1994).

In 1996 the mean income per person was US $960 and the inflation rate was 40%.

In 1996 the infant mortality rate was 24.2 per 1000 live births and the average life expectancy at birth was 72.7 years.

In 1996 total health expenditure accounted for 3.3% of GDP.

Health care is delivered at the national, regional, district and village levels by institutions managed centrally by the Ministry of Health. In addition, there is a network of therapeutic facilities operated by other departments, as well as private medical facilities. Uzbekistan has inherited quite a well developed and rather elaborate health care system but now lacks the means to support it. Its hierarchical top-heavy infrastructure is expensive and in many cases does not meet modern requirements.

Approach towards achieving health for all

A purposeful reform of the health system is under way in Uzbekistan that includes maintaining and modernizing the existing infrastructure, especially at the primary level; introducing a new system of financing health care services; decentralization of the development of national pharmaceutical and biotechnological products; and emphasis on family planning and the control of infectious diseases. Programmes are currently under way to privatize some hospitals, dental services, pharmacies and retail opticians' outlets.

The Constitution guarantees that the state will take steps to ensure citizens' rights to health care.

Uzbekistan has considerable legislation on health care. The most important is the Law on Protecting the Health of Citizens of the Republic of Uzbekistan of 29 August 1996. It was drawn up with the participation of international experts and meets international standards. The Law ensures that citizens have equal rights to accessible and high-quality medical care. It also declares that citizens are responsible for preserving public and personal health. The Law envisages the extension of public participation by the population and individual communities (such as villages and small towns) as well as by local authorities, in matters related to sanitation, health and health education.

In addition, a Law on AIDS Prevention has been in force since 1991, and a Law on State Sanitary Surveillance since 1992. The Cabinet of Ministers has also adopted a number of decrees defining the intersectoral and interdepartmental nature of efforts to protect people's health in Uzbekistan.

The Concept of Health Care Development in the Republic of Uzbekistan (1992) is in final form and envisages long-term plans for modernization of health care. The document has been endorsed by the Ministry of Health but has not been reviewed or discussed in Parliament. The Concept envisages the attainment, in the long term, of the following goals:

- forming new economic mechanisms to use resources more effectively;
- decentralizing the state health care system; and
- improving people's health and setting priorities in health development.

The programme of health care development for 1996–1998 makes provision for efforts to protect people's health in the short term. In view of the population's health status and the unusual demographic situation, the allocation of priorities is designed to meet women's and children's needs for better health and emphasizes efforts to control infectious diseases and protect the environment.

Since the development of the Concept and programme, an intersectoral steering group has been established to oversee their implementation under the umbrella of the World Bank Health Reform Project. This committee also has responsibility for work in preventing AIDS and HIV infection.

Focus on health outcomes and reorientation towards primary health care

One of the main objectives of current reforms is to make primary health care more effective. The new system is based on the introduction of a general practitioner system. Training doctors as general practitioners has been initiated, and the process of establishing rural polyclinics staffed with general and family practitioners has begun. This should precipitate a shift from inpatient to outpatient activities and day care centres. The number of inpatient beds has already been substantially reduced and a further reduction is planned.

Considerable information on the health status and needs of the population is already available in regular reports from the Ministry of Health, regional health departments and international bodies and elsewhere. Steps are being taken to make appropriate use of information in the process of policy formulation and to disseminate it widely at various levels.

Promotion of equity, public participation and intersectoral action

Equity

The transition to independence was peaceful, without much of the political and social instability that occurred in several other newly independent states. Uzbekistan is rich in natural resources, including gold, oil, natural gas, coal, silver and copper, and agriculture provides 40% of the GDP. The economy was severely affected, however, by the deterioration of trade relations with the Russian Federation and other newly independent states, and real household incomes have declined, especially among vulnerable groups.

Under the former Soviet system, the centrally funded social programmes were a source of considerable income for families. The current Government is trying to maintain a support system for vulnerable groups, but equity tends to be interpreted as equal access to health care and is not interpreted in its wider context as one of the determinants of health.

A number of measures are being taken to promote equity, including the provision of free health services for socially vulnerable groups, especially in rural areas. Certain geographical areas are given priority for additional support, such as rural areas, where the poor quality of drinking-water and lack of sewage facilities promotes communicable diseases. Special measures are being taken to support victims of tuberculosis and their families; for example, they are exempted from taxes on farm income and are provided with free housing, travel costs to treatment centres and, for high-risk groups, free meals.

Public participation

According to the state health programme, a new interface needs to be developed between the people and the state, with both sharing responsibility for health. This will require participation from various bodies, including other ministries, regional representatives and nongovernmental organizations. The Ministry of Health will assume responsibility for coordination but intends to continue with its policy of decentralizing and strengthening local care structures.

Intersectoral action

The programme for health care development 1996–1998 does not explicitly refer to intersectoral action for health. Examples of intersectoral initiatives have been confined to the traditional areas of lifestyles and environment. To promote healthy lifestyles, campaigns against alcohol and substance abuse are planned. A broader health promotion message will be spread through the various health centres established throughout the country. In an effort to reduce the increase in cancer incidence, a diet rich in vegetables with low fat content is being promoted.

Thirty years of rapid expansion in cotton production has had a strong negative effect on environmental conditions. Waste of water resources and massive use of fertilizers and pesticides have led to pollution, soil degradation and the gradual desiccation of the Aral Sea, causing severe deterioration of the health situation in adjacent areas. A major health problem is the poor and declining quality of drinking-water, especially in rural areas. A national environment and health action plan has been prepared to address this situation.

A number of environmental health measures have been introduced to reduce the increase in cancer incidence, including using gas instead of other types of fuel, developing safe, nutritious and high-quality foodstuffs, and regulating the use of fertilizers. Effective implementation of environmental health measures will require collaboration between the Ministries of Health, Transport, Power and Agriculture.

Uzbekistan has always accorded high priority to training its physicians and public health staff, but concepts such as intersectoral action and community participation are new. One recent development has been the training of occupational health workers.

04186809